Basics of Drug Analysis

Basics of Drug Analysis

G. Vidya Sagar

Professor & Principal,
Veerayatan Institute of Pharmacy, Jhakamia, Bhuj-Mandvi Road,
Tal. Mandvi - Kutch, 370 460, Gujarat
and
Dean, Faculty of Pharmaceutical Sciences,
K.S.K.V. Kachchh Univeristy, Bhuj, Kutch, Gujarat

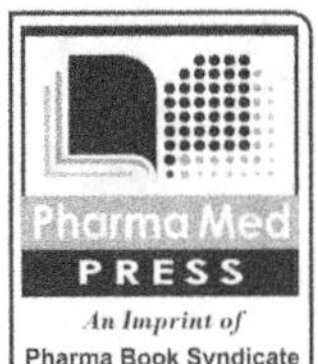

PharmaMed Press
An imprint of Pharma Book Syndicate

A unit of BSP Books Pvt., Ltd.

4-4-309/316, Giriraj Lane,
Sultan Bazar, Hyderabad - 500 095.

Published by :

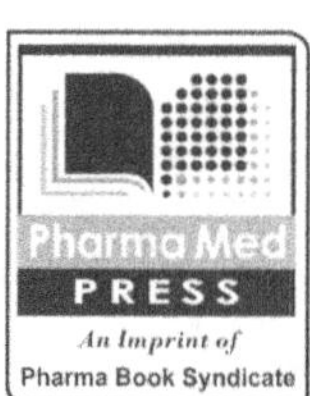

PharmaMed Press
An imprint of Pharma Book Syndicate

A unit of BSP Books Pvt., Ltd.

4-4-309/316, Giriraj Lane, Sultan Bazar, Hyderabad - 500 095.
Phone: 040-23445605, 23445688; Fax: 91+40-23445611
E-mail: info@pharmamedpress.com
www.pharmamedpress.com/pharmamedpress.net

ISBN : 978-93-89974-58-4 (HB)

Foreword

It gives me pleasure to write the foreword for the textbook written by Dr. G. Vidya Sagar. With the rapid development that took place during last few years, all the subjects of Pharmaceutical Sciences have undergone metamorphosis. Lot of new techniques have come into practice in Pharmaceutical Analysis, more so in the case of Laboratory practice. In this context "Basics of Drug Analysis" by Dr. G. Vidya Sagar is a boon to the pharmacy student community as well as to the practicing analysts. The book deals with fundamental aspects of Pharmaceutical Analysis viz., various methods like gravimetry, titrimetry, diazotization, qualitative and quantitative analytical techniques.

The subject matter is written with adequate theoretical background and presented in a simple manner for better understanding among the student community. The book serves as a text for undergraduate pharmacy students of Indian Universities in Pharmaceutical Analysis.

I deem it privilege to recommend this textbook which is well conceived and lucidly presented and I wish the author all success in his efforts.

Prof. Dr. Kantibhai Gor
Vice-chancellor
KSKV Kachchh University,
Bhuj, Kutch, Gujarat.

Preface

The hand notes I have prepared for teaching undergraduates of Pharmacy over the last 20 years helped me in preparing this textbook. Much care has been taken to present the contents in a simple language without much jargon.

The purpose of this book is to review several important analytical techniques that find wide applications in Pharmaceutical Analysis. The theory and principle of each technique is discussed with special emphasis on applications in Pharmaceutical analysis. This book will be useful to students of B.Pharm. and also for analysts, quality control chemists and those employed in Pharmaceutical Industry.

This book is not meant for exhaustive reading but is well suited for undergraduates in understanding the fundamental aspects easily and for the examination point of view. The text serves as lucid exposition for introductory Pharmaceutical Analysis.

Critical comments and suggestion are welcome for the betterment of qualitative aspect of the book. I hope my efforts will help to fulfil the objectives.

-Author

Mandvi, Kutch, Gujarat

Acknowledgements

To write a book of this magnitude, one requires a lot of patience and perseverance. My teaching the subject over the last 20 years helped me to get the experience and skills to write this book. I gratefully acknowledge the unstinted support by the following friends and academicians. They helped me in going through the manuscript and offering their valuable comments.

1. Prof. Dr. B. Suresh, Principal, JSS College of Pharmacy, Ooty.
2. Prof. Dr. K.P.R. Choudhary, Principal, University College of Pharmaceutical Sciences, Andhra University, Vishakapatnam.
3. Prof. Dr. Ashok Vitthal Bhonsale, Professor and Principal, Sheth Govind Raghunath Sable College of Pharmacy, Saswad, Pune.
4. Prof. R.V. Shete, Principal, Rajgadh Dhyanpeeth College of Pharmacy, Bhor, Pune District.
5. Prof. Dr. Harish N. More, Principal, Bharati Vidyanpeeth College of Pharmacy, Bhor, Kolhapur.

I gratefully acknowledge the sustained support of the management, staff and students of Veerayatan Institute of Pharmacy in writing this textbook. I thank Shri Ojas M. Suroo for his meticulously computerizing the entire manuscript.

The successful compilation of this book was possible with the cooperation and help of my wife, Mrs. Swapna Sagar and my daughter Hasitha.

Finally I would like to place on record the services of Shri Anil Shah, PharmaMed Press in bringing out this book in a most beautiful way.

-Author

Contents

Contents

CHAPTER 1

QUALITY ASSURANCE

A. Statistical Quality Control

Introduction

It has been the constant endeavor of Pharmacists to strive at higher and higher accuracy but absolute accuracy is unattainable. No two things can be made exactly alike. In Pharmaceutical production, no attempts are made to attain absolute perfection but to control the degree of variability of production so that the variation is within the prescribed statutory tolerance limits. There are two types of causes responsible for the variation of Pharmaceutical product manufactured.

(i) Inherent source of variation (Indeterminate or accidental variation)

(ii) Assignable causes of variation (determinate or constant variation)

(i) Inherent Source of Variation

These variations or errors manifest themselves by the slight variations that occur in successive measurements by the same observer with the greatest care under as nearly identical conditions as possible. This natural variability can't be controlled and it occurs even under the best of methods and circumstances. These variations cannot be predicted and hence cannot be eliminated.

(ii) Assignable Causes of Variation

These are the variations which can be avoided or whose magnitude can be determined and hence can be checked and controlled. The assignable variations if present must be detected and corrected before defective results and products are produced. Some of the determinate errors are:

1. *Operational and personal errors:* these mostly physical in nature. These errors are due to factors for which the individual is responsible and are not connected with the method or procedure. These errors may arise from the constitutional inability of an individual to make certain observations accurately. An example for this kind is – some persons are unable to judge color changes sharply in visual titrations which may result in slight overlapping of the end point.

2. *Instrumental and reagent errors:* these variations arise due to defective instruments and improper chemicals.

3. *Errors of method or variations due to the process:* these arise from the incorrect sampling and from the incompleteness of the reaction.

4. *Additive and proportional variations:* the absolute value of an additive error is independent of the amount of the constituent present in the determination. Some examples of additive errors are loss in weight of a crucible in which a precipitate is ignited and errors in weights. The absolute value of a proportional error depends upon the amount of the constituents. An example of proportional error is impurity in a primary standard which leads to an incorrect value for the normality of a standard solution.

The science of quality control is largely statistical in nature. The statistical quality control technique is based on the theory of probability and sampling and is extensively used in Pharmaceutical industries and quality control labs. Quality control is a powerful productivity technique for effective diagnosis of lack of quality or conformity to settle standards in any of the materials, processes, machines or end products. Statistical quality control is a key factor in process validation and the manufacture of Pharmaceutical products. The technique attempts to locate the variability or error while the Pharmaceutical work is in process or progress.

In statistical quality control techniques, the actual physical measurements are first secured by inspection. Then the degree of variation among the measurements is analysed by statistical methods in terms of a standard value of variation among acceptable limits. By such comparisons, quality control is made to predict the significance of the variation analysed. This type of prediction can then be used to exert a positive influence over the control of product quality by studying the assignable causes. The quality control is thus directly associated with inspection and for statistical quality control, control charts are maintained. In order that things may be economical and quick, 100% inspection is not desirable. Rather 100% inspection leads to fatigue of human brain and faulty results are likely to be accepted. Control charts tell immediately whether the product is satisfactory or not.

The important objectives of statistical quality control in Pharmaceutical practice are as follows:

   (i)   Better quality level

   (ii)   Better uniformity of quality

   (iii)   Better utilization of raw materials

   (iv)   Most efficient utilization of equipments

   (v)   Less scrap and rework

   (vi)   Better inspection

   (vii)   Improved producer consumer relations and

   (viii)   Better specifications

Attributes and Variables

Attributes

Those measurements in which a quality characteristic is present or absent or falls into a limited number of discrete categories are referred to as attribute measurements. Here the examination leads to the result being satisfactory or unsatisfactory. Measurements by attributes are generally less expensive but many more measurements have to be taken in such cases as there is no way of telling to what extent an item fails to meet the desired quality level when it is rejected on a attribute basis.

Variability

Two things are said to be alike when the differences among them are so small that we do not care about them. But generally two things are considered to be identical vary from each other when sufficiently precise measuring equipment or process is available. Measurement by variable involved the use of a scale which can be theoretically subdivided infinitely and the results of the quality can be expressed quantitatively i.e. in numbers. The measures of size, weight, surface etc. are the examples of measurement by variables.

Control Charts

The statistical quality control is mainly classified into process control and product control. The aim of process control is to maintain satisfactory quality level in production. The process control should ensure that the product conforms with the specified quality standards. The process control is achieved through the technique of control charts. Controlling the quality of product by critical examination at strategic points is known as product control and is achieved through sampling inspection plans. Random samples of work in process are taken and inspected, data collected are then presented graphically in chart form and chart method is an essential part of quality control systems.

A control chart is a statistical device principally used for the study and control of repetitive processes. It is a device to measure the extent of variation or defects in a process and to identify where there is an assignable cause for the variation. Dr. Walter A. Shewhart, its originator suggested that control chart may serve, first to define the goal or standard for the process that the management might strive to attain and secondly it may be used as an instrument to attain that goal and thirdly it may serve as a means of judging whether the goal is being achieved. The charts provide a very simple but powerful graphic method or finding whether a process is in statistical control or not. The control charts are simple to construct and easy to interpret and they tell the manager at a glance whether the process is in control or not. It is a graphic device for presenting data so as to directly reveal the frequency and extent of variations from established standards of goals.

The control charts help to easily identify the assignable causes of quality variation and these should be controlled or eliminated economically whenever detected. In gathering data for preparation of control charts the following points should be borne in mind:

1. We should be sure that we are measuring the thing we want to measure.
2. Measuring equipment and computing equipment should be operated properly.
3. The operator should be properly trained and instructed and free from bias.
4. Transcription errors should be avoided by adequate checking.
5. At least 40 to 100 observations should be taken.

It is necessary that the control chart limits be based on only the variability that is inherent in the process. If the standard deviation is computed on the basis of individual measurements, it will include the determination of all the assignable causes as well as chance causes of variation.

Important Points to be Observed in Drawing the Quality Control Chart

As the quality control charts form important documents and have to be examined by senior personnel, these should be drawn in convenient manner and the following points should be considered:

1. The size of the chart should be handy one.
2. The chart should be as neat as possible.
3. There should be provision for accommodating additional information on the charts in future.
4. The chart should be labeled properly and sufficiently.
5. When it becomes necessary to draw revised control chart limits on the basis of additional data, they should not be drawn over the original limits but after these.
6. Plotted point should be legible.
7. The average lines are drawn by solid and control limits by dotted lines.

8. There should be minimum number of background lines on the graph paper selected for drawing the control charts. Such charts are often plotted on rectangular cross section paper. Some times profile paper may also be used. The vertical scale is used for the statistical measures and the horizontal scale is used for subgroup numbers, dates, hours or lot numbers etc.

Objectives of Control Charts

1. To determine whether a process can meet the specifications or to collect further information for establishing or changing the specifications.
2. To get information for changing the production procedures.
3. To get information for changing the inspection techniques or acceptance procedures.
4. Determination as to when to find causes of variation and take action to correct them and when to leave the process alone.
5. To take decision on acceptance or rejection of manufactured or purchased products.

Types of Quality Control Charts

Broadly speaking, control charts can be divided under tow heads:

(i)   Control Charts for attributes

(ii) Control Charts for Variables

(i)   Control Charts for Attributes

Control charts for attributes can be used for quality characteristics which can be observed only as attributes by classifying an item as defective or non defective, i.e. confirming to specifications or not. The following are the three main attribute charts:

1. p-chart or chart for fraction defectives
2. np-chart or chart for number of defectives
3. c-chart or chart for number of defects per unit

(ii) Control Charts for Variables

Control charts for variables are used for any quality characteristic that is measurable. Usually $\overline{X}$ and R charts used to control the mean (location) and standard deviation (dispersion) respectively of the quality characteristics.

(i)   Control Charts for Attributes

1. *The Shewhart control chart for fraction defective*: This is also described as p-chart in technical language. In most of the routine inspection work (either

100% inspection or sampling inspection), the products are classified as either accepted or rejected. In such inspection it is a common practice to make a record of the number of items rejected. The ratio of the number of items rejected to the number of items inspected is the fraction of defective which is commonly expressed as a decimal fraction. The control limits of the chart which easily detect the presence of assignable and chance causes are set by simple statistical calculations. The p-chart is somewhat less sensitive than $\overline{X}$ and R charts and it does not have a great diagnostic value, but it serves to point out those situations needing diagnosis of trouble by the control chart for variables.

Nevertheless, it is an extremely useful to production supervision in giving information as to when and where to exert pressure for quality improvement. It results in the reduction of the average fraction defective and in the improvement of inspection practices by disclosing erratic fluctuations in the quality of inspection. The p-chart serves as a very good tool in dealing with outside vendors by pointing out whether the vendors differ in quality level or in the variability of quality level.

2. *The Shewhart control chart for number of defectives:* This chart is also described as np-chart or the chart for the number of defectives in the sample. The control chart for this is drawn by taking *m* samples, each of size *n* are drawn at regular intervals of time from a production process and for each sample the number of defectives *d* is found out. *d* follows the binomial distribution with parameters *n* and *p*, where *n* is total the total number of items in the sample and *p* is the fraction defectives of the sample.

The control limits for np-chart:

$$CL = n\,\overline{P}$$

$$LCL = n\,\overline{P} - 3\,[n\,p\,(1-\overline{P})]^{1/2}$$

$$UCL = n\,\overline{P} - 3\,[n\,p\,(1-\overline{P})]^{1/2}$$

3. *The Shewhart control chart for defects per unit:* In technical language of the subject, it is described as c-chart. This type of chart applies to a limited number of manufacturing situations involving quality, e.g., inspection of a fairly complex assembled unit in which there are a great many opportunities for occurrences of defects of various types, and the total number of defects or all types found by inspection are recorded for each unit.

In c-chart also, the control limits are set in a way to detect the presence or absence of assignable causes of variations; thereby telling when to take action on the process

(ii) Control Charts for Variables ($\overline{X}$ Chart and R Chart)

These charts help in trouble shooting of the manufacturing process by providing information on three matters, all of which need to be known as a basis for action.

(a) Basis variability of the quality characteristic.

(b) Consistency of Performance.

(c) Average level of the quality characteristic.

No production process can produce identical objects. Some variability is unavoidable which depends upon the various characteristics of the production process such as the machines, the materials, the operators. When both upper and lower values (e.g. dimensional tolerances) are specified and control chart shows that the process variability is great, then it is necessary to make change in the process or to take the trouble of sorting good product from bad. Sometimes it may be observed that tolerances are tighter than necessary for the functioning of the product and they can be widened instead of choosing a very precise and costly process.

The control limits on the charts are so placed as to disclose the presence or absence of the assignable causes. The control charts tell when to leave process alone and when to take action to correct trouble. The elimination of assignable causes of erratic fluctuation is described as bringing a process under control and is responsible for many of the cost savings resulting from statistical quality control.

In some instances the process variability is such that the natural tolerance range is narrower than the specified tolerance range, still the products are unsatisfactory because the average level of the quality characteristic is too high or too low. This will also be disclosed by control charts and correction of the average level can be taken by changing machine setting or taking some suitable action.

Once the control chart shows that a process is brought under control at a satisfactory level and with satisfactory limits of variability, one may feel confident that the product meets specifications. This suggests the possibility of basing acceptance procedures on the control charts and thereby result in substantial savings in costs related to inspection.

$\overline{X}$ chart is used to show the quality averages of the samples drawn from a given process. Let X denote the quality characteristic of a manufactured product. m samples each of size n are drawn from the production process at regular intervals of time.

Let $\overline{X}_i$ be the mean and R_i be the range of the ith sample, ($I = 1, 2, \ldots, n$).

Calculate $\overline{\overline{X}}_i$ and $\overline{R}$ using

$$\overline{\overline{X}} = \frac{\Sigma \overline{X}_i}{m} \qquad \text{and} \qquad \overline{R} = \frac{\Sigma \overline{R}_i}{m}$$

The control limits of $\overline{X}$ chart are set at

Central line (CL) = $\overline{\overline{X}}$

Lower control limit (LCL) = $\overline{\overline{X}} - A_2 \overline{R}$

Upper control limit (UCL) = $\overline{\overline{X}} - A_2 \overline{R}$

The values of the constant A_2 are computed and tabulated for different values of *n*.

The control limits for R – Chart are set at

Central line (CL) = $\overline{R}$

Lower control limit (LCL) = $D_3 \overline{R}$

Upper control limit (UCL) = $D_4 \overline{R}$

Here D_3 and D_4 are constants which depend on the sample size n.

For $\overline{X}$ chart the sample numbers are taken on the X-axis and the values of $\overline{X}$ are taken on the Y-axis. The central line and both the control limits are drawn parallel to the X-axis. The value of $\overline{X}$ for each sample is plotted on the graph paper. On joining these points in order, $\overline{X}$ chart is obtained.

For R – chart the sample numbers are taken on the X-axis and the values of R are taken on the Y-axis. The central line, LCL and UCL for R – chart are drawn parallel to the X-axis. The values of R obtained from each sample are plotted on the graph paper. On joining these points in order, R – chart is obtained.

Acceptance Sampling

Acceptance inspection (generally done by sampling techniques) is a necessary part of manufacturing and is applied at various stage in a factory, e.g. it can be applied to incoming materials, to partially finished products at various intermediate stages of the manufacturing process and to final product, by the purchaser of the product.

It may be emphasized here that the best protection against the acceptance of defective product is in having the product made right in the first place and that the good sampling acceptance often contribute to this objective through more effective pressure for quality improvement which can be exerted with 100% inspection.

The modern sampling acceptance producers are based on the laws of probability and through much superior but some defectives are likely to be passed by it if a part of the stream of product submitted for acceptance is defective. It attempts to evaluate the risk assumed with alternative sampling procedures and to make a decision as to the degree of protection needed in any instance. It is then possible to choose a sampling acceptance scheme that gives a desired degree of protection with due consideration for the various costs involved.

B. Validation – Analytical Instruments & Analytical Methods

Introduction

The pharmaceutical industry relies on the precision and accuracy of analytical instruments to obtain valid data for research, development, manufacturing, and quality control. Indeed, advancements in the automation, precision, and accuracy of these instruments parallel those of the industry itself. Through published regulations, regulatory agencies require pharmaceutical companies to establish procedures assuring that the users of analytical instruments are trained to perform their assigned tasks. The regulations also require the companies to establish procedures assuring that the instruments that generate data supporting regulated product testing are fit for use. The regulations, however, do not provide clear and authoritative guidance for validation/qualification of analytical instruments. Consequently, competing opinions abound regarding instrument validation procedures and the roles and responsibilities of the people who perform them. On the latter point, many believe that the users (analysts), who ultimately are responsible for the instrument operations and data quality, were not sufficiently involved when the various stakeholders attempted to establish criteria and procedures to determine the suitability of instruments for their intended use. The objectives of Analytical Instrument Qualification are:

- Review and propose an effective and efficient instrument validation process that focuses on outcomes, and not only on generating documentation.
- Propose a risk-based validation process founded on competent science.
- Define the roles and responsibilities of those associated with an instrument's validation
- Determine whether differences exist between validations performed in laboratories that adopt Good Laboratory Practice (GLP) regulations vs those that adopt Good Manufacturing Practice regulations (GMP).
- Establish the essential parameters for performing instrument validation.
- Establish common terminology.
- Publish a white paper on analytical instrument validation that may aid in the development of formal future guidelines and submit it to regulatory agencies.

Components of Data Quality

Analytical instrument qualification helps justify the continued use of equipment, but it alone does not ensure the quality of data. Analytical instrument qualification is 1 of the 4 critical components of data quality. Analytical Instrument Qualification forms the base for generating quality data. The other essential components for generating quality data are the following:

Analytical Methods Validation, System Suitability Tests, and Quality Control Checks. These quality components are described below.

Analytical Instrument Qualification (AIQ) is documented evidence that an instrument performs suitably for its intended purpose and that it is properly maintained and calibrated. Use of a qualified instrument in analyses contributes to confidence in the veracity of generated data

Analytical methods validation is documented evidence that an analytical method does what it purports to do and delivers the required attributes. Use of a validated method should instill confidence that the method can generate test data of acceptable quality.

Various user groups and regulatory agencies have defined procedures for method validation. Among some common parameters generally obtained during method validations are the following:

- accuracy
- precision
- sensitivity
- specificity
- repeatability
- linearity
- analyte stability

Typically conducted before the system performs samples analysis, system suitability tests verify that the system works according to the performance expectations and criteria set forth in the method, assuring that at the time of the test the system met an acceptable performance standard.

Most analyses are performed using reference or calibration standards. Single- or multipoint calibration or standardization correlates instrument response with a known analyte quantity or quality. Calibrators/standards are generally prepared from certified materials suitable for the test. Besides calibration or standardization, some analyses also require the inclusion of quality control check samples, which provide an in-process assurance of the test's performance suitability.   The extent of system suitability tests or quality control checks varies for individual analyses. For example, chemical analyses, which are largely subject to GMP regulations, may require more system suitability tests than bioanalytical work. The bioanalytical work, largely subject to GLP regulations, requires more quality control checks during sample analysis. In summary, AIQ and analytical method validation assure the quality of analysis conducting the tests. System suitability tests and quality control checks assure the high quality of analytical results *immediately before or during* sample analysis.

Analytical Instrument Qualification

The following sections address in detail the analytical instrument qualification process. The other 3 components of building quality into analytical data—analytical methods validation, system suitability tests, and quality control checks—are not within the scope of this report.

Qualification Phases

Qualification of instruments is not a single, continuous process but instead results from many discrete activities. For convenience, these activities have been grouped into 4 phases of qualification.

- Design Qualification (DQ)
- Installation Qualification (IQ)
- Operational Qualification (OQ)
- Performance Qualification (PQ)

These qualification phases were used for AIQ because of their wide acceptance within the community of users, manufacturers, and quality assurance. Some of these qualification phases have their roots in manufacturing process validation. Note, however, that adoption of process validation terms does not imply that all process validation activities are necessary for AIQ. Some AIQ activities could arguably be performed within one or the other qualification phase. It is important that required AIQ activities are performed, but it should not be important under which qualification phase the individual activity is performed or reported.

Design Qualification (DQ)

The Design Qualification activity is most suitably performed by the instrument developer/manufacturer. Since the instrument design is already in place for the commercial off-the-shelf (COTS) systems, the user does not need to repeat all aspects of DQ. However, users should ensure that COTS instruments are suitable for their intended applications and that the manufacturer has adopted a quality system for developing, manufacturing, and testing. Users should also establish that manufacturers and vendors adequately support installation, service, and training. Methods for ascertaining the manufacturer's design qualification and an instrument's suitability for its intended use depend on the nature of the instrument, the complexity of the proposed application, and the extent of users' previous interaction with the manufacturer. Vendor audits or required vendor-supplied documentation satisfy the DQ requirement. The required scope and comprehensiveness of the audits and documentation vary with users' familiarity with the instrument and their previous interactions with the vendor.

Informal personal communications and networking with peers at technical or user group meetings significantly inform users about the suitability of instrument design for various applications and the quality of vendor support services. Informal site visits to other user and/or vendor facilities to obtain data on representative samples using the specified instruments also are a good source of information regarding the suitability of the instrument design for intended use. In many instances an assessment of the quality of vendor support, gleaned from informal discussions with peer users, significantly influences instrument selection.

Installation Qualification (IQ)

Installation Qualification is a documented collection of activities needed to install an instrument in the user's environment. IQ applies to a new, pre-owned or an existing on-site—but not previously qualified—instrument. The activities and documentation associated with IQ are as follows:

- **System Description:** Provide a description of the instrument, including its manufacturer, model, serial number, software version, etc. Use drawings and flowcharts where appropriate.

- **Instrument Delivery:** Ensure that the instrument, software, manuals, supplies, and any other accessories arrive with the instrument as the purchase order specifies and that they are undamaged. For a pre-owned or existing instrument, manuals and documentation should be obtained. Verify that the installation site satisfactorily meets vendor-specified environmental requirements. A commonsense judgment for the environment suffices; one need not measure the exact voltage for a standard-voltage instrument or the exact humidity reading for an instrument that will operate at ambient conditions.

- **Network and Data Storage:** Some analytical systems require users to provide network connections and data storage capabilities at the installation site. If this is the case, connect the instrument to the network and check its functionality.

- **Assembly and Installation:** Assemble and install the instrument and perform any initial diagnostics and testing. Assembly and installation of a complex instrument are best done by the vendor or specialized engineers, whereas users can assemble and install simple ones. For complex instruments, vendor-established installation tests and guides provide a valuable baseline reference for determining instrument acceptance. Any abnormal event observed during assembly and installation merits documenting. If the pre-owned or unqualified existing instrument requires assembly and installation, perform the tasks as specified here, and then perform the installation verification procedure described below.

- **Installation Verification:** Perform the initial diagnostics and testing of the instrument after installation. On obtaining acceptable results, the user and (when present) the installing engineer should confirm that the installation was successful before proceeding with the next qualification phase.

Operational Qualification (OQ)

After a successful IQ the instrument is ready for OQ testing. The OQ phase may consist of these test parameters:

- **Fixed Parameters:** These tests measure the instrument's nonchanging, fixed parameters such as length, height, weight, etc. If the vendor-supplied specifications for these parameters satisfy the user, he or she may waive the test requirement. However, if the user wants to confirm the parameters, testing can be performed at the user's site. Fixed parameters do not change over the life of the instrument and therefore never need redetermining.

- **Secure Data Storage, Backup, and Archive:** When required, secure data handling, such as storage, backup, and archiving should be tested at the user site according to written procedures.

- **Instrument Functions Tests:** Test important instrument functions to verify that the instrument operates as intended by the manufacturer and required by the user. The user should select important instrument parameters for testing according to the instrument's intended use. Vendor-supplied information is useful in identifying specifications for these parameters. Tests should be designed to evaluate the identified parameters. Users, or their qualified designees, should perform these tests to verify that the instrument meets vendor and user specifications.

OQ tests can be modular or holistic. Modular testing of individual components of a system may facilitate interchange of such components without requalification and should be done whenever possible. Holistic tests, which involve the entire system, are acceptable in lieu of modular testing. Having successfully completed OQ testing, the instrument is qualified for use in regulated samples testing.

The extent of OQ testing that an instrument undergoes depends on its intended applications. We therefore offer no specific OQ tests for any instrument or application. Nevertheless, as a guide to the type of tests possible during OQ, consider these, which apply to a high-performance liquid chromatography (HPLC) unit

- pump flow rate
- gradient linearity
- detector wavelength accuracy
- detector linearity
- column oven temperature
- peak area precision
- peak retention time precision

Routine analytical tests do not constitute OQ testing. OQ tests specifically designed to determine operation qualification should verify the instrument's operation according to specifications in the user's environment. OQ tests may not be required to be repeated at a regular interval. Rather, when the instrument undergoes major repairs or modifications, relevant OQ tests should be repeated to verify whether the instrument continues to operate satisfactorily.

Performance Qualification (PQ)

After the IQ and OQ have been performed, the instrument's continued suitability for its intended use is proved through performance qualification. The PQ phase includes these parameters:

- **Performance Checks:** Set up a test or series of tests to verify an acceptable performance of the instrument for its intended use. PQ tests are usually based on the instrument's typical on-site applications. Some tests may resemble those performed during OQ, but the specifications for their results can be set differently if required. PQ tests are performed routinely on a working instrument, not just on a new instrument at installation. Therefore, PQ specifications can be slightly less rigorous than OQ specifications. Nevertheless, user specifications for PQ tests should evince trouble-free instrument operation vis-à-vis the intended applications. PQ tests should be performed independent of the routine analytical testing performed on the instrument. Like OQ testing, the tests can be modular or holistic. Since many modules within a system interact, holistic tests generally prove more effective by evaluating the entire system and not just the system's individual modules. Testing frequency depends on the ruggedness of the instrument and criticality of the tests performed. Testing may be unscheduled—for example, each time the instrument is used. Or it may be scheduled to occur at regular intervals; eg, weekly, monthly, yearly. Experience with the instrument can influence this decision. Generally, the same PQ tests are repeated each time so that a history of the instrument's performance can be compiled. Some system suitability tests or quality control checks that run concurrently with the test samples also imply that the instrument is performing suitably. However, though system suitability tests can supplement periodic PQ tests, they cannot replace them.

- **Preventive Maintenance and Repairs:** When PQ test(s) fail to meet specifications, the instrument requires maintenance or repair. For many instruments a periodic preventive maintenance may also be recommended. Relevant PQ test(s) should be repeated after the needed maintenance or repair to ensure that the instrument remains qualified.

- **Standard Operating Procedure for Operation, Calibration, and Maintenance:** Establish standard operating procedures to maintain and calibrate the instrument. Use a logbook, binder, or electronic record to document each maintenance and calibration activity.

Roles and Responsibilities

Users are ultimately responsible for the instrument operations and data quality. Users group includes analysts, their supervisors, and the organizational management. Users should be adequately trained in the instrument's use, and their training records should be maintained as required by the regulations. Users should be responsible for qualifying their instruments. Their training and expertise in the use of instruments make them the best-qualified group to design the instrument test(s) and specification(s) necessary for successful AIQ. Consultants, validation specialists, and quality assurance personnel can advise and assist as needed, but the final responsibility for qualifying instruments lies with the users. The users must also maintain the instrument in a qualified state by routinely performing PQ.

The quality assurance (QA) role in AIQ remains as it is in any other regulated study. QA personnel should understand the instrument qualification process, and they should learn the instrument's application by working with the users. Finally, they should review the AIQ process to determine whether it meets regulatory requirements and that the users attest to its scientific validity.

The manufacturer is responsible for DQ when designing the instrument. It is also responsible for validating relevant processes for manufacturing and assembly of the hardware and for validating software associated with the instrument as well as the stand-alone software used in analytical work. The manufacturer should test the assembled instrument prior to shipping to the user.

The manufacturer should make available to the users a summary of its validation efforts and also the results of final instrument and software tests. It should provide the critical functional test scripts used to qualify the instrument and software at the user site. For instance, the manufacturer can provide a large database and scripts for functional testing of the network's bandwidth for laboratory information management system (LIMS) software. Finally, the manufacturer should notify all known users about hardware or software defects discovered after a product's release, offer user training and installation support, and invite user audits as necessary

Software Validation

Software used for analytical work can be classified into following categories:

- firmware
- instrument control, data acquisition, and processing software
- stand-alone software

The computerized analytical instruments contain integrated chips with low-level software (firmware). Such instruments will not function without properly operating firmware, and users usually cannot alter the firmware's design or function. Firmware is thus considered a component of the instrument itself. Indeed, qualification of the hardware is not possible without operating it via its firmware. So when the hardware; ie, analytical instrument, is qualified at the user's site, it essentially qualifies the integrated firmware. No separate on-site qualification of the firmware is needed. Any changes made to firmware versions should be tracked through change control of the instrument

Software for instrument control, data acquisition, and processing for many of today's computerized instruments is loaded on a computer connected to the instrument. Operation of the instrument is then controlled via the software, leaving fewer operating controls on the instrument. Also, the software is needed for data acquisition and post acquisition calculations. Thus, both hardware and software, their functions inextricably intertwined, are critical to providing analytical results.

The manufacturer should perform the DQ, validate this software, and provide users with a summary of validation. At the user site, holistic qualification, which involves the entire instrument and software system, is more efficient than modular validation of the software alone. Thus, the user qualifies the instrument control, data acquisition, and processing software by qualifying the instrument according to the AIQ process defined earlier.

An authoritative guide for validating stand-alone software, such as LIMS, is available. The validation process is administered by the software developer, who also specifies the development model appropriate for the software. It takes place in a series of activities planned and executed through various stages of the development cycle.

The software validation guidance document indicates that user-site testing is an essential part of the software development cycle. Note, however, that user-site testing, though essential, is only part of the validation process for stand-alone software and does not constitute complete validation. Refer to the guide for activities needed to be performed at the user site for testing stand-alone software used in analytical work.

Change Control

Changes to the instrument and software become inevitable as manufacturers add new features and correct known defects. However, implementing all such changes may not always benefit users. Users should therefore adopt only the changes they deem useful or necessary. The Change Control process enables them to do this.

Change Control follows the DQ/IQ/OQ/PQ classification process. For DQ, evaluate the changed parameters, and determine whether the need for the change warrants implementing it. If implementation of the change is needed, install the changes to the system during IQ. Evaluate which of the existing OQ and PQ tests need revision, deletion, or addition as a result of the installed change. Where the change calls for additions, deletions, or revisions to the OQ or PQ tests, follow the procedure outlined below:

- **OQ:** Revise OQ tests as necessitated by the change. Perform the revised OQ testing. If the OQ did not need revision, repeat only the relevant tests affected by the change. This procedure ensures the instrument's effective operation after the change is installed.

- **PQ:** Revise PQ tests as necessitated by the change. Perform the PQ testing after installation of the change if similar testing is not already performed during OQ. In the future, perform the revised PQ testing.

For changes to the firmware and the instrument control, data acquisition, and processing software, Change Control is performed through DQ/IQ/OQ/PQ of the affected instrument. Change Control for the stand-alone software requires user-site testing of the changed functionality

AIQ Documentation

Two types of documents result from AIQ: Static and Dynamic

Static documents are obtained during the DQ, IQ, and OQ phases and should be kept in a "Qualification" binder. Where multiple instruments of one kind exist, common documents should go into one binder or section, and documents specific to an instrument should go into that instrument's binder or section. During Change Control, additional documents can be placed with the static ones, but previous documents should not be removed. When necessary, such documents may be archived.

Dynamic documents are generated during the OQ and PQ phase, when the instrument is maintained, or when it is tested for performance. Arranged in a binder or logbook, they provide a running record for the instruments and should be kept with them, available for review by any interested party. These documents may also be archived as necessary.

Instrument Categories

Modern laboratories typically include a suite of tools. These vary from simple spatulas to complex automated instruments. Therefore, applying a single set of principles to qualify such dissimilar instruments would be scientifically inappropriate. The users are the most qualified to establish the level of qualification needed for an instrument. Based on the level of qualification needed, it is convenient to categorize instruments into 3 groups: A, B, and C, as defined below. Each group is illustrated by some example instruments. The list of instruments provided below as illustration is not meant to be exhaustive, nor can it provide the exact category for an instrument at a user site. The exact category of an instrument should be determined by the user for their specific instrument or application.

Conformance of *Group A* instruments to user requirements is determined by visual observation. No independent qualification process is required. Example instruments in this group include light microscopes, magnetic stirrers, mortars and pestles, nitrogen evaporators, ovens, spatulas, and vortex mixers.

Conformance of *Group B* instruments to user requirements is performed according to the instruments' standard operating procedures. Their conformity assessments are generally unambiguous. Installation of Group B instruments is relatively simple and causes of their failure readily discernable by simple observations. Example instruments in this group include balances, incubators, infrared spectrometers, melting point apparatus, muffle furnaces, pH meters, pipettes, refractometers, refrigerator-freezers, thermocouples, thermometers, titrators, vacuum ovens, and viscometers

Conformance of *Group C* instruments to user requirements is highly method specific, and the conformity bounds are determined by their application. Installing these instruments can be a complicated undertaking and may require the assistance of specialists. A full-qualification process, as outlined in this document, should apply to these instruments. Example instruments in this group might include the following:

- atomic absorption spectrometers
- differential scanning calorimeters
- densitometers
- diode-array detectors
- electron microscopes
- elemental analyzers
- flame absorption spectrometers
- gas chromatographs
- high-pressure liquid chromatographs
- inductively coupled argon plasma emission spectrometers
- mass spectrometers
- micro-plate readers
- near infrared spectrometers
- Raman spectrometers
- thermal gravimetric analyzers
- UV/Vis spectrometers
- x-ray fluorescence spectrometers

The purpose of the use of analytical instruments is to generate reliable data. Instrument qualification helps fulfill this purpose. No authoritative guide exists that considers the risk of instrument failure and combines that risk with users' scientific knowledge and ability to use the instrument to deliver reliable and consistent data. In the absence of such a guide, the qualification of analytical instruments has become a subjective and often fruitless document-generating exercise.

Analytical Method Validation

Testing of drugs has to be done at several stages for standardization and quality control. For this purpose analytical techniques like chromatography, chemical assay, microbiological assay etc. are employed.

Management of Quality

Quality must be assured, not assumed! Quality does not happen by itself. Quality must be achieved by work processes that are carefully planned, properly operated, optimally controlled, appropriately measured and continuously improved.

- **Management of Quality:** Standard, Standard process, Standard of Quality, a standard process for managing quality and priorities for developing standard quality management processes.

- **Standard:** known value for calibration of a testing process and represents purity, truth and correctness.

- **Standard Process:** Standard analytical process provides a well defined protocol for performing a laboratory test or experiment.

- **Standard of Quality:** a criterion or statement that describes the acceptable level of something. For an analytical test, we need to know how quickly a test result needs to be reported as well as how close the result must be to the true or correct value.

A Standard Process for Managing Quality

- **QP** (Quality Planning) – the best way to get the work done (selection and evaluation of the analytical method, equipment, reagents and procedures used to perform the experiment.

- **QLP** (Quality Laboratory Processes) – Standard work processes to utilize the policies, procedures, protocols and personnel of the laboratories.

- **QC** (Quality Control) – Quantitative measures of process performance using statistical process control techniques.

- **QA** (Quality Assessment) – Measures how well the work is getting done (the effectiveness of specimen acquisition procedures, turn around time for laboratory services, appropriate formats for reporting results etc.

- **QI** (Quality Improvement) – problem solving mechanism to determine root causes which can then be eliminated through QP

Validation of Analytical Procedures used in Standardization of Drugs

- **Validation:** the process of demonstrating that the analytical procedure is suitable for its intended purpose, e.g. identification, determination of impurities, assay of active or other ingredients.

- **Analytical Procedure:** refers to the way of performing the analysis. It should describe in detail the steps necessary to perform each analytical test. This may include but is not limited to the sample, the reference standard and the reagents preparations, use of the apparatus, generation of the calibration curve, use of the formulae for the calculation etc.

  If the analytical procedure for product testing is included in the official Pharmacopoeias or the official methods of analysis of the association of Analytical Chemists (AOAC international) then validation of that procedure is not required.

Determining the Need for Validation

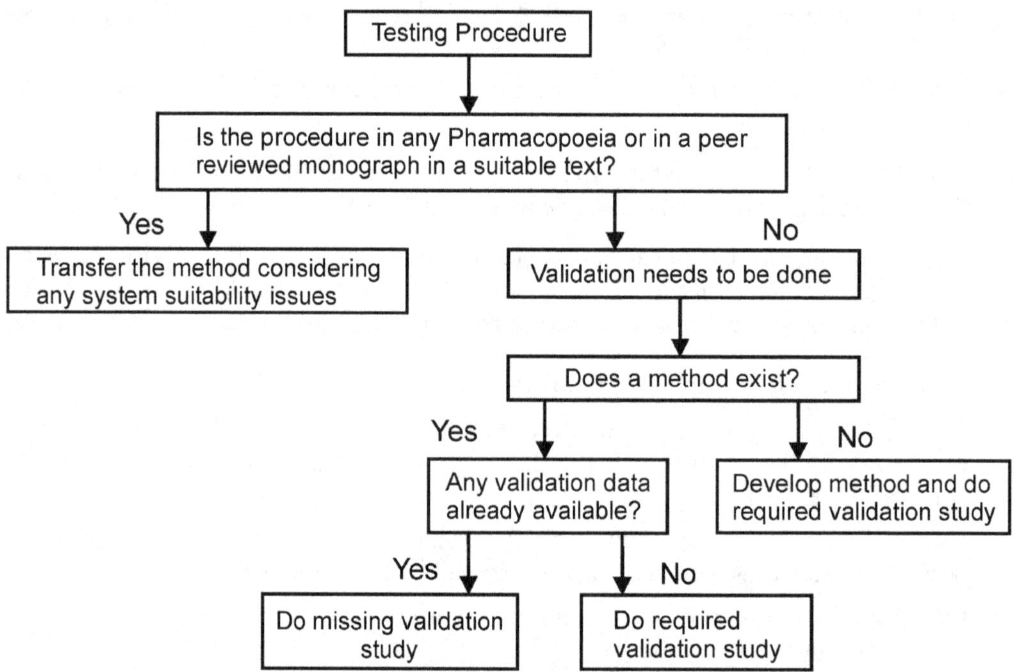

Types of Analytical Procedures to be Validated

Identification tests, quantitative tests for impurities' content, limit test for the control of impurities and quantitative tests for the active molecule in samples of substance or medicinal product or other selected component(s) in the medicinal product.

- Identification Tests – to ensure the identity of an analyte in a sample. Achieved by comparison of a property of sample like spectrum, chromatographic behavior, chemical reactivity etc. to that of a reference standard.

Testing for impurities can be either a quantitative test or a limit test for the impurity in a sample. Either test is intended to accurately reflect the purity characteristics of the sample.

Assay procedures are intended to measure the analyte present in a given sample. The assay represents a quantitative measurement of the major component(s) in the substance.

Validation of Analytical Procedures used in Standardization of Drugs

Validation Characteristics for Analytical Procedures

- Accuracy
- Precision
- Specificity
- Detection limits
- Quantitation limit
- Linearity
- Range
- Robustness
- System Suitability testing

Revalidation may be necessary in the following circumstances:

- Changes in the synthesis of the active substance
- Changes in the composition of the medicinal product
- Changes in the analytical procedure

Accuracy

The accuracy of an analytical procedure expresses the closeness of agreement between the value which is accepted either as a conventional true value or an accepted reference value and the value found. This is sometimes termed trueness.

Accuracy should be established across the specified range of the analytical procedure.

1. Assay and

2. Impurities (Quantitation)

3. Recommended Data

1. **Assay**

- **Active Substance**
  - Application of an analytical procedure to an analyte of known purity (Reference)
  - Comparison of the results of the proposed analytical procedure with those of a second well characterized procedure
  - Accuracy may be inferred once precision, linearity and specificity are established

- **Medicinal product**
  - Application of the analytical procedure to synthetic mixtures of the product components to which known quantities of the substance to be analyzed have been added.
  - In cases where it is impossible to obtain samples of all product components, it may be acceptable either to add known quantities of the analyte to the product or to compare the results obtained from a second well characterized procedure, the accuracy of which is stated or defined.
  - accuracy may be inferred once precision, linearity and specificity are established.

2. Impurities (Quantitation)

Accuracy should be assessed on samples (substance/product) spiked with known amounts of impurities.

In cases where it is impossible to obtain samples of certain impurities or degradation products, it is considered acceptable to compare results obtained by an independent procedure. The response factor of the drug substance can be used.

3. Recommended Data

Accuracy should be assessed using a minimum of 9 determinations over a minimum of 3 concentration levels covering the specified range. (i.e. 3 concentrations / 3 replicates each of the total analytical procedure).

Accuracy should be reported as percent recovery by the assay of known added amount of analyte in the sample or as the difference between the mean and the accepted true value together with the confidence intervals.

Precision: The precision of an analytical procedure expresses the closeness of agreement (degree of scatter) between a series of measurement obtained from multiple sampling of the same homogeneous sample under the prescribed conditions. Precision may be considered at three levels: repeatability, intermediate precision and reproducibility.

Precision should be investigated using homogeneous, authentic samples. However, if it is not possible to obtain a homogenous sample it may be investigated using artificially prepared samples or a sample solution.

The precision of an analytical procedure is usually expressed as the variance, standard deviation or coefficient of variation (ANOVA) of a series of measurements.

(a) Repeatability

(b) Intermediate precision

(c) Reproducibility

Repeatability: Expresses the precision under the same operating conditions over a short interval of time. Repeatability is also termed intra-assay precision.

a minimum of 9 determinations covering the specified range (3 conc. / 3 replicates each)

or a minimum of 6 determinations at 100% of the test conc.

Intermediate Precision: Expresses within laboratory variation: different days, different analysts, different equipment etc.

Reproducibility: Assessed by means of an inter-laboratory trial. Reproducibility should be considered in case of standardization of an analytical procedure, for instance, for inclusion of procedure in pharmacopoeias.

Specificity: Specificity is the ability to assess unequivocally the analyte in the presence of components which may be expected to be present. Typically these might include impurities, degradants, matrix, etc.

Lack of specificity of a individual analytical procedure may be compensated by other supporting analytical procedure(s).

This definition has the following implications:

Identification: to ensure the identity of an analyte.

Purity Tests: to ensure that all the analytical procedures performed allow an accurate statement of the content of impurities of an analyte. i.e. related substances test, heavy metals, residual solvents content etc.

Assay (Content or Potency): to provide an exact result which allows an accurate statement on the content or potency of the analyte in a sample.

Detection Limit: The detection limit of an individual analytical procedure is the lowest amount of analyte in a sample which can be detected but not necessarily quantitated as an exact value.

Several approaches for determining the detection limit are possible depending on whether the procedure is a non instrumental or instrumental.

1. Based on visual evaluation
2. Based on signal to noise
3. Based on the standard deviation of the response and the slope
   (a) Based on the standard deviation of the blank
   (b) Based on the calibration curve

1. **Based on Visual Evaluation:** visual evaluation may be used for non-instrumental methods but may also be used with instrumental methods.

The detection limit is determined by the analysis of samples with known concentration of analyte and by establishing the minimum level at which the analyte can be reliably detected.

2. **Based on Signal-to-Noise:** This approach can only be applied to analytical procedures which exhibit baseline noise.

Determination of the signal-to-noise ratio is performed by comparing measured signals from samples with known low concentrations of analyte with those of blank samples and establishing the minimum concentration at which the analyte can be reliably detected. A signal-to-noise ratio between 3 or 2:1 is generally considered acceptable for estimating the detection limit.

3. **Based on the Standard Deviation of the Response and the Slope**

The detection limit (DL) may be expressed as:

$$DL = 3.3 \, \sigma / S$$

where σ = the standard deviation of the response

S = the slope of the calibration curve

The slope S may be estimated from the calibration curve of the analyte. The estimate of σ may be carried out in a variety of ways, for example:

(a) **Based on the Standard Deviation of the Blank:** Measurement of the magnitude of analytical background response is performed by analyzing an appropriate number of blank samples and calculating the standard deviation of these responses.

(b) **Based on the Calibration Curve:** A specific calibration curve should be studied using samples containing an analyte in the range of DL. The residual standard deviation of a regression line or the standard deviation of y-intercepts of regression lines may be used as the standard deviation.

Quantitation Limit

The quantitation limit of an individual analytical procedure is the lowest amount of analyte in a sample which can be quantitatively determined with suitable precision and accuracy. The quantitation limit is a parameter of quantitative assays for low levels of compounds in sample matrices, and is used particularly for the determination of impurities and/or degradation products.

1. Based on visual evaluation
2. Based on signal to noise
3. Based on the standard deviation of the response and the slope
   (a)   Based on the standard deviation of the blank
   (b)   Based on the calibration curve

1. **Based on Visual Evaluation:** visual evaluation may be used for non-instrumental methods but may also be used with instrumental methods.

   The Quantitation limit is determined by the analysis of samples with known concentration of analyte and by establishing the minimum level at which the analyte can be quantified with acceptable accuracy and precision.

2. **Based on Signal-to-Noise Approach:** This approach can only be applied to analytical procedures which exhibit baseline noise.

   Determination of the signal-to-noise ratio is performed by comparing measured signals from samples with known low concentrations of analyte with those of blank samples and establishing the minimum concentration at which the analyte can be reliably quantified. A signal-to-noise ratio is 10:1.

3. **Based on the Standard Deviation of the response and the slope**

   The Quantitation Limit (QL) may be expressed as:

   $$QL = 10\,\sigma / S$$

   where $\quad\quad\sigma$ = the standard deviation of the response

   $\quad\quad\quad\quad\quad$ S = the slope of the calibration curve

The slope S may be estimated from the calibration curve of the analyte. The estimate of σ may be carried out in a variety of ways, for example:

   (a) **Based on the Standard Deviation of the Blank:** Measurement of the magnitude of analytical background response is performed by analyzing an appropriate number of blank samples and calculating the standard deviation of these responses.

   (b) **Based on the Calibration Curve:** A specific calibration curve should be studied using samples containing an analyte in the range of QL. The residual standard deviation of a regression line or the standard deviation of y-intercepts of regression lines may be used as the standard deviation.

Linearity: The linearity of analytical procedure is its ability (within a given range) to obtain test results which are directly proportional to the concentration (amount) of analyte in the sample.

A linear relationship should be evaluated across the range of the analytical procedure. It may be demonstrated directly on the active substance by dilution of standard stock solution using the proposed procedure. Linearity should be evaluated by visual inspection of a plot of signals as a function of analyte concentration or content.

For the establishment of linearity, the correlation coefficient, y-intercept, slope of the regression line and the residual sum of squares should be submitted. A minimum of five concentrations is recommended for proving linearity.

Range

The range of an analytical procedure is the interval between the upper and lower concentration (amounts) of analyte in the sample (including these concentration) for which it has been demonstrated that the analytical procedure has a suitable level of precision, accuracy and linearity.

Minimum specified Ranges:

- for the assay of an active substances or a finished product: normally from 80 to 120 percent of the test concentration;
- for content uniformity, covering a minimum of 70 to 130 percent of the test concentration, unless a wider more appropriate range, based on the nature of the dosage form (e.g., metered dose inhalers) is justified;
- for dissolution testing: ± 20% over the specified range; e.g., if the specifications for a controlled released product cover a region from 20%, after 1 hour, up to 90%, after 24 hours, the validated range would be 0-110% of the label claim;
- for the determination of an impurity: from the reporting level of an impurity to 120% of the specification; for impurities known to be unusually potent or to produce toxic or unexpected pharmacological effects, the detection/ quantitation limit should be commensurate with the level at which the impurities must be controlled. Note: for validation of impurity test procedures carried out during development, it may be necessary to consider the range around a suggested (probable) limit;
- if assay and purity are performed together as one test and only a 100% standard is used, linearity should cover the range from the reporting level of the impurities to 120% of the assay specification.

Robustness: The robustness of an analytical procedure is a measure of its capacity to remain unaffected by small, but deliberate variations in method parameters and provides an indication of its reliability during normal usage.

If measurements are susceptible to variations in analytical conditions, the analytical conditions should be suitably controlled or a precautionary statement should be included in the procedure. One consequence of the evaluation of the evaluation of robustness should be that a series of system suitability parameters (e.g., resolution test) is established to ensure that the validity of the analytical procedure is maintained whenever used.

Examples of typical variations are:

- Stability of analytical solutions
- Extraction time

In the case of liquid chromatography, examples of typical variations are:

- Influence of variation of pH in a mobile phase
- Influence of variation in mobile phase composition
- Different columns (different lots and/or suppliers)
- Temperature
- Flow rate

In the case of gas-chromatography, examples of typical variations are:

- Different columns (different lots and/or suppliers)
- Temperature
- Flow rate.

System Suitability Testing: System suitability testing is an integral part of many analytical procedures. The tests are based on the concept that the equipment, electronics, analytical operations and samples to be analyzed constitute an integral system that can be evaluated as such. System suitability test parameters to be established for a particular procedure depend on the type of procedure being validated.

System suitability tests and requirements are often included in the validated methods. The ability to achieve these system suitability requirements is a key step in ensuring method transfer, but is not the only step.

The effectiveness of transferring a validated method from the original laboratory to another laboratory needs to be verified. Differences in instrumentation and other equipment e.g., chromatography columns of different brands, age etc., capability of detectors, quality of reagents used, different filter materials etc.

It is possible that the analytical test procedure being transferred has been partially or fully validated by someone else. If this is the case it should be possible to obtain a summary statement of validation. This statement must include the following:

- Which aspects of validation have been addressed (such as specificity, accuracy, precision etc.)
- The extent of compliance of analytical procedure
- Documented details of the equipment used in the validation activities
- Details of the equipment that was used in the validation activity

C. Good Laboratory Practices (GLP)

Introduction and Objectives and Key Requirements

Good Laboratory Practice (GLP) deals with the organization, process and conditions under which laboratory studies are planned, performed, monitored, recorded and reported. GLP practices are intended to promote the quality and validity of test data.

Published GLP regulations and guidelines have a significant impact on the daily operation of an analytical laboratory.

GLP is a regulation. It is not only good analytical practice. Good analytical practice is important, but it is not enough. For example, the laboratory must have a specific organizational structure and procedures to perform and document laboratory work. The objective is not only quality of data but also traceability and integrity of data. But the biggest difference between GLP and Non-GLP work is the type and amount of documentation.

For a GLP inspector it should be possible to look at the documentation and to easily find out

- who has done a study,
- how the experiment was carried out,
- which procedures have been used,
- whether there has been any problem and if so
- how it has been solved.

And this should not only be possible during and right after the study has been finished but also 5 to 10 or more years later.

Frequently the question comes: how much does this cost? It has been estimated that these additional organizational and documentation requirements increase operational costs of up to 30% compared to non-GLP operation.

The key requirements of a GLP type works are:
- Responsibilities should be defined for the sponsor management, for study management and for the quality assurance unit.
- All routine work should follow written standard operating procedures.
- Facilities such as laboratories should be large enough and have the right construction to ensure the integrity of a study, for example, to avoid cross contamination.

- Test and control articles should have the right quality and instruments should be calibrated and well maintained
- People should be trained or otherwise qualified for the job
- Raw data and other data should be acquired, processed and archived to ensure integrity of data.

Unfortunately most laboratories are in situations where they have had to interpret the regulations. Procedures have been developed on an ad hoc basis, in isolation, in response to inspections by both their company's Quality Assurance Unit and regulatory bodies.

Under such duress, many scientists in industry have developed procedures to validate their instrumentation even though the same approach will already have been applied at the instrument manufacturer's site. Standard operating procedures written to accompany such validation efforts often duplicate extracts from operation manuals —why don't the manufacturers provide the SOPs directly? When it comes to validating the instrument's application software, the person responsible has to take the manufacturer's word for it that the software has been validated and hope that supporting documents, such as test results and source code are available to regulatory agencies upon request.

GLP vs. GCP, GMP

Figure 1 illustrates how so called Good Practices regulations correlate to the life of a drug, starting from basic research and drug discovery on the left side through preclinical development in the middle and clinical trials and manufacturing at the right

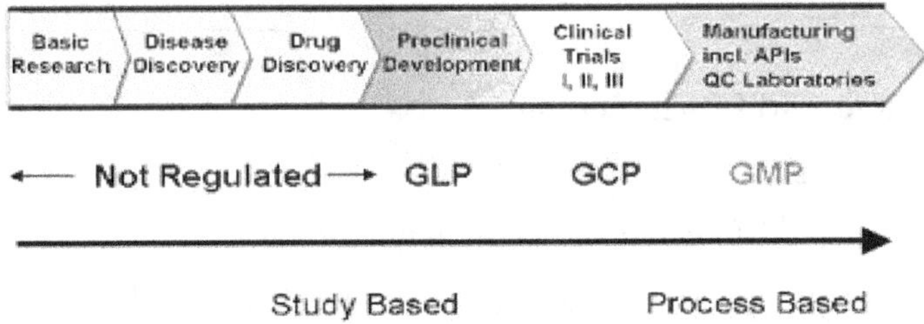

Figure 1 GLP vs. GCP, GMP.

Typically research and drug discovery are not regulated at all. GLP starts with preclinical development, for example toxicology studies. Clinical trials are regulated by good clinical practice regulations and manufacturing through GMPs. There is a frequent misunderstanding that all laboratory operations are regulated by GLP. This is not true. For example, Quality Control laboratories in manufacturing are regulated by GMPs and not by GLPs. Also Good laboratory Practice regulations are frequently mixed up with good analytical practice. Applying good analytical practices is important but not sufficient, as we will see in this presentation. When small quantities of active ingredients are prepared in a research or development laboratory for use in samples for clinical trials or finished drugs, that activity has be covered by GMP and not by GLP.

Independent from Location and Duration of a Study

GLPs regulate all non-clinical safety studies that support or are intended to support applications for research or marketing permits for products regulated by the Regulatory Authority, or by similar other national agencies. This includes drugs for human and animal use but also aroma and color additives in food, biological products and medical devices. The duration and location of the study is of no importance. For example GLP applies to short term experiments as well as to long term studies. And if a pharmaceutical company subcontracts part of a study to a university, that university still must comply with the same requirements as the sponsor company. Some laboratories tried to get away from GLP through outsourcing, but I can tell you this does not work.

GLP is needed for:	GLP is not needed for:
• Non clinical safety studies of development of drugs	• Basic research
• Agricultural pesticide development	• Studies to develop new analytical methods
• Development of toxic chemicals	• Chemical tests used to derive the specifications of a marketed food product
• Food control (food additives)	
• Test of substance with regard to explosive hazards	

Facility Management and Other Personnel

Qualification of Personnel

Like all regulations also GLPs have chapters on personnel.

The assumption is that in order to conduct GLP studies with the right quality a couple of things are important. Number one there should be sufficient people and second, the personnel should be qualified.

Qualification can come from education, experience or additional trainings, but it should be documented. This also requires a good documentation of the job descriptions, the tasks and responsibilities.

Facility Management

Responsibilities of facility management are well defined. They include to designate a study director and also to monitor the progress of the study and if it is not going well to replace the study director.

The management is responsible for many things, basically they should assure that a quality assurance unit is available, test and control articles are characterized, and that sufficient qualified personnel is available for the study.

Because it is obvious that management can not take care personally about all this, they have to rely on other functions, for example GLPs require that the QA should give a regular report on the compliance status of the study.

Study Director

The position of a study director is unique for GLP. He/she has overall responsibility for the technical conduct of the safety studies, as well as for the interpretation, analysis, documentation and reporting of the results. He or she is designated by and receives support from management. The study director serves as the single point of study control. It is important that this is a single individual person and not a department or any other grouping of people. An assistant study director is not permitted but there may be an alternate study director who serves as study director only in that person's absence.

The study director may be the laboratory manager and may be responsible for more than one study. However, he or she should not be over-burdened—an auditor could otherwise get the impression that the study director cannot monitor all studies carefully.

Quality Assurance Unit

The quality assurance unit (QAU) serves an internal control function. It is responsible for monitoring each study to assure management that facilities, equipment, personnel, methods, practices, records, controls, SOPs, final reports (for data integrity), and archives are in conformance with the GLP/GALP regulations. For any given study, the QAU is entirely separate from and independent of the personnel engaged in the direction and conduct of that study.

As well as immediately reporting of any problems, GLP/GALP regulations require the QAU to maintain and periodically submit to laboratory management comprehensive written records listing findings and problems, actions recommended and taken, and scheduled dates for inspection. A designated representative from the Regulatory Authority or EPA may ask to see the written procedures established for the QAU's inspection and may request the laboratory's management to certify that inspections are being implemented, and followed-up in accordance with the regulations governing the QAU.

Part-time or full-time personnel may be used depending on whether the volume of work is sufficient to justify employing one or more full-time quality assurance professionals. Full-time professionals are the preferred arrangement, because such an arrangement provides a degree of independence and removes the possibility that the demands of the person's second job will interfere with his or her performance of the QA function. For small organizations it might not be possible to designate a full-time person.

The Regulatory authorities mandate that responsibilities and procedures applicable to the QAU, the records maintained by the QAU, and the method of indexing such records be in writing and be maintained. The agencies further require that these items, including inspection dates, the description of the study inspected, the phase or segment of the study, and the name of the individual performing the inspection, be made available for review by an authorized Regulatory Authority.

Main Responsibilities of the Quality Assurance Unit

Maintain copy of master schedule sheet of all studies conducted. These are to be indexed by test article and must contain the test system, nature of study, date the study was initiated, current status of each study, identity of the sponsor, and name of the study director.

Maintain copies of all protocols pertaining to the studies for which QAU is responsible.

Inspect studies at intervals adequate to assure the integrity of the study and maintain written and properly signed records of each periodic inspection. These records must show the date of the inspection, the study inspected, the phase or segment of the study inspected, the person performing the inspection, findings and problems, action recommended and taken to resolve existing problems, and any scheduled date for re-inspection. Any problems discovered which are likely to affect study integrity are to be brought to the attention of the study director and management immediately.

Periodically submit to management and the study director written status reports on each study, noting problems and corrective actions taken.

Determine whether deviations from protocols and SOPs were made with proper authorization and documentation.

Review the final study report to assure that it accurately describes the methods and SOPs and that the reported results accurately reflect the raw data of the study.

Prepare and sign a statement to be included with the final study report that specifies the dates of audits and dates of reports to management and to the study director.

Audit the correctness of the statement, made by the study director, on the GLP compliance of the study.

Facilities

All GLP regulations also have requirements for facilities, for example, animal care facilities are listed as well as animal supply facilities, facilities for handling test and control articles, and laboratories and storage facilities. The main purpose of this is to ensure integrity of the study and of study data. Three main requirements for facilities are

1. Limited access to buildings and rooms
2. Adequate size and
3. Adequate construction.

For example, if a testing facility is to small to handle the specified volume of work there may be a risk to mix incompatible functions. Or if the air conditioning system is wrongly designed, there may be cross contamination between different areas.

Equipment and Computer Systems

All GLP regulations also have requirements for equipment. They are related to design, calibration, maintenance and validation. This includes analytical equipment such as chromatographs, spectrophotometers, and computerized equipment for instrument control and direct data capture, data evaluation, printing, archiving and retrieval. .

Design

Equipment used in generation, measurement, or assessment of data and equipment used for facility environmental control shall be of appropriate design and adequate capacity to function according to the protocol and shall be suitably located for operation, inspection, cleaning, and maintenance. The equipment should undergo a validation process to ensure that it will consistently function as intended. Examples are analytical equipment such as chromatographs, spectrophotometers, computerized equipment for direct data capture, and computers for statistical analysis of data.

Maintenance, Calibration, Testing and Validation

Equipment shall be adequately inspected, cleaned, and maintained. Equipment used for generation, measurement, or assessment of data shall be adequately tested, calibrated and/or standardized. These activities are frequently called qualification for equipment hardware and single modules and validation for software and complete systems. A laboratory shall establish schedules for such operations based on manufacturer's recommendations and laboratory experience.

Time interval for Calibration, Re-Validation and Testing

The frequency for calibration, re-validation and testing (performance verification) depends on the instrument itself, the recommendations from manufacturers of equipment, laboratory experience, and the extent of use. For instance, a pH meter should be calibrated before each use and the wavelength of an HPLC variable wavelength detector should be calibrated about every month or whenever the cell is removed and reinstalled. Typically proof of chromatographic instrument performance should be done every 6 to 12 months.

Equipment Records and Other Documents

Written records shall be maintained of all inspection, maintenance, testing, calibrating and/or qualification / validation operations. These records, containing the date of operation, shall describe whether the maintenance operations followed written SOPs. Written records shall be kept of non-routine repairs performed on equipment as a result of failure and malfunction. Such records shall document the nature of the defect, how and when the defect was discovered, and any remedial action taken in response to the defect. Written records may be in log books especially designed for that purpose. A log book should accompany the instrument when it is moved. Remedial action should include a review of effects on data generated before the defect was discovered. Such equipment records should be maintained as long as the data generated by the equipment.

Equipment records should include:

- name of the equipment
- name of the manufacturer,
- model or type for identification
- serial number
- date equipment was received in the laboratory
- condition when received (new, used)
- details of checks made for compliance with relevant calibration or test standard specification
- date equipment was placed in service by the laboratory
- current location in the laboratory, if appropriate
- copy of manufacturer's operating instruction(s)
- details of maintenance carried out
- history of any damage, malfunction, modification or repair
- person responsible for the equipment

Important Questions to be Answered for any Analytical Instrument

For an auditor there are several important questions to be answered for any analytical instrument:

1. What is the equipment being used for and are there specifications?
2. Is the instrument within specification and is the documentation to prove this available?
3. If the instrument is not within specifications, how much does it deviate by?
4. If the instrument is not within specifications, how long has this been the case?
5. If the instrument is not within specifications what action has been taken to overcome the defect?
6. Can the standards used to test and calibrate the instruments be traced back to national standards?

Standard Operating Procedures

Standard operating procedures (SOPs) are written procedures for a laboratorie's program. They define how to carry out protocol-specified activities. Most often they are written in a chronological listing of action steps.

- Routine inspection, cleaning, maintenance, testing, calibration and standardization of instruments
- Actions to be taken in response to equipment failure
- Analytical methods
- Definition of raw data
- Data handling, storage, and retrieval
- Health and safety precautions
- Receipt, identification, storage, mixing, and method sampling of test and control articles
- Record keeping, reporting, storage, and retrieval of data
- Coding of studies, handling of data, including the use of computerized data systems
- Operation of quality assurance personnel in performing and reporting study audits, inspections, and final study report reviews

SOPs should preferably be written in the laboratory close to the instrument, and not in an office. It should be either written or thoroughly reviewed by the instruments' operators. SOPs should not be written to explain how procedures are supposed to work, but how they work. This ensures that the information is adequate and that the document invites rather than discourages routine use.

SOPs are frequently mentioned as deviations in Regulatory Authority warning letters where three major deviations come up:

- SOPs are not available
- They are not adequate or
- They are not followed.

One of the first procedures should be an SOP on writing SOPs. This is important for consistency and efficiency. For example, it should be defined who is responsible for initiating, authoring, and approving SOPs and how procedures are distributed and how the use of SOPs is enforced.

GLPs allow to deviate from SOPs but deviations should be approved and documented.

Reagents and Solutions

To ensure ongoing quality of reagents and solutions used for GLP studies, purchasing and testing should be handled by a quality assurance program. That also should include qualification of suppliers.

All reagents and solutions in the laboratory areas shall be labeled to indicate identity, titer or concentration, storage requirements, and expiration date. Deteriorated or outdated reagents and solutions shall not be used. If reagents and solutions used for non-GLP regulated work are stored in the same room as reagents for GLP-regulated studies, all reagents must be labeled. Reagents that are not adequately labeled, even if not intended for use in GLP-regulated studies, may have an adverse effect on GLP regulated laboratory work. It is also good practice to include the Date opened:. This can be critical for some chemicals such as ether.

Many reagents can be stored under ambient temperature: does this mean we have to put a label on all these? One practical recommendation to avoid too much paper work is to have a procedure that has a sentence like this: "You don't need to label environmental conditions on each reagent if it is stored under ambient temperature." So everybody in your lab should know: reagents and solutions without storage temperature do not require cooling for storage

Expiration Date

The expiration date depends on the nature of the chemical. Sodium chloride has practically no expiration date. In these cases it might be acceptable to indicate NONE or Not applicable (N/A) on the label for expiration date. The laboratory must be prepared to justify this designation. Formal studies are not always required to justify assigned expiration dates. It is sufficient to assign expiration dates based on literature references and/or laboratory experience.

Test and Control Articles

Control articles or reference substances as they are called in the OECD principles are of utmost importance because they are commonly used to calibrate the instrument. The accuracy of the reference substances also determines the accuracy of the analytical method. In other words, if the reference standard is wrong, also the test result.

Main requirements for control articles are: The identity, strength, purity, composition and other characteristics should be determined for each batch and documented. Methods of synthesis, fabrication, or derivation of test and control articles should also be documented. Copies of this documentation must be stored with the study data and must be available for Regulatory Authority inspection.

In addition, the stability of each test or control article should be determined. This can be done either before study initiation, or simultaneously according to written SOPs which provide for periodic reanalysis of each batch.

Each storage container for a test or control article should be labeled by name, chemical abstract number or code number, batch number, expiration date, and, where appropriate, storage conditions necessary to maintain the identity, strength, purity and composition.

Furthermore, storage containers should be assigned to a particular test article for the length of the study.

Certified reference standards can be purchased from appropriate suppliers. If standards are not available, the recommendation is to take a lot of your own material, and analyze, certify and use it as the standard. However, they should be made from high purity material and be compared against the primary standard to ensure the traceability chain. For the comparison, validated test methods should be used.

Conduct of a Study, Study Protocol and Study Report

Study Protocol

Each GLP study should be conducted according to a study protocol. The study director writes the study protocol to document what should be done and when, it also describes anticipated exceptions from SOPs. Most important is the description of the experimental design, the type, frequency of tests and analyses. The study protocol also documents which records should be archived and available for inspections.

As a minimum the study protocol should include:

- Title and statement of the purpose of the study
- Identification of test and control article
- Identification of test system
- Name of the sponsor
- Description of experimental design
- Type and frequency of tests and analyses
- Records to be maintained

Conduct of a Study

The study should follow strictly the protocol and any deviations should be documented, if there are any. This section also includes requirements on how hand-recorded data and data captured from automated equipment should be recorded. For example, hand written data must be recorded in ink and not with a pencil. Changes must not obscure the original entry but and must be dated and signed together with a reason for the change.

When data are acquired from an automated system, the person responsible for the system and the system itself should be identified and documented.

Records

GLP regulations specify what should be recorded. Examples include:

- Name and address of the laboratory
- Objectives and procedures

- Statistical methods
- Test and control articles, including stability data
- Description of methods
- Description of test system
- Description of dosage, route of administration, duration
- Name of the study director
- Location where raw specimens and data are stored
- Descriptions of transformations and calculations

Most of requirements are quite obvious, but let's look at the last bullet: GLP inspectors want to see on how final results have been derived from raw data. This means to document it on paper when you use a calculator, it also can mean to store the formulas as part of an Excel spreadsheet, or for commercial systems formulas are included in the operation manual. Sometimes software companies don't disclose calculations used in their software to protect intellectual proprietary. This usually did not appear to be a big problem as long as you document it.

Retention and Retrieval of Records

GLPs have several paragraphs with details on how to store and retrieve records and data, for example, what should be archived and retention time.

What should be Archived

The list of documents that should be archived includes everything from raw data to final results, but also protocols from meetings, if decisions related to the integrity of a study have been made.

GLPs require the position of an archivist. This is either a part time or full time person who is responsible for the archive. Some companies have a procedure that requires documents from an archive to only be checked out by the archivist or his designate. Whenever documents are taken out of the archive this should be documented, and the person who requests it should sign a statement that nothing has been changed, added or deleted.

Retention Periods

GLPs also specify for how long records and specimens should be retained. For example, in the US material supporting Regulatory Authority submissions should be retained until

- 2 years after Regulatory Authority approval or
- 5 years after Regulatory Authority submission

For wet specimens may be shorter: they should only be retained as long as the quality affords evaluation. However, this is only for US Regulatory Authority and retention times in other countries may be different.

The numbers such as 2 and 5 years don't look as a long time. However, two years are after Regulatory Authority approval and 5 years are after Regulatory Authority submission can be a long time. Sometimes it may take ten or more years between the time GLP studies have been conducted and approved by the Regulatory Authority.

GLP says you can keep either the original or an exact copy of a record. An exact copy can be a copy of an instable thermo paper to durable plain paper or when paper records are scanned into TIF or PDF files.

Responsibility for Archiving

The sponsor company is responsible for the records. When a sponsor company outsources studies or also just the archiving part, the sponsor company must make sure that archiving of records complies with GLP regulations and in case the contractor goes out of business the sponsor company has access to all data. Long archiving time as require by GLP typically is no problem for normal paper records, but it may be one for electronic records, especially when records are archived as original records in the proprietary applications format. Examples are chromatographic or spectroscopic data. So the question is always whether electronic records can be printed and the original records can be deleted. For this discussion we take a closer look into the definition of raw data.

Raw Data

GLPs also have specific requirements for raw data. They are defined as any laboratory worksheets, records, memoranda, notes, or exact copies thereof, that are the results of original observations and activities of a study. The term covers all data necessary for the reconstruction of the report of the study. Raw data may include hand-written notes, photographs, microfilm copies, computer print-outs, magnetic media, dictated observations, and recorded data from automated instruments.

Examples also include records of animal receipt, results of environmental monitoring, instrument calibration records, and integrator output from analytical equipment. Raw data may also be entries in a worksheet used to read and note information from an LED display of an analytical instrument.

Electronic Records

Raw data are well defined as long as information is recorded on paper. For example original observations are recoded on paper and exact copies can be made if necessary. A more frequently discussed question is what is an exact copy of a paper print-out that comes from an electronic record. Most important here is to look again at the definition of an exact copy: as long as the print-out includes everything that is necessary to reconstruct the study, there should not be a problem. Or as an Regulatory Authority professional explained to a conference audience: as long as you can demonstrate compliance with the regulation.

For example, one requirement of GLP is to document in an audit trail when data have been changed. So look if the print-out includes the audit trail information, for example when data on the computer have been changed. An other question would be if all chromatographic peak in the print-out are on scale?

GLP Inspections and Enforcement

It is Regulatory Authority' responsibility to enforce the federal Food, drug and Cosmetic Act to ensure safety and effectiveness of drugs and medical devices. This is enforced through regulations, guidance documents and Regulatory Authority inspections. The Regulatory Authority has the responsibility to inspect GLP studies related to products that are marketed in the United States, it does not matter where the products are developed or manufactured.

Inspection Program

The Regulatory Authority has developed an inspection program with two types of inspections: Routine inspections and 'For cause' inspections. Routine inspections should be conducted at least every second year. It is an on-going evaluation of a laboratory's compliance with GLP regulation.

For cause inspections are less frequent, they constitute only about 20% of all GLP inspections. Reasons for such inspections could be a follow up of an inspection with serious deficiencies or when the Regulatory Authority suspect non-compliance when investigating NDA applications. It also may happen that the Regulatory Authority gets some hints from external sources about non-compliance in laboratories.

Typically the Regulatory Authority does not announce GLP inspections. If a laboratory refuses to accept Regulatory Authority inspections, either in full or also part of it, the Regulatory Authority will not accept studies in support of new drug applications.

Basic Safe Laboratory Practices

1. Eye protection (minimum: chemical splash goggles) must be worn at all times in the laboratory.
2. Students should wear durable clothing that covers the arms, legs, torso and feet. (note: sandals, shorts, tank-tops etc. have no place in the lab. Students inappropriately dressed for lab, could be denied access)
3. To protect clothing from chemical damage, wear a lab apron or lab coat. Long hair should be tied back to keep it from coming into contact with lab chemicals or flames.

4. An open flame may be ignited only when no flammable solvents are in the vicinity. The person lighting the flame must check with students in the vicinity to see if they are working with flammable solvents.

5. Exercise great caution in handling volatile, flammable solvents such as ether, acetone and methanol. Never evaporate these solvents on a hot plate in an open system. An efficient condenser system must be used.

6. In case of injury (cut, burn, fire etc.) notify the instructor immediately

7. In case of a fire or imminently dangerous situation, notify everyone who may be affected immediately, be sure the lab instructor is also notified.

8. If chemicals splash into someone's eyes, act quickly and get them into the eye wash station, do not wait for the instructor.

9. In case of a serious cut, stop blood flow using direct pressure using a clean towel, notify the lab instructor immediately.

10. Know the location and operation of :
    - Fire Extinguishers
    - Safety showers and Eye Wash Stations
    - Fire Alarm Boxes
    - Exit Doors
    - Telephones

11. Eating, drinking and smoking are prohibited in the laboratory at all times

12. Never work in the laboratory without proper supervision by an instructor.

13. Never carry out unauthorized experiments. Come to the laboratory prepared. If you are unsure about what to do, please ask the instructor.

14. Never pipette using mouth suction. Avoid inhaling and never taste any chemical in the lab.

15. Never force glass tubing through a rubber stopper. If glass tubing must be inserted into a rubber stopper, be sure to lubricate both the stopper and the tubing (glycerol or soapy water). Protect your hands, wrap the glass tubing in a towel while inserting.

16. Always remember, HOT glassware looks exactly the same as COLD glassware, be careful what you touch. $100°C = 212°F$ (boiling point of water).

Preparing for Lab

The student laboratory plays an important role in allowing the student a "hands on" opportunity to verify chemical principles and learn important techniques for safe chemical manipulation. In order to get the most out of the laboratory this list of simple suggestions has been prepared.

- Read the laboratory experiment and any suggested additional reading (s), *before* coming to lab.

- Do the assigned pre-lab exercises (if any). These generally cover any calculations or important observations which need to be made.

- Make a list of questions regarding the experiment. A simple question can save hours of time in the lab.

- All data should be recorded in a sturdy laboratory notebook. Do not use sheets of paper or 3 ring binders, as these pages can become quickly lost.

- Make a brief outline of the experiment in your notebook as a way of speeding up getting started, including calculations for needed reagents.

- It is sometimes necessary to modify lab procedures on the day of the lab to obtain better results. If you are prepared these changes should be easy to make.

- Prepare data tables ahead of time. Well prepared data tables not only speed up the recording of data, but also aid greatly during report writing.

- Clean your glassware at the end of the period so it will be ready the next lab. Many students waste time washing and drying glassware only to find out the large beaker they just cleaned and dried will be used to boil water. THINK!!!!!

- Many students are so busy trying to get *done* they *forget* to write down their observations. Color changes, endothermic or exothermic changes, physical state changes, boiling points, melting points, freezing points, etc.

- Look at the data, does it look reasonable for the type of experiment? When in doubt repeat a portion of the experiment, there is no better teacher than finding your own mistake. If you are still unsure, the lab instructor should be able to help, ask him or her.

- Lab instructors will sometimes discuss the important aspects of the lab with students individually or in small groups in an effort to help them get more out of the experiment. Keep your ears open and you may hear something that will help you out.

- Lastly, it is important to follow the safety do's and don'ts of the laboratory, not only for your own safety but also your fellow classmates. Report the dangerous lab practices of others, you will be doing them (and yourself) a big favor.

Report Writing

A key ingredient for writing a good laboratory report is taking good lab notes and writing down observations.

Experiment Title: Although self explanatory, the title helps you, as the student, define your understanding of the laboratory experiment.

Purpose: A brief description of what scientific principle is to be tested or verified.

Procedure: A brief outline of the experimental procedure. By including a procedure outline in the report your attention is focused on the what happened during the experiment.

Data Collection: This is one of the most critical portions of the lab report. Without good data recording in the laboratory note book, completion of the lab write up beyond this point futile or will certainly seem so. Presentation of data in tables allows easy following of the coming data manipulations. Tables should be clearly labeled as to their content and numbered for ease of referral in the discussion section.

Part of the data may involve making observations (color changes, temperature changes, melting point, boiling point, the physical appearance of a chemical substance, etc.). The observations requested in the lab experiment are the bare minimum needed to perform the experiments. Sometimes extra observations you make may provide extra clues.

As an example: You are given a metal sample and told it was either pure gold (Au) or pure silver (Ag). The lab asks you to perform a series of chemical tests, wouldn't the metal's color give you a clue as to the its identity? Keep your eyes open.

Calculations: One clear example of each different type of calculation should be presented as a check of your work. Do not include pages full of each and every calculation, it just wastes your time and paper. Who wants to read 3 pages of the same calculations with different numbers?

Uncertainty/Error Analysis: We all generally regard our answers as absolute. This is fine for expressions such as $4 + 5 = 9$, where the exact solution is known. However, in the real world of experimental chemistry no results (or very few, if any) are absolute. Therefore, some estimation of the experimental uncertainty is necessary to help explain the results and to verify if the scientific principle tested holds.

Discussion and Conclusion: This is an area which gives many students trouble. It requires looking at the experimental title, the purpose, the data and calculation sections of the lab report and briging them all together. Sometimes it involves the comparison of the student's experimentally derived answer to a known literature value. Other times, it requires the student to identify an unknown from a list of unknowns based on the information gathered during the experiment.

Often these 'known values' are provided for the student. When the answers are not provided it is up to the student to seek out the truth The World Wide Web (WWW or W3) has become an electronic super highway of information, with more data added daily.

Table Samples

Often, tables show up in student lab reports like the example below. While the student knows what the numbers mean, anyone (usually the lab instructor) reading the table needs to search the lab report and interpret their meaning.

49.8	158.709
56.8	179.089
63.2	199.679
68.5	222.135

The numbers in this table represent data for the determination of the density of an unknown solid. Let me show you how this can be improved with a few minutes of work.

In order to make the data more meaningful, tables should be drawn using these basic guidelines.

Draw tables using a straight edge (such as a ruler, if drawn by hand) or prepare on a computer using any number of word processing or graphing programs. Neat data tables not only look good, but also keep the data organized in an easy to follow format.

Each table should have a short title and/or be numbered.

Columns and rows for each table should also have identifying titles if needed.

Units (i.e. mL, g, mm) are usually placed in the column heading inside ()'s.

For all measurements there is some degree of uncertainty, this may be added to the table after each entry, included in the column heading or listed below the table.

Here are four examples of the same table prepared according to the guide lines.

V0 is the volume of water in a graduated cylinder, M0 is the mass of the cylinder plus the water V0. The values V1-V3 and M1-M3 represent the additions of the unknown solid to the water and the resulting new volumes and new masses.

Computer programs (i.e. Microsoft Word, etc.) are capable of generating attractive table borders and dividers. Only basic table examples are shown here, more elaborate tables are possible, experiment and see what looks good.

Table Example 5.1 Data for unknown # 7

Volume		Mass	
V0	49.8mL	M0	158.709g
V1	56.8mL	M1	179.089g
V2	63.2mL	M2	199.679g
V3	68.5mL	M3	222.135g

Table Example 5.2 Data for unknown # 7

Volume (mL)		Mass (g)	
V0	49.8	M0	158.709
V1	56.8	M1	179.089
V2	63.2	M2	199.679
V3	68.5	M3	222.135

Table Example 5.3 Data for unknown # 7

Volume (mL $\pm$ 0.2mL)		Mass (g $\pm$ 0.001g)	
V0	49.8	M0	158.709
V1	56.8	M1	179.089
V2	63.2	M2	199.679
V3	68.5	M3	222.135

Table Example 5.4 Data for unknown # 7

Volume (mL)		Mass (g)	
V0	49.8	M0	158.709
V1	56.8	M1	179.089
V2	63.2	M2	199.679
V3	68.5	M3	222.135
Mass $\pm$ 0.001 g Volume $\pm$ 0.2 mL			

Calculations: Now that you have your data table(s) set up it's time to see how calculations are to be presented in the lab report.

Your calculation section should contain the following

1. Title this section of the lab report "CALCULATIONS".

2. Provide one (1) example of each different type of mathematical calculation performed. Please, do not include page after page of all your calculations. It wastes a lot of your time which could be better spent doing other "homework assignments". (If you absolutely need to write all the calculations out, keep them for your records).

3. Clearly label the calculations being performed, be sure to include the units associated with any numbers.

4. Error analysis and/or uncertainty calculations may be included in this section.

5. Put the results in a well ordered table. By putting the results in a table, you can more easily spot results that don't make sense. Quite often these turn out to be simple math errors which can easily be fixed before turning in the lab report.

Table 1 Data for Unknown # 7

Volume (mL)		Mass (g)	
V0	49.8	M0	158.709
V1	56.8	M1	179.089
V2	63.2	M2	199.679
V3	68.5	M3	222.135
Mass $\pm$ 0.001 g Volume $\pm$ 0.2 mL			

Sample Calculations

Change in Volume

$V_x = V_x - V_0$, where x = 1, 2, 3

$V1 = V_1 - V_0 = 56.8$ mL - 49.8 mL = 7.0 mL

Change in Mass

$M_x = M_x - M_0$; where x = 1, 2, 3

$M1 = M_1 - M_0 = 179.089g - 158.709g = 20.380g$

Density Calculations

$dx = M_x / V_x$, where x = 1, 2, 3

$d_1 = M_1 / V_1$; 20.380g/7.0 mL = 2.911 g/mL (round to 2 significant figures d1 = 2.9 g/mL)

Average Density

$d_{ave} = (d_1 + d_2 + d_3)/3$

d= (2.9 g/mL + 3.1 g/mL 3.4 g/ml)/3= 3.1 g/mL

Table 2 Data for Unknown # 7

Mass		Volume		Density	
ΔM_x (g)		ΔV_x (mL)		d_x (g/mL)	
ΔM_1	20.380	ΔV_1	7.0	d_1	2.9
ΔM_2	40.970	ΔV_2	13.4	d_2	3.1
ΔM_3	63.326	ΔV_3	18.7	d_3	3.4

The data has been presented, sample calculations have been given. Now it is time to go to the next step, Uncertainty Analysis.

Uncertainty Analysis

What is Uncertainty Analysis?

Uncertainty can be described as that portion of the measurement beyond which we are not sure of its true value.

Each time a measurement is taken (mass, volume, length etc.) we rely upon a mechanical or visual point of reference in order to assign the appropriate value. These values, no matter how carefully they are obtained contain some degree of what is referred to as *uncertainty*.

The Denver 300 balance used to obtain data for this experiment reads to 0.001 g (1 mg). The true value could be as low as 0.0005g or as high as 0.0014g. The fourth decimal place (which cannot be read on this balance) causes us to be uncertain about the true value of the third decimal place. To account for this we assign an uncertainty to the balance reading obtained as ± 0.001g (e.g. 158.709 ± 0.001 g). Similarly a balance which reads 0.01g would have an assigned uncertainty of ± 0.01 g.

For volumetric (graduated cylinders, Mohr pipettes and burettes) and length measurements a general rule is to assign an uncertainty of one half of the smallest scale division. For example, the smallest division on a 100 mL graduated cylinder is 1 mL, a prudent uncertainty would be ± 0.5 mL. This may vary for each person and some what depends on the person's eye sight, some will be able to estimate 0.2 mL others will do well to estimate 1.0 mL. Be consistent, use values you believe are appropriate for your ability.

Uncertainty Calculations

The Student Laboratory Manual contains an introductory section on the propagation of error. Examples are given to illustrate how the High-Low method is used to estimate errors. The following is another example applied to the table below.

Note: While the calculations shown here are dealt with as a separate topic, they may be included in the Calculations section of the lab report. Only one example of each calculation is illustrated.

Table 5.3 Data for unknown # 7

Volume (mL ± 0.2 mL)		Mass (g ± 0.001 g)	
V0	49.8	M0	158.709
V1	56.8	M1	179.089
V2	63.2	M2	199.679
V3	68.5	M3	222.135

Using the High-Low Method

Look at the data for V_0. V_0 can be as high as 50.0 mL or as low as 48.6 mL, similarly the masses M0 can also be as high as 158.710g or as low as 159.708g. Using the high-low method we obtain the results in Table 5.4.

Table 5.4 Data for unknown # 7

ΔM_1	ΔV_1
High 179.090-158.708 = 20.382g	High 57.0mL-49.6mL = 7.4mL
Mid 179.089-158.709 = 20.380g	Mid 56.8mL-49.8mL = 7.0mL
Low 179.088-158.0710 = 20.378g	Low 56.6mL-50.0mL = 6.6mL
ΔM_1 = 20.380g $\pm$ 0.002g	ΔV_1 = 7.0g $\pm$ 0.4mL

Once the uncertainty is calculated for each mass and volume change, a similar set of calculations may be performed when determining the density, shown in Table 5.5.

Table 5.5 Density Uncertainity

d_1
High 20.382g/6.6mL = 3.088g/mL
Mid 20.380g/7.0mL = 2.911g/mL
Low 20.378g/7.4mL = 2.754g/mL
d_1 = 2.9g/mL $\pm$ 0.17g/mL

Table 5.6 Uncertainity Summary for all the experimental data

ΔM_x (g)		ΔV_x (mL)		d_x (g/mL)	
ΔM_1 (g)	20.380 $\pm$ 0.002	ΔV_1	7.0 $\pm$ 0.4	d_1	2.9 $\pm$ 0.2
ΔM_2 (g)	40.97 $\pm$ 0.002	ΔV_2	13.4 $\pm$ 0.4	d_2	3.1 $\pm$ 0.1
ΔM_3 (g)	63.326 $\pm$ 0.002	ΔV_3	18.7 $\pm$ 0.4	d_1	3.4 $\pm$ 0.1

Error Calculations using Standard Deviation

A better method used to estimate the spread of the data is called standard deviation and denoted by the Greek Letter σ (lower case, sigma). It is calculated using the formula shown to the right. Fortunately many scientific calculators have this function built in.

$$\sigma = \sqrt{\frac{(X_1 - \bar{X})^2 + (X_2 - \bar{X})^2 + (X_3 - \bar{X})^2 ... (X_n - \bar{X})^2}{(N-1)}}$$

Where

$X_1, X_2, X_3 \ldots X_n$ are the individual values

$$\bar{X} \text{ (average value of X)} = \sqrt{\frac{X_1 + X_2 + X_3 + \ldots X_n}{N}}$$

N = the number of experimental trials

The standard deviation is calculated using the density values 2.9 g/mL, 3.1 g/mL and 3.4 g/mL and found to be 0.3 g/mL. The average density is then expressed as 3.1 g/mL ± 0.3g/mL. (Although I have used values rounded off to 2 significant figures, care must be taken, round off final answers, only after all chain calculations are done.)

Calculation of Confidence Limits

A more advanced approach is to calculate the data spread based on a confidence limit. The confidence limit is a statistical evaluation of the data spread and is calculated using the following formula

$$\text{Confidence Limit} = \pm \frac{t\sigma}{\sqrt{N}}$$

The standard deviation σ described in the previous is the same value used to determine the confidence limit for the specific data set. The Factor t values are obtained from a statistical table, note that the values of t vary for not only the number of observations but also to the level we wish to express our confidence. N is the number of observations made. The normally accepted confidence level is 95%.

Thus for the density data std. dev. = 0.25, for the 95% confidence level and 3 observations (the number of times the density was determined) the Factor t = 4.30. This leads to a confidence limit = 0.62. The result is then expressed as 3.1 ± 0.6 which means we are 95% confident the true value of the density lies some where between 3.7 and 2.5.

Results and Discussion

In this section the student describes the results of the experiment (calculations, observations, error analysis etc.) and discusses any important findings (such as, the density of a metal unknown matching the density from a given list of possibilities). Here are some suggested questions the student might think about. Always remember the KISS principle (keep it simple student) when writing up the lab discussion. Too little written suggests not caring or understanding the lab report, too much written looks like trying to bluff your way through.

What was the experiment about?

What did I do?

What was (were) the result(s)?

How do these results compare with known values?

Would my answer have been closer with better equipment, better preparation on my part, performing the experiment more carefully, etc.?

Here is an example of how a results and discussion section might be written

The object of this experiment was to determine the density of an unknown metal sample. While the weight of a sample of the metal could easily be determined by using a scale (balance), the volume of the sample could not be determined directly.

Since the metal pieces were of odd sizes, the metal was poured into a known volume of water in a graduated cylinder. The change in volume then represents the volume of the metal sample. This was repeated three times, the density for each trial and the average density were calculated using the formula Mass/Volume = Density.

The result was an average density of 3.1 g/mL ± 0.6 g/mL (95% confidence level). We were given the following list of possible metals:

- Copper (Cu) d = 8.92 g/mL
- Zinc (Zn) d = 7.14 g/mL
- Lead (Pb) d = 11.34 g/mL
- Aluminum (Al) d = 2.7 g/mL
- Magnesium (Mg) 1.74 g/mL
- Silver (Ag) d = 10.49 g/mL
- Gold (Au) d = 19.3 g/mL

Since the metal sample used had a silver/grey color, copper and gold can both be eliminated. Based on calculations an error analysis the density spread for this experiment was between 2.5g/mL to 3.7g/mL. From the list above the only metal sample falling in this range is Aluminum at 2.7g/mL. Therefore within experimental error, unknown metal sample was Aluminum.

Organic Tips

Laboratory Tips for Organic Chemistry Lab

- Organic Lab is the one lab where water can be the death of a reaction. Many students make the mistake of beginning each lab by washing their glassware. Soon, they find out, too much time has been wasted, their glassware is wet and they have no way to dry it. Clean your glassware at the end of a lab period so that it has time to dry for the next lab period.

- There will be times when stand and wait and watch a reaction are required. While waiting, why not prepare for the next step? Obtain needed reagents (provided, working in a fume hood is not required), set up/lay out glassware and review the next step.

- Always label reagents and flask contents. Many organic liquids are clear and colorless just like water, so are many aqueous solutions such as acids and bases.

- Liquid organic reagents are best measured by volume. Most common organic liquids have their densities reported in one or more of the reference books. (mass/volume = density)

- Speaking of liquids - Some clothing items (nylons, rayon etc.) dissolve when coming in contact with solvents such as acetone, ethyl acetate. Sulfuric acid (same acid used in car batteries) will leave holes in cotton clothing, yes even the dilute acid!!! Don't wear your best clothes to lab.

- Cooling water always enters the bottom of the condenser and flows out the top at a gentle pace, no need to blow off hoses and soak you lab mates. Check to see if the water is running before heating starts.

- Hot glass looks exactly the same as cold glass. This becomes especially important when disassembling distillation and reflux equipment.

- Many organics don't mix or dissolve in water and thus require special waste containers. Do not pour organics down the sink!!!!!!!

- When performing extractions, SAVE BOTH LAYERS (organic and water) until you are sure which contains the desired product. Can't remember which layer is which? Add a few drops of water to both from your wash bottle, the rest will be obvious.

- Always stop distillations before the boiling flask goes dry. Residues concentrated to dryness or near dryness during distillation may be unstable and explode. (This is particularly important with ethers and some alcohols which can form organic peroxides)

- Use enough grease on joints to prevent "freezing" but not so much that it drips from the joints, except for Teflon stopcocks, which are never greased. Glass joints which come in contact with "Strong Bases" (KOH, NaOH etc.) need to be greased. Failure to clean them promptly after use will result in permanent sealing of the glass surfaces. (Many labs are changing to microscale labware which by design does not require grease).

- Never leave a reaction unattended. If you need to leave the lab for a few min. (restroom break, etc.) ask one of your classmates or the instructor to watch your reaction.

D. ISO 9000

Introduction

ISO is the International Organization for Standardization. It was set up in 1947 and is located in Geneva, Switzerland. Its purpose is to facilitate and support International trade by developing standards that people everywhere would recognize and respect. ISO achieves this purpose through the participation and support of its members. These members come from 158 National Standards Organizations. ISO standards are developed by Technical Committees. The people who serve on these Technical Committees come from many National Standards Organizations. Consequently, ISO standards have worldwide support.

ISO 9000 is sweeping the world. It is rapidly becoming the most important standard. Thousands of companies in over 100 countries have already adopted it and many more are in the process of doing so. ISO 9000 applies to all types of organizations. It does not matter what size they are or what they do. It can help both product and service oriented organizations achieve standards of quality that are recognized and respected throughout the world.

What is ISO 9000?

The term ISO 9000 refers to a set of quality management standards. ISO 9000 currently includes three quality standards ISO 9000: 2005, ISO 9001: 2000 and ISO 9004: 2000. ISO 9001: 2000 presents requirements, while ISO 9000: 2005 and ISO 9004: 2000 present guidelines. All of these are process standards but not product standards.

According to ISO the new ISO 9000: 2000 standards are based on eight quality management principles. ISO chose these principles because they can be used to improve organizational performance and achieve success. If we want to improver performance of our organization, we need to develop and implement an ISO 9000: 2000 quality management system that applies the eight principles listed below.

ISO 9000 : 2000 Quality Management Principles

1. Focus on your customers

   - Organizations rely on customers. Therefore Organizations must understand customer needs.

   - Organizations must meet customer requirements.

   - Organizations must exceed customer expectations.

2. Provide Leadership
   - Organizations rely on leaders therefore leader must establish a unity of purpose and set the direction that the organization must take.
   - Leaders must create an environment that encourages people to achieve organizations objectives.

3. Involve your people
   - Organizations rely on people. Therefore, Organizations must encourage the involvement of people at all levels.
   - Organizations must help people to develop and use their abilities.

4. Use a Process approach
   - Organizations are more efficient and effective when they use a process approach. Therefore, Organizations must use a process approach to manage activities and related resources.

5. Take a systems approach
   - Organizations are more efficient and effective when they use a systems approach. Hence, they should identify interrelated processes and treat them as a system.

6. Encourage continuous improvement
   - Organizations must make a permanent commitment to continuously improve their overall performance.

7. Get the facts before you decide
   - Generally the decisions are best when they are based on facts. Hence, the organizations must base decisions on the analysis of factual information and data.

8. Work with your suppliers
   - Organizations depend on their suppliers to help them create value.
   - Organizations must maintain a mutually beneficial relationship with their suppliers.

Fields of Application

The ISO 9000: 2000 standards apply to all kinds of organizations in all kinds of areas, some of the important are manufacturing, processing, servicing, printing, forestry, electronics, steel, computing, legal services, financial services, accounting, trucking, banking, retailing, drilling, recycling, aerospace, construction, exploration, textiles, pharmaceutical, oil & gas, pulp & paper, petrochemicals, publishing, shipping, energy, telecommunications, entertainment and so on. From this it is clear that there is no sphere of human activity where these standard principles can not be applied.

How does ISO 9000 Work?

Every organization needs to develop a quality management system that meets the new quality standard. This is imperative to control or improve the quality of the products and services and to reduce the cost associated with poor quality or to become more competitive. Today technological innovations are taking place very fast. Hence, it is necessary that the customers expectations are fulfilled or a governmental body mandatory requirements are to be fulfilled. In such cases a quality management system should be developed that meets the requirements specified by ISO 9001: 2000. The quality management system developed must meet ISO requirements but not its guidelines.

A quality management system can be developed by two approaches 1. Gap Analysis and 2. Follow a detailed system development plan. If already a quality management system exists in the organization and is working well, then Gap Analysis can be used to upgrade to the new ISO 9001:2000 standard. A Gap Analysis will tell you exactly what you need to do to meet the ISO 9001: 2000 quality management standard. It will help you identify the gaps that exist between the ISO standard and your organization's processes. Once you know where the gaps are, you can take steps to fill your gaps. By following this incremental approach, you will not only comply with the new ISO 9001 standard but you will also improve the overall performance of your organization's process.

ISO 9001: 2000 Process Oriented Quality Management System Development Plan

These standards are provided by ISO and if the detailed steps provided in the plan are followed, quality management system can be achieved which meet the needs of the organization and ISO's requirements. Once the quality management system has been fully developed and implemented, internal audit is carried out to ensure that the organization fulfills every single ISO 9001: 2000 requirement. When the process is complete a Registrar is asked to audit the effectiveness of the quality management system of the organization. If the auditors like what they see, they certify the quality system to meet the ISO's requirement and then an official certificate is issued to the organization and recorded in the registry.

Then the organization announces to the world that the quality of their products and services is managed, controlled and assured by a registered ISO 9001 quality management system.

Why is ISO 9000 Important?

ISO 9000 is important because of its orientation. While the content itself is useful and important, the content alone does not account for its widespread appeal. Currently ISO 9000 is supported by National Standards bodies from more than 120 countries. This makes it the logical choice for any organization that does business internationally or that serves customers who demand an international standard of quality.

ISO is also important because of its systemic orientation. The standards of quality can be achieved only by institutionalizing the right attitude of the employees by supporting it with the right policies, procedures, records, technologies, resources and structures. Unless a quality attitude is established by creating a quality system it is impossible to achieve a world class standard of quality. Simply a quality attitude comes from a quality system. This is what ISO recognizes and this is why ISO 9000 is important.

E. Total Quality Management

Introduction

Total quality management (TQM) refers to management methods used to enhance quality and productivity in organizations, particularly businesses. TQM is a comprehensive system approach that works horizontally across an organization, involving all departments and employees and extending backward and forward to include both suppliers and clients/customers.

TQM is only one of many acronyms used to label management systems that focus on quality. Other acronyms that have been used to describe similar quality management philosophies and programs include CQI (continuous quality improvement), SQC (statistical quality control), QFD (quality function deployment), QIDW (quality in daily work), and TQC (total quality control). Despite the ambiguity of the popularized term "TQM," that acronym is less important than the substance of the management ideology that underlies it. TQM provides a framework for implementing effective quality and productivity initiatives that can increase the profitability and competitiveness of organizations.

Origins of TQM

Although TQM techniques were adopted prior to World War II by a number of organizations, the creation of the total quality management philosophy is generally attributed to Dr. W. Edwards Deming (1900-1993). In the late 1920s, while working as a summer employee at Western Electric Company in Chicago, he found worker motivation systems to be degrading and economically unproductive; incentives were tied directly to quantity of output, and inefficient postproduction inspection systems were used to find flawed goods.

Deming teamed up in the 1930s with Walter A. Shewhart (1891-1967), a Bell Telephone Company statistician whose work convinced Deming that statistical control techniques could be used to supplant traditional management methods. Using Shewhart's theories, Deming devised a statistically controlled management process that provided managers with a means of determining when to intervene in an industrial process and when to leave it alone. Deming got a chance to put Shewhart's statistical quality-control techniques, as well as his own management philosophies, to the test during World War II. Government managers found that his techniques could easily be taught to engineers and workers, and then quickly implemented in overburdened war production plants.

One of Deming's clients, the U.S. State Department, sent him to Japan in 1947 as part of a national effort to revitalize the war-devastated Japanese economy. It was in Japan that Deming found an enthusiastic reception for his management ideas. Deming introduced his statistical process control, or statistical quality control programs into Japan's ailing manufacturing sector. Those techniques are credited with instilling a dedication to quality and productivity in the Japanese industrial and service sectors that allowed the country to become a dominant force in the global economy by the 1980s.

While Japan's industrial sector embarked on a quality initiative during the middle 1900s, most American companies continued to produce mass quantities of goods using traditional management techniques. America prospered as war-ravaged European countries looked to the United States for manufactured goods. In addition, a domestic population boom resulted in surging U.S. markets. But by the 1970s some American industries had come to be regarded as inferior to their Asian and European competitors. As a result of increasing economic globalization during the 1980s, made possible in part by advanced information technologies, the U.S. manufacturing sector fell prey to more competitive producers, particularly in Japan.

In response to massive market share gains achieved by Japanese companies during the late 1970s and 1980s, U.S. producers scrambled to adopt quality and productivity techniques that might restore their competitiveness. Indeed, Deming's philosophies and systems were finally recognized in the United States, and Deming himself became a highly sought-after lecturer and author. The "Deming Management Method" became the model for many American corporations eager to improve. And total quality management, the phrase applied to quality initiatives proffered by Deming and other management gurus, became a staple of American enterprise by the late 1980s. By the early 1990s, the U.S. manufacturing sector had achieved marked gains in quality and productivity. By the late 1990s several American industries had surpassed their Japanese rivals in these areas.

Total Quality Management (TQM)

Total = Quality involves everyone and all activities in the company.

Quality = Conformance to Requirements (Meeting Customer Requirements).

Management = Quality can and must be managed.

TQM = A process for managing quality; it must be a continuous way of life; a philosophy of perpetual improvement in everything we do.

TQM Compared to ISO 9001

ISO 9000 is a Quality System Management Standard. TQM is a philosophy of perpetual improvement. The ISO Quality Standard sets in place a system to deploy policy and verifiable objectives. An ISO implementation is a basis for a Total Quality Management implementation. Where there is an ISO system, about 75 percent of the steps are in place for TQM. The requirements for TQM can be considered ISO plus. Another aspect relating to the ISO Standard is that the proposed changes for the next revision (1999) will contain customer satisfaction and measurement requirements. In short, implementing TQM is being proactive concerning quality rather than reactive.

TQM as a Foundation

TQM is the foundation for activities which include;

- Meeting Customer Requirements
- Reducing Development Cycle Times
- Just In Time/Demand Flow Manufacturing
- Improvement Teams
- Reducing Product and Service Costs
- Improving Administrative Systems Training

Ten Steps to Total Quality Management (TQM)

The Ten Steps to TQM are as follows:

1. Pursue New Strategic Thinking
2. Know your Customers

3. Set True Customer Requirements

4. Concentrate on Prevention, Not Correction

5. Reduce Chronic Waste

6. Pursue a Continuous Improvement Strategy

7. Use Structured Methodology for Process Improvement

8. Reduce Variation

9. Use a Balanced Approach

10. Apply to All Functions

Principles of TQM

The Principles of TQM are as follows

1. Quality can and must be managed.

2. Everyone has a customer and is a supplier.

3. Processes, not people are the problem.

4. Every employee is responsible for quality.

5. Problems must be prevented, not just fixed.

6. Quality must be measured.

7. Quality improvements must be continuous.

8. The quality standard is defect free.

9. Goals are based on requirements, not negotiated.

10. Life cycle costs, not front end costs.

11. Management must be involved and lead.

12. Plan and organize for quality improvement.

Processes must be Managed and Improved

Processes must be managed and improved! This involves:

- Defining the process

- Measuring process performance

- Reviewing process performance

- Identifying process shortcomings

- Analyzing process problems

- Making a process change
- Measuring the effects of the process change
- Communicating both ways between supervisor and user

Key to Quality

The key to improving quality is to improve processes that define, produce and support our products.

All people work in processes.

People

- Get processes "in control"
- Work with other employees and managers to identify process problems and eliminate them

Managers and/or Supervisors Work on Processes

- Provide training and tool resources
- Measure and review process performance
- Improve process performance with the help of those who use the process

Planning a Change

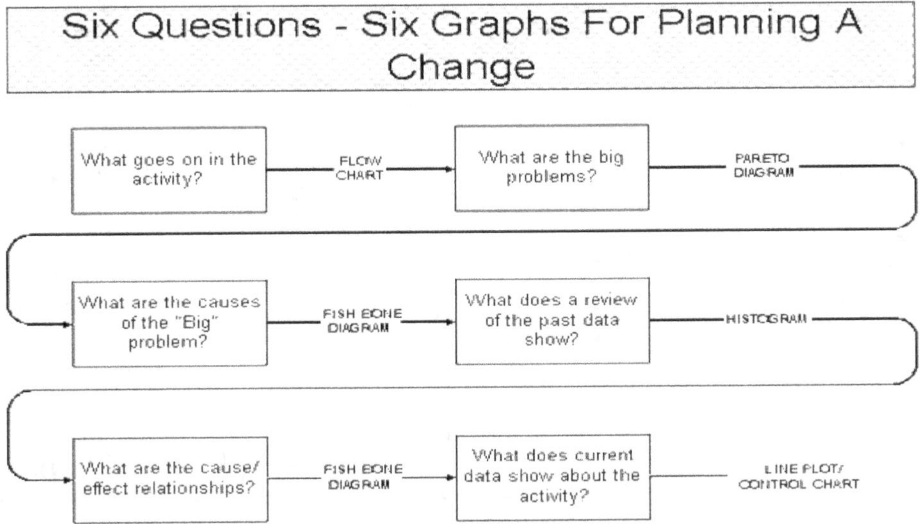

TQM Process Improvement and Problem Solving Sequence					
PLAN (PLAN A CHANGE)			DO (IMPLEMENT THE CHANGE)	CHECK (OBSERVE THE EFFECTS)	ACTION (EMBED THE FIX INTO THE PROCESS FOR GOOD)
DEFINE THE PROBLEM	**IDENTIFY POSSIBLE CAUSES**	**EVALUATE POSSIBLE CAUSES**	**MAKE A CHANGE**	**TEST THE CHANGE**	**TAKE PERMANENT ACTION**
1. Recognize that what you are doing is a "PROCESS" 2. Identify the commodity being processed. - Process Inference 3. Define some measurable characteristics of value to the commodity. 4. Describe the "PROCESS" • Process Flow Analysis's • Flow charts • List of steps 5. Identify the "Big" problem •Brainstorming • Checklists • Pareto analysis	6."BRAINSTORM" what is causing the problem. 7. Determine what past data shows. • Frequency distribution • Pareto charts • Control charts - sampling	8.Determine the relationship between cause and effect • Scatter diagrams • Regression analysis 9. Determine what the process is doing now • Control charts - sampling	10.Determine what change would help • Your knowledge of the process • Scatter diagrams • Control Charts • sampling • Pareto analysis ****Then make the change.	11. Determine what change worked (confirmation). • Histograms • Control charts • sampling •Scatter diagrams	12. Ensure the fix is embedded in the process and that the resulting process is used. Continue to monitor the process to ensure: A. The problem is fixed for good. B. The process is good enough • Control charts - sampling ****To ensure continuous improvement, return to step 5.

Making TQM Work

Joseph Jablonski, author of *Implementing TQM,* identified three characteristics necessary for TQM to succeed within an organization: participative management; continuous process improvement; and the utilization of teams.

Participative management refers to the intimate involvement of all members of a company in the management process, thus deemphasizing traditional top-down management methods. In other words, managers set policies and make key decisions only with the input and guidance of the subordinates who will have to implement and adhere to the directives. This technique improves upper management's grasp of operations and, more importantly, is an important motivator for workers who begin to feel as if they have control and ownership of the process in which they participate.

Continuous process improvement, the second characteristic, entails the recognition of small, incremental gains toward the goal of total quality. Large gains are accomplished by small, sustainable improvements over a long term. This concept necessitates a long-term approach by managers and the willingness to invest in the present for benefits that manifest themselves in the future. A corollary of continuous improvement is that workers and management develop an appreciation for, and confidence in, TQM over time.

Teamwork, the third necessary ingredient for the success of TQM, involves the organization of cross-functional teams within the company. This multidisciplinary team approach helps workers to share knowledge, identify problems and opportunities, derive a comprehensive understanding of their role in the overall process, and align their work goals with those of the organization.

Jablonski also identified six attributes of successful TQM programs

- Customer focus (includes internal customers such as other departments and coworkers, as well as external customers)
- Process focus
- Prevention versus inspection (development of a process that incorporates quality during production, rather than a process that attempts to achieve quality through inspection after resources have already been consumed to produce the good or service)
- Employee empowerment and compensation
- Fact-based decision making
- Receptiveness to feedback

In addition to identifying three characteristics that need to be present in an organization and six attributes of successful TQM programs, Jablonski offers a five-phase guideline for implementing total quality management: preparation, planning, assessment, implementation, and diversification. Each phase is designed to be executed as part of a long-term goal of continually increasing quality and productivity. Jablonski's approach is one of many that has been applied to achieve TQM, but contains the key elements commonly associated with other popular total quality systems.

TQM in the Future

Total quality management—first popularized in the 1950s in Japan—swept through American businesses in the 1980s and resulted in significant improvements in quality, productivity, customer satisfaction, and competitiveness in many companies by the 1990s. The basic principles of TQM are intended to achieve continuous organizational improvement through the participation and commitment of workers throughout a company. TQM focuses all the resources of an organization upon meeting the needs of customers (both internal and external), using statistical tools and techniques to measure results and aid decision making.

Despite the impressive results many companies have achieved through TQM, its future popularity is still in doubt. By the late 1990s some experts began to question whether TQM was a fad that would soon be superseded by yet another management technique. At the same time, however, other experts sought to apply TQM to emerging business problems, such as making computer systems compliant in the year 2000. It appears as if the underlying principles of TQM may find continued applications in business, even if they are eventually incorporated into a new movement for management innovation and organizational change.

PRINCIPLES OF QUALITY MANAGEMENT & QUALITY REVIEW

Principle 1. Segmentation

A. Divide an object or system into independent parts.

- Quality system elements.
- Customized marketing - complete market segmentation.
- Autonomous region sales centers.
- Sales splitting between customers.
- Four quality costs categories.
- Five steps of '5S' technique for continuous improvement: sort, set in order, shine, standardize, sustain.
- Eight steps of 8D problem solving technique.

B. Make an object or system easy to disassemble.

- Project team.
- Concurrent engineering team.
- Process improvement and problem solving teams.
- Material Review Board.

C. Increase the degree of fragmentation or segmentation

- Break down strategic quality goals into tactical goals.
- Quality goals and objectives deployment.
- Mass customization - each customer is a market.
- Scientific management - breaking down work into simple, repetitive tasks.
- Project milestones.
- Work breakdown structure (PERT/Gantt) for projects.
- Quality costs breakdown.
- Cause and effects diagram.
- Affinity diagram - breaking down complicated issues into easier to understand categories and patterns.
- Tree diagram.
- FMEA, FMECA, FTA.
- Pareto diagram categories.
- Histogram intervals.
- Stratified sampling for heterogeneous population.

Principle 2. Taking out

A. Separate an interfering part or property from an object or system, or single out the only necessary part or property.

- External accredited body approval.
- External laboratory testing.
- Supplier selection.
- Outsourcing.
- Lean manufacturing - elimination of non-value added activities.
- Containment action (D3 from 8D).
- Root cause analysis (D4 from 8D).
- Analysis of special cause of variation.
- Removal of defective parts at screening inspection.
- Segregation of non-conformant product, material, equipment.
- Cluster analysis - distill qualitative customer feedback into quantitative data.
- Separate problem from people.
- 'Drive out fear' (W. E. Deming).
- Make quality audit function independent.
- Discrete personal interviews, reviews, etc.

Principle 3. Local quality

A. Change an object or system structure from uniform to non-uniform, change an external environment (or external influence) from uniform to non-uniform.

- Strength, Weakness, Opportunity and Threat (SWOT) analysis.
- Develop strategy for each market segment.
- Design for specific market niches.
- Use different (individual) marketing approach, advertising and promotions for each customer sector.
- Customize marking, packaging, labeling, etc.
- Benefit best customers.
- Business and quality goals prioritization.
- Unequal resource allocation.
- Individual budgets for different departments.
- Pareto principle of unequal distribution.
- 'Vital few and trivial many' concept (J.M.Juran).
- Prioritize projects through the use of gap analysis, Pareto analysis, etc.
- Weight importance of customer needs in Quality Functional Deployment (QFD).
- Three levels of problem criticality: critical, major, minor.
- Classification of product characteristics and defects: critical, major,minor.
- Identify non-random patterns at trend analysis.
- Identify non-random pattern of variation (special cause) at SPC.
- Quantify customer preferences for product features at forced allocation survey.

B. Make each part of an object or system function in conditions most suitable for its operation.

- Locate distribution centers near to customers.
- Match personality types to the task to be performed.
- Educational modules - different in content and duration for different organizational levels.

C. Make each part of an object or system fulfil a different and useful function.

- Organizational division by function rather than product.
- Hire different specialists for different functions.

Principle 3 (inverted). Generic quality

- Mass marketing - market with no segmentation.
- Census instead of sampling survey.
- Random sampling.
- Random pattern of variation (common cause) at SPC.
- Audit randomly selected procedures.
- Random access quality data storage.

Principle 4. Asymmetry

A. Change the shape of an object or system from symmetrical to asymmetrical

B. If an object or system is asymmetrical, change its degree of asymmetry

- Use asymmetry for mismatching at mistake-proofing (Poka-Yoke).
- Asymmetrical statistical distributions.
- One-tail Student's test.
- Process performance index C_{pk} as a measure of parameter distribution asymmetry around the target.

Principle 4 (inverted). Symmetry

- Symmetrical normal distribution.
- Two-tail Student's test.

Principle 5. Merging

A. Bring closer together (or merge) identical or similar objects, assemble identical or similar parts to perform parallel operations.

- Transcontinental corporations.
- Business partnership, alliance, merging.
- Bring customers and suppliers into design loop.
- Professional associations.
- Quality function - collection of activities.
- As a project manager - develop network of alliances that reach all project stakeholders.
- Unanimous concurrence of all MRB members at decision of nonconforming material acceptance.
- 'Break down barriers between departments'
- Consensus style decision making at Theory Z management.
- 5S technique for continuous improvement.

- 8D problem solving technique.
- Team approach at problem solving.
- Bring collective judgment to project problems and opportunities at team meetings.
- Storyboarding - merging both creative and analytical thinking.
- Merged categories and patterns at affinity diagram.

B. Make operations contiguous or parallel; bring them together in time.

- Concurrent engineering.
- Use PERT/Gantt chart for project management.
- Institute parallel processes for cycle time reduction.
- Groupware: mail, e-mail, Intranet, meetings, phone and video conferencing, etc.

Principle 6. Universality

A. Make an object or system perform multiple functions; eliminate the need for other parts.

- Awareness of universality and integration as global marketing and business driving forces.
- Facilitate skill diversification at matrix organization.
- Hire multi-skilled personnel for complex jobs.

B. Use standardizes features

- International standards.
- Market based cost standards.
- Company procedures.
- Product and process specifications.
- Work instructions and workmanship standards.
- Measurement, inspection and test equipment calibration versus national standards.
- Material specifications.
- Specifications for incoming, in-process and final quality inspection.
- Specifications for functional, mechanical and environmental reliability testing.
- Standard record forms.
- Templates.
- Interchangeable work-force.

Principle 6 (inverted). Specialization

- In-depth skill development at hierarchical organization.

Principle 7. Nesting

A. Place one object inside another; place each object, in turn, inside the other.

- Hierarchy of ISO 9000 standards - 9001 embraces 9002 which in turn embraces 9003.
- Organization structure - several levels with several people within each organizational unit.
- Maslow's hierarchy of employee needs - basic, environment, simple individual, complex individual, transcendent.
- Hierarchy of customer expectations - basic, expected, desired, unanticipated.
- Market niches for new products.
- Store-in-store.
- Match personalities when assembling a team.

B. Make one part pass through a cavity in the other.

- Allow anyone in organization to communicate directly to any higher level.
- Expose traditionally inward facing employees to external events.

Principle 7 (inverted). Mutual exclusivity

- Mismatching at mistake-proofing.

Principle 8. Anti-weight

A. To compensate for the weight (downward tendency) of an object or system, merge it with other object or system that provide lift.

- Business partnership, alliance, merger - combining unique strengths.
- Company wide quality effort.
- Breakthrough benchmarking.
- Finding sponsors for a project.
- As a project manager - get top management ongoing support.
- Deliver management presentation before implementation of new initiative (e.g. quality cost system).
- Hitch-hike on others ideas at brainstorming sessions.

B. To compensate for the weight (downward tendency) of an object or system, make it interact with the environment (e.g. use global lift forces).

- Attach product marketing to customer and business driving forces (miniaturization, integration, universality, etc.).

Principle 9. Preliminary anti-action

A. If it will be necessary to do an action with both harmful and useful effects, this action should be replaced with anti-actions to control harmful effects.

- Proactive approach.
- Customer perception survey.
- b-Site customer trials - provide information on reliability of high risk new product prior to distribution to general public.
- Use PERT during project management - eliminate the need in crisis management.
- Process decision program chart (PDCA) - planning countermeasures to avoid undesirable situations.
- Failure analysis and prevention techniques.
- Mistake-proofing - design for foreseeable unintended use.
- Prevent wear-out failures by replacing short life parts.

B. Create beforehand stresses in an object or system that will oppose known undesirable working stresses later on.

- Self-assessment, correction of non-conformances before starting ISO 9000 registration process.
- Pre-award survey for potential supplier approval.
- Robust design - design for reliability.
- Design verification and validation.
- Design reviews.
- Prototype and pre-launch stages of Advanced Product Quality Planning (APQP) process.
- Field reliability testing, reliability data package.
- Burn-in, voltage stress, thermal shock, etc. accelerated testing for sorting out parts prone to failure at infant mortality period.
- Process certification.
- Entrance applicant screening, testing, interview.
- Key process employee certification.
- Amplification of human senses at product control.
- Quality system audits.
- Indicate unfavorable trend or potential problem at audit report.
- Run and update anti-virus software.

Principle 9 (inverted). Afterward anti-action

- Post-project evaluations and reviews.
- Lost customers survey and analysis.

Principle 10. Preliminary action

A. Perform, before it is needed, the required change of an object or system (either fully or partially).

- Strategic business planning and programming.
- Strategic quality planning.
- Marketing research.
- Project pre-planning.
- Product pre-advertising.
- Concurrent engineering.
- Capability study.
- Preventive maintenance.
- Early Supplier Involvement (ESI).
- Procedure writing.
- Training and qualification.
- Timely supply of information.

B. Pre-arrange objects such that they can come into action from the most convenient place and without losing time for their delivery.

- Project PERT/Gantt chart.
- Process flow chart.
- Batch route card.
- Decrease setup time using Single Minute Exchange of Die (SMED) techniques.
- Just-In-Time (JIT) delivery concept.
- First Expired First Out (FEFO) storage concept.
- First In First Out (FIFO) storage and delivery concept.
- Prepare questionnaire before survey.
- Prepare quality audit checklist.
- Distribution agenda before meeting.

Principle 11. Beforehand cushioning

A. Prepare emergency means beforehand to compensate for the relatively low reliability of an object or system.

- Business interruption contingency planning.
- Back-up functions.
- Split sales between customers.
- Institute recovery system for response to customer complaint and conflict resolution.
- Redundancy.
- Troubleshooting.
- Project contingency planning.
- Emergency quality planning.
- Second source suppliers.
- Excess inventory.
- Back-up power generator.
- Back-up computer data.

Principle 12. Equipotentiality

A. In a potential field, limit position changes (e.g. change operating conditions to eliminate the need to raise or lower objects in a gravity field).

- For quality costs trend analysis - compare quality costs to proper measurement bases (dollars per unit of production, % of manufacturing cost, relation to net sales, etc.).
- Time weighted inflows and outflows at benefit-cost analysis.
- Resource leveling at project management - smoothing peaks and valleys, minimizing effect of conflict in demand for the same resources, scheduling activities during slack periods.
- Homogeneous customer sectors (clusters).
- Homogeneous training groups.
- Nominal group technique.

Principle 13. Inverse

A. Invert the action(s) used to solve the problem (e.g. instead of cooling an object, heat it).

- 'A people-building philosophy will make the program successful, a people-using philosophy will make the program fail'.

- Blame the process not the person.
- Proactively encourage customers to complain.

B. Make movable parts (or the external environment) fixed, and fixed parts movable.

- Overcome reluctance of dissatisfied customers to complain.
- Pursue the full story from dissatisfied customers, get them to really talk.
- Management By Walking Around (MBWA).

C. Turn the object or system 'upside down'.

- Product-based vs function-based organization structure.
- Upward vs downward communication flow.
- Make survey and analysis of lost customers.
- Provocation technique at brainstorming sessions - turn the problem upside down.

Principle 14. Spheroidality

A. Instead of using rectilinear parts, surfaces, or forms, use curvilinear ones; change flat surfaces to spherical ones; parts shaped as a cube (parallelepiped) to ball-shaped structures.

- Rounded personalities provide customer service.
- Smoothing technique for conflict resolution - emphasizing areas of agreement, de-emphasizing areas of disagreement, seeking a joint problem solving opportunity.
- Deviation request procedure - formal method for circumventing the rules.

B. Use rollers, balls, spirals, domes

- Quality circle.
- Round-robin fashion of idea submission at nominal group technique.

C. Change from linear to rotary motion, use centrifugal forces.

- Team leadership rotation.
- Rolling forecast of customers purchase requirements.
- Customer survey questionnaires circulation.

Principle 14 (inverted). Linearity

- Aspiration for steeper operating characteristic curve at sampling inspection.

Principle 15. Dynamics

A. Allow (or design) the characteristics of an object, external environment, or process to change to be optimal or to find an optimal operating condition

- Address variation as a fact of life in external and internal environment.
- Adapt to highly competitive business environment.

- Adapt to dynamic customer wants, needs and expectations.
- Project management - ad hoc activity needed to effect change.
- 'Project by project' approach.
- Optimum quality cost model.
- Engineering change procedure.
- Update documentation periodically.
- Adjust internal quality audits frequency.
- Adjust calibration schedule on the basis of results.
- As a project manager - identify team members who have the ability to adapt to a changing situation in which they report to multiply mangers.

B. Divide an object or system into parts capable of movement relative to each other.

C. If an object or system is rigid or inflexible, make it movable or adaptive.

- Quality is a moving target.
- Flexible organization structure ('chaocracy').
- Flexible staff - use of temporary workers and overtime.
- Control charts, run charts, trend charts for displaying dynamic picture of process behavior.
- Continuous ranking change of jobs to be completed.

Principle 15 (inverted). Statics

- 'Reduce variation'.
- Take no actions as the best choice in order not to tamper with an object or system.
- Awareness of organizational roadblocks for change.

Principle 16. Partial or excessive actions

A. If 100 percent of an objective is hard to achieve using a given solution method then, by using 'slightly less' or 'slightly more' of the same method, the problem may be considerably easier to solve.

- Under-promise and over-deliver to achieve customer satisfaction.
- Stretching internal versus external specification requirements.
- Safety margins.
- Use stretch goals and objectives for employees.
- Vital few categories at Pareto diagram.
- Tolerance - permitted range of deviation from standard.
- Measurement accuracy - indication of closeness to the true value.
- Accuracy of quality costs estimates (typically 85%).

- Acceptable Quality Level (AQL) - percent of defectives that is considered satisfactory as a process average.
- Waiver - written authorization to release product that does not conform to specified requirements.
- Compromise at conflict resolution.

Principle 16 (inverted). All or nothing

- 'All or nothing' approach .
- 'Zero defects' quality goal.
- 100% Inspection - visual, dimensions go/no-go, non-destructive.
- 100% On-time delivery goal.
- 'Six Sigma' quality goal.

Principle 17. Another dimension

A. Move an object or system in two- or three-dimensional space.

- Matrix (product vs function) organization structure.
- Matrix (project vs line) management system.
- Multi-dimensional organization hierarchy charts.
- Parallel structures (quality council, etc.).
- Cross-functional collaboration at project management.
- Multi-disciplinary cross-functional teams.
- Multi-dimensional customer satisfaction surveys.
- Interrelationship diagram.
- Matrix diagram for FMEA, FTA, 8D Summary, DOE.
- L, T, Y, X, C types of matrices.
- House of quality (QFD).

B. Use a multi-story arrangement of objects instead of a single-story arrangement.

- Multi-layers hierarchy at vertical organization.

C. Tilt or re-orient the object or system, lay it on its side.

- Horizontal flow of work at project management.
- Horizontal communication.
- Shift from line to project management dominance in matrix organization and vice-versa - depending on prevailing market conditions.
- Excursion technique at brainstorming sessions - approach to problem from a different angle.

D. Use 'another side' of a given area.

- Commitment - internalizing the values of customer focus by all employees.
- Organizational assessment - viewing organization from the other side - either directly or using external consultants.
- Extensive two-way communication.

Principle 17 (inverted). Decreased dimensionality

- Flat organization structure advantage - fewer layers between leadership and customer.

Principle 18. Mechanical vibration

A. Cause an object or system to oscillate or vibrate.

- Frequently communicate in multiple modes.

B. Increase its frequency (even up to the ultrasonic).

C. Use an object or system resonant frequency.

- Use strategic planning to select right frequency and get organization resonating to accomplish breakthrough strategy.

D. Use piezoelectric vibrators instead of mechanical ones.

E. Use combined ultrasonic and electromagnetic field oscillations. (Use external elements to create oscillation/vibration).

- Periodically re-energize continuous improvement initiatives ('enthusiasm injections').
- Initiate third party external assessment.
- Bring new-blood/new challenge into a team.

Principle 19. Periodic action

A. Instead of continuous action, use periodic or pulsating actions.

- Shewhart - Deming PDCA cycle.
- 'Project by project' approach.
- Project life cycle concept - most projects pass through similar phases from start to finish.
- Periodical project reviews.
- Payback period method - measure of project liquidity.
- Batch manufacture - small customized series.
- Multiple process runs.
- Periodical in-process control, analysis, inspection.
- Periodical reliability testing.
- Periodical quality auditing, metrics, reporting.

B. If an action is already periodic, change the periodic magnitude or frequency

- Monthly and weekly feedback reporting instead of annual reviews.
- Adjustable internal quality audits frequency.

C. Use pauses between impulses to perform a different action.

- Perform preventive maintenance during vacations.
- Conduct training during pauses in work.
- Use slack time at PERT.

Principle 20. Continuity of useful action

A. Carry on work continuously; make all parts of an object or system work at full load, all the time.

- 'Constancy of purpose' .
- 'Continual survival at the marketplace'
- Long-term strategic business planning.
- Long-term strategic quality planning - road map for directions of continuous improvement.
- Quality control - preservation of status-quo.
- Kaizen - continuous improvement.
- Build customer retention.
- Nurture customer loyalty.
- Adapt to steady increasing customer expectations.
- Be aware that satisfaction of customer needs is never ending challenge.
- Introduce self-competing.
- Create company brand and trademark.
- Use stable and predictable historical perspective as a basis for establishing quality objectives.
- Single source supplier advantages - long-term commitment, reduced variation.
- Written procedures and specifications as perpetual coordination device.
- Configuration control.
- Traceability system.
- Calibration - comparison against instrument with verified accuracy in order to promote consistency of measurement.
- Life-long learning.
- 'Do it all over again'.

B. Eliminate all idle or intermittent actions or work.

- Resource leveling - smoothing peaks and valleys, minimizing effect of conflict in demand for the same resources, scheduling activities during slack periods.
- Streamline both internal and external setups to reduce total setup time (SMED).
- Use multi-skilled bottleneck functions to improve workflow.
- Preventive and predictive maintenance.

Principle 21. Skipping

A. Conduct a process, or certain stages (e.g. destructive, harmful or hazardous operations) at high speed.

- 'Fast Cycle - Full Participation' - method of involving the whole organization simultaneously and rapidly in a major change, such as reengineering.
- Get through painful processes quickly (e.g. conflict resolution).
- Promptly remove invalid or obsolete documents.

Principle 22. "Blessing in disguise"

A. Use harmful factors (particularly, harmful effects of the environment or surroundings) to achieve a positive effect.

- Use customer complaints as opportunities for improvement.
- Customers whose complaints are handled properly are more loyal than customers who never had a complaint.

B. Eliminate the primary harmful action by adding it to another harmful action to resolve the problem.

- Eliminate fear of change by introducing fear of competition.

C. Amplify a harmful factor to such a degree that it is no longer harmfull

- Reduce resource levels to such an extent that new ways of doing the job have to be discovered.
- Apply burn-in, voltage stress, thermal shock, etc. accelerated testing for sorting out parts prone to failure at infant mortality period.

Principle 22 (inverted). "Cursing in disguise"

- Absence of customer complaints may indicate lack of customer candor and unwillingness to share information.
- Expenditures under project budget may serve as evidence of 'cutting corners'.
- 'Quality is everybody's job, but because it is everybody's job, it can become nobody's job'.

Principle 23. Feedback

A. Introduce feedback (referring back, cross-checking) to improve a process or action.

- 'C' (check) at PDCA cycle.
- Management reviews.
- Budget variance measurements.
- Voice of the customer - survey, visit, report, focus group, interview, mail, feedback form, customer satisfaction checklist.
- Customer complaints and suggestions system.
- Product returns and field failures analysis system.
- Product guarantees - provide feedback data on how products fail to meet customer needs.
- Enlist customers into design process.
- Ongoing feedback loop for project evaluation - schedule, technical objectives, strategic fit.
- Periodical project reviews.
- Prototype testing.
- Periodical reliability testing.
- Failure analysis.
- b-Site customer trials.
- Supplier surveys.
- Supplier performance evaluation process.
- Quality audits and reviews.
- Corrective actions and follow-up.
- Quality reporting and information system.
- Annual employee reviews.

B. If feedback is already used, change its magnitude or influence.

- Monthly, weekly and daily business reviews.
- Continuous feedback communication at project management.
- Test run for process parameters adjustment.
- First article inspection.
- Statistical Process Control (SPC).

- Nonconforming product control system - monitoring, reporting and corrective actions.
- Incoming, in-process and final quality inspection and testing.
- Quality costs monitoring.
- For making training program effective - feed back to employee meaningful measures of his performance.

Principle 23 (inverted). Feedforward

- 'Predict and compare'
- Long-term strategic business planning and programming.
- Strategic quality planning.
- Leadership vision.
- Marketing forecast.
- Anticipating customer future needs.
- Technology road map.
- Trend analysis.
- Predictability within limits as output of SPC.
- Reliability prediction.
- Anticipatory Failure Determination.

Principle 24. Intermediary

A. Use an intermediary carrier article or intermediary process.

- Third-party external quality auditing.
- External laboratory testing.
- Top management representative for quality system implementation and management.
- Change agent at reengineering.
- Region sales offices.
- Customer service, customer contact person.
- Intermediate customers - wholesaler, distributor, retailer.
- Export/import, transportation and delivery agencies.
- Facilitator at nominal group, brainstorming, problem solving team.
- Transfer calibration standard.

B. Merge one object temporarily with another (which can be easily removed).

- Implement interim containment action.
- Hire temporary employees.
- Introduce specialist to trouble-shooting/fire-fighting team.
- Hire consultant.
- Use impartial body during difficult negotiation.
- Use arbitrator for sensitive discussion.
- Introduce moderator to a focus group.
- Hitch-hike on others ideas at brainstorming sessions.

Principle 24 (inverted). Direct contact

- Management By Walking Around (MBWA).

Principle 25. Self-service/Self-organization

A. Make an object or system serve itself by performing auxiliary helpful functions.

- Self-benchmarking.
- Self-competing.
- Self-assessment.
- Self-auditing (internal quality audits and corrective actions system).
- Self-directed work team.
- Self-inspection.
- Self-improvement (process improvement teams).

B. Use waste (or lost) resources, energy, or substances.

- Re-hire retired workers for jobs where their experience is needed.
- Use scrapped or dummy parts for experiments.
- Re-cycle materials.

Principle 26. Copying

A. Instead of an unavailable, expensive, or fragile object or system, use simpler inexpensive copies.

- Use customer satisfaction as a measure of an organization's business well-being.
- Lead by example.
- Use models of excellence.
- Benchmark competitors.
- Benchmark similar projects in order to identify improvement opportunities.

- Design and process modeling.
- Rapid prototyping.
- Using reference at experiments.
- Quality tests - designed to approximate conditions at customer's application.
- Quality metrics - any critical and useful performance measurement.

B. Replace an object or system with optical copies.

- Using electronic database instead of paper records.
- Numerical simulation - virtual business development, strategic planning modeling, etc.
- Drawing conclusion about population on the basis of sampling statistics.
- Video-conferencing instead of physical travel.

C. If optical copies are used, change to IR or UV. (Use an appropriate, out-of-the-ordinary illumination and viewing situation).

Evaluate customer satisfaction using multiple techniques.

- Respond to perceived customer needs.
- Use simulations, games, case-studies instead of lecture-style training.

Principle 27. Cheap short-living objects

A. Replace an expensive object with a multiple of inexpensive objects, compromising certain qualities (such as service life, for instance).

- Subcontract non-core business.
- Hire temporary employees for non-critical positions.
- By no-brand equipment and materials for non-critical processes.
- Use disposable miscellaneous and packaging materials.

Principle 28. Mechanics substitution

A. Replace a mechanical means with a sensory (optical, acoustic, taste or smell) means.

B. Use electric, magnetic and electromagnetic fields to interact with the object or system.

- Electronic communication.
- Electronic data processing.
- Electronic data transmission.
- Electronic bar coding.
- Electronic tagging.
- Electronic voting.

C. Change from static to movable fields, from unstructured fields to those having structure.

- Force field analysis.

Principle 29. Pneumatics and hydraulics

A. Use gas and liquid parts of an object or system instead of solid parts (e.g. inflatable, filled with liquids, air cushion, hydrostatic, hydro-reactive).

- Flexible (fluid) organization structure versus fixed hierarchical structure.
- Liquidation of assets.
- Introduction of 'breathing spaces' into contracts

Principle 30. Flexible shells and thin films

A. Use flexible shells and thin films instead of three-dimensional structures.

- Flat organization structure advantage - fewer layers between leadership and customer.

B. Isolate the object or system from the external environment using flexible shells and thin films.

- Use 'trade secret' methods to separate company proprietary knowledge from general knowledge.

Principle 31. Porous materials

A. Make an object or system porous or add porous elements (inserts, coatings, etc.).

B. If an object or system is already porous, use the pores to introduce a useful substance or function.

- Customer-facing layer of a company - porous membrane which filters information flow both into and out of the organization.
- Improve internal communications by creating Intranet accessible by all hierarchical layers, giving workers access to CEO and vice-versa.
- Encourage open-mindedness of employees to new ideas.

Principle 32. Color changes

A. Change the color of an object or its external environment.

- 'Corporate colors' - create a strong brand image through use of colors.
- Foster employee diversity.

B. Change the transparency of an object or its external environment.

- Clear, concise vision and mission statement.
- Use smoke-screen misinformation to disguise confidential (e.g. R&D) activities.

Principle 33. Homogeneity

A. Make objects interact with a given object of the same material (or material with identical properties).

- Hire local people to acquire cultural knowledge of local customers.
- Treat employees as external customers.
- Common data transfer protocols between different organizations.

Principle 34. Discarding and recovering

A. Make portions of an object or system that have fulfilled their functions go away or modify them directly during operation.

- Eliminate duplicated, redundant and non value-added activities (lean manufacturing, cycle time reduction).
- Reduce duplication with supplier.
- Downsizing.
- Using contract labor for capacity balance.
- Temporary team members on short-term projects.

B. Conversely, restore consumable parts of an object or system directly in operation.

- Warranty - commitment of manufacturer to repair or replace any part that fails during the life of product.
- Periodically re-energize continuous improvement initiatives.
- Introduce periodical re-training.
- Rework of nonconforming product.

Principle 35. Parameter changes

A. Change an object's physical state (e.g. to a gas, liquid, or solid).

Virtual prototyping.

Numerical simulation.

B. Change the concentration or consistency.

- Team structure change.

C. Change the degree of flexibility.

- Different (individual) marketing approach for each customer sector.
- Customized marking, packaging, labeling, etc.
- Flexible, variable-sized team.

D. Change the temperature.

- Get customers excited about the product by giving them ownership of the change.
- Get employees excited about the future of the company by using full involvement strategic planning, stock options, etc.

Principle 36. Phase transitions

A. Use phenomena occurring during phase transitions.

- Project stages - conception, birth, development, maturity, retirement.
- Design reviews - preliminary, specification, critical, final, etc.
- Phases of QFD - organization, descriptive, breakthrough, implementation.
- Phases of PERT - planning, scheduling, improvement, controlling.
- Phases of team development - forming, storming, norming, performing.
- 'Stages of learning - unconscious incompetence, conscious incompetence, conscious competence, unconscious competence'.

Principle 37. Thermal expansion

A. Use thermal expansion (or contraction) of materials.

B. If thermal expansion is being used, use multiple materials with different coefficients of thermal expansion.

- Expand or contract marketing efforts depending on the product's 'hotness' - rate of sales and profitability.
- Empowerment (power expansion) - authority transfer to individuals.

Principle 38. Boosted interactions

A. Replace common air with oxygen-enriched air (enriched atmosphere).

- Necessity is the mother of invention.
- 'Commitment to mission' (TQM).
- Establish sense of urgency for need to change - the first step in transforming an organization.
- Obsession with customer-perceived quality, desire to delight customer.
- Get customers excited about the product by giving them ownership of the change.
- Periodically re-energize continuous improvement initiatives ('enthusiasm injections').
- Hire highly creative individuals who understand the voice of the customer.
- Build staff with high performers.
- Use internal subject matter experts.
- Inject new-blood/new challenge into a team.

- Consider personal chemistry issues when assembling a team.
- Find people who will spark-off interesting reactions with each other.
- Foster mutual stimulation at brainstorming sessions.

B. Replace enriched air with pure oxygen (highly enriched atmosphere).

C. Expose air or oxygen to ionizing radiation.

D. Use ionized oxygen.

E. Replace ozonized (or ionized) oxygen with ozone (atmosphere enriched by 'unstable' elements).

- Venture capital.
- Reengineering - radical change.

Principle 39. Inert atmosphere

A. Replace a normal environment with an inert one.

- Nominal group technique.
- Maintain atmosphere free of criticism at brainstorming sessions.

B. Add neutral parts, or inert additives to an object or system.

- Use neutral third parties during difficult negotiations.
- Invite outsider/guest to brainstorming sessions.
- Introduce 'quiet areas' into the workplace.
- Use time-out during negotiations.
- Use rest breaks/pauses for reflection in meetings.

Principle 40. Composite structures

A. Change from uniform to composite (multiple) structures.

B. Combine high risk and low risk investment strategy.

- Multi-disciplinary cross-functional teams.
- Mix of thinking skills in a team.
- Hard person/soft person negotiating team.
- Hybrid audit staff - full-time employees and volunteers.
- Multi-channel communication with supplier.
- Combine multiple modes (newsletter, Intranet, staff meetings, etc.) for effective communication.

- Introduce training with a combination of lecture, simulations, on-line learning, video, etc.
- Hire Renaissance people.

International Conference on Harmonisation (ICH) – Guidelines

A Brief History of ICH

The Need to Harmonise

The history of medicinal product registration, in much of the industrialised world, has followed a similar pattern which could be described as: Initiation, Acceleration, Rationalisation and Harmonisation.

The realisation that it was important to have an independent evaluation of medicinal products before they are allowed on the market was reached at different times in different regions. In the United States a tragic mistake in the formulation of a children's syrup in the 1930s was the trigger for setting up the product authorisation system under the Food and Drug Administration. In Japan, government regulations requiring all medicinal products to be registered for sale started in the 1950s. In many countries in Europe the trigger was the thalidomide tragedy of the 1960s, which revealed that the new generation of synthetic drugs, which were revolutionising medicine at the time, had the potential to harm as well as heal.

For most countries, whether or not they had initiated product registration controls earlier, the 1960s and 1970s saw a rapid increase in laws, regulations and guidelines for reporting and evaluating the data on safety, quality and efficacy of new medicinal products. The industry, at the time, was becoming more international and seeking new global markets, but the registration of medicines remained a national responsibility. Although different regulatory systems were based on the same fundamental obligations to evaluate the quality, safety and efficacy, the detailed technical requirements had diverged over time to such an extent that industry found it necessary to duplicate many time-consuming and expensive test procedures, in order to market new products, internationally.

The urgent need to rationalise and harmonise regulation was impelled by concerns over rising costs of health care, escalation of the cost of R&D and the need to meet the public expectation that there should be a minimum of delay in making safe and efficacious new treatments available to patients in need.

Initiation of ICH

Harmonisation of regulatory requirements was pioneered by the European Community, in the 1980s, as the EC (now the European Union) moved towards the development of a single market for pharmaceuticals. The success achieved in Europe demonstrated that harmonisation was feasible. At the same time there were bilateral discussions between Europe, Japan and the US on possibilities for harmonisation. It was, however, at the WHO Conference of Drug Regulatory Authorities (ICDRA), in Paris, in 1989, that specific plans for action began to materialise. Soon afterwards, the authorities approached IFPMA to discuss a joint regulatory-industry initiative on international harmonisation, and ICH was conceived.

The birth of ICH took place at a meeting in April 1990, hosted by the EFPIA in Brussels. Representatives of the regulatory agencies and industry associations of Europe, Japan and the USA met, primarily, to plan an International Conference but the meeting also discussed the wider implications and terms of reference of ICH. The ICH Steering Committee which was established at that meeting has since met at least twice a year, with the location rotating between the three regions.

Structure of ICH

ICH is a joint initiative involving both regulators and industry as equal partners in the scientific and technical discussions of the testing procedures which are required to ensure and assess the safety, quality and efficacy of medicines.

The focus of ICH has been on the technical requirements for medicinal products containing new drugs. The vast majority of those new drugs and medicines are developed in Western Europe, Japan and the United States of America and therefore, when ICH was established, it was agreed that its scope would be confined to registration in those three regions.

ICH is comprised of Six Parties that are directly involved, as well as three Observers and IFPMA. The Six Parties are the founder members of ICH which represent the regulatory bodies and the research-based industry in the European Union, Japan and the USA. These parties include the EU, EFPIA, MHLW, JPMA, FDA and PhRMA.

The Observers are WHO, EFTA, and Canada (represented by Health Canada). This important group of non-voting members acts as a link between the ICH and non-ICH countries and regions.

ICH is operated via the ICH Steering Committee, which is supported by ICH Coordinators and the ICH Secretariat.

ICH Observers

Since ICH was initiated, in 1990, there have been observers to act as a link with non-ICH countries and regions. The ICH Observers are:

The World Health Organisation (WHO), The European Free Trade Association (EFTA), Swissmedic Switzerland and Health Products & Food Branch, Health Canada

The ICH Secretariat

The Secretariat operates from the IFPMA offices, in Geneva, and is primarily concerned with preparations for, and documentation of meetings of the Steering Committee as well as coordination of preparations for Working Group (EWG, IWG, Informal WG) and Discussion Group meetings. The ICH Secretariat also provides administrative support for the GCG and MedDRA.

At the time of ICH Conferences, the Secretariat is responsible for the technical documentation and for liaison with the speakers for the Conference. Organisational aspects of the Conferences are handled by the industry and regulatory parties in the country where the Conference takes place.

ICH Steering Committee

ICH is administered by the ICH Steering Committee which is supported by the ICH Secretariat. The ICH Steering Committee (SC) was established in April 1990, when ICH was initiated. The Steering Committee, working with the ICH Terms of Reference, determines the policies and procedures for ICH, selects topics for harmonisation and monitors the progress of harmonisation initiatives. The Steering Committee meets at least twice a year with the location rotating between the three regions.

Since the beginning, each of the six co-sponsors has had two seats on the ICH Steering Committee (SC) which oversees the harmonisation activities. IFPMA provides the Secretariat and participates as a non-voting member of the Steering Committee.

The ICH Observers, WHO, Health Canada, and the European Free Trade Association (EFTA) nominate non-voting participants to attend the ICH Steering Committee Meetings.

ICH Coordinators

Fundamental to the smooth running of ICH has been the designation, by each of the six co-sponsors, of an ICH Coordinator to act as the main contact point with the ICH Secretariat and ensure that ICH documents are distributed to the appropriate persons within the area of their responsibility.

Each party has also established a Contact Network of experts within their own organisation or region in order to ensure that, in the discussions, they reflect the views and policies of the co-sponsor they represent. The way in which this network operates differs according to the administrative structure of the party concerned.

Due to the structural differences within the EU and MHLW, ICH Technical Coordinators are also designated from the EMEA and PMDA respectively. They support the ICH Coordinator and facilitate every action of the Steering Committee members in the region, mainly by applying their scientific knowledge. Their roles include acting as a contact point between the experts within EMEA and PMDA and the ICH Coordinator at the main regulatory body, and as a contact point with the ICH Secretariat.

Contact names and addresses for both the ICH Coordinators and Technical Coordinators are given on the About Us page.

The Early Meetings

At the first SC meeting of ICH the Terms of Reference were agreed and it was decided that the Topics selected for harmonisation would be divided into Safety, Quality and Efficacy to reflect the three criteria which are the basis for approving and authorising new medicinal products. It was also agreed that six-party Expert Working Groups (EWGs) should be set up to discuss scientific and technical aspects of each harmonisation Topic. Eleven such Topics were selected for discussion at the First International Conference on Harmonisation.

The "pattern" of ICH work was also established in those early Steering Committee meetings, that is, that the EWGs meet in the same week as the Steering Committee and report on their progress to the Committee.

Commitment and Process

Key factors in the success of ICH have been the commitment of the parties to the objectives and outcome of ICH and the development of the "ICH Process" for developing harmonised guidance on technical issues. The commitment to ICH was set out in a Steering Committee Statement from the meeting in Tokyo, October 1990.

The ICH "Process" was first drawn up at the Steering Committee meeting in Washington, March 1992 and amended in Tokyo, September 1992. The defined process with "decision points" at Step 2 and Step 4 has enabled the Steering Committee to monitor the progress of the topics selected for harmonisation.

Format of Applications

The Steering Committee has given priority to harmonising the technical content of the sections of the reporting data where significant differences have been identified between regulatory requirements across the three regions: Europe, Japan and the USA. The first ICH Guideline to deal with harmonising the format of reporting data was E3, Content and Format of Clinical Study Reports. This Guideline describes a single format for reporting the core clinical studies that make up the clinical section of a registration dossier.

A target for the first phase of ICH activities was to remove redundancy and duplication in the development and review process, such that a single set of data could be generated to demonstrate the quality, safety and efficacy of a new medicinal product. The long-term goal of developing a harmonised format has led to the creation of the ICH Guideline M4, The Common Technical Document (CTD). The CTD provides a harmonised format and content for new product applications. ICH achieved Step 4 status of the CTD at the ICH5 Conference in San Diego, California, in November 2000. The agreed upon implementation date for the CTD, in the three regions, was July 2003.

The Electronic Common Technical Document (eCTD) was developed subsequently by the M2 Expert Working Group. This specification document allows for the electronic submission of the CTD from applicant to regulator and provides a harmonised technical solution to implementing the CTD electronically. The eCTD has begun to be implemented across the ICH partner and observer regions.

Continuation of Harmonisation Activities

ICH has been successful in achieving harmonisation, initially of technical guidelines and more recently on the format and content of registration applications. All parties agree that there is a need to maintain this harmonisation in the interest of the patient and public health to prevent unnecessary duplication without compromising the regulatory obligations of safety, quality and efficacy. New approaches to the maintenance of the products of harmonisation is needed. In addition, further harmonisation activities should be continued in a focused manner.

- **Implementation and monitoring:** The current magnitude of successful harmonisation actions and the need for these to remain current in a rapidly changing international environment calls for focusing more effort on the implementation and monitoring of ICH commitments. These will be key to the success, in particular, of the Common Technical Document (CTD), in which the creation of implementation groups or task forces will be important.

- **Selection of new topics:** The Steering Committee agrees that it is important to continue with the work of harmonisation after ICH 5, provided that the selection of possible new topics continues to be carried out in a systematic and focused manner. Experience with recent harmonisation activities have identified a need for an even more careful advance examination of a potential topic for future harmonisation in order to ensure that it is feasible, able to be implemented in a timely manner, and provides a high added value for all of the ICH partners. New activities will most likely be in areas where there are new technological advances, new innovative medicines, or in post marketing areas. Topic selection should be preceded, where necessary, by a feasibility study and/or a scientific pre-screening.

Recent interactions between the regulators involved in ICH have identified post marketing activities as a future area where increased regulatory co-operation can help to contribute to the enhancement of the protection of the health of citizens on a more international basis.

Global co-operation

The recent emphasis on global co-operation actions by ICH acknowledges the important role of WHO in disseminating information and providing input beyond the ICH regions. The Steering Committee recognizes the need to expand its communication and dissemination of information with non-ICH parties.

New ways of Working Together

There is a need to explore alternate approaches to the traditional ICH model of expert working groups (EWGs), particularly in areas where constantly changing scientific information has been identified. The possibility of making better use of techniques such as videoconferencing and electronic communication can only serve to enhance the communication between the ICH parties, as well as with other involved parties.

Revised ICH Terms of Reference

- To maintain a forum for a constructive dialogue between regulatory authorities and the pharmaceutical industry on the real and perceived differences in the technical requirements for product registration in the EU, USA and Japan in order to ensure a more timely introduction of new medicinal products, and their availability to patients;

- To contribute to the protection of public health from an international perspective (added upon revision in 2000);

- To monitor and update harmonised technical requirements leading to a greater mutual acceptance of research and development data;

- To avoid divergent future requirements through harmonisation of selected topics needed as a result of therapeutic advances and the development of new technologies for the production of medicinal products;

- To facilitate the adoption of new or improved technical research and development approaches which update or replace current practices, where these permit a more economical use of human, animal and material resources, without compromising safety;

- To facilitate the dissemination and communication of information on harmonised guidelines and their use such as to encourage the implementation and integration of common standards

Categories of Ich Harmonisation Activities

The ICH harmonisation activities fall into 4 categories (see Table below). The original Formal ICH Procedures involved a step-wise progression of guidelines. This process has evolved to include maintenance activities (Maintenance Procedure), as an essential part of the ICH procedure.

In addition to the maintenance activity, it is also important to have procedures in place to enable the modification of existing guidelines (Revision Procedure), as well as to assist in their implementation (Q&A Procedure).

Category	Type of procedure	Technical Discussion Group	Explanation	Example
1	Formal ICH Procedure	EWG	Development of a new guideline	M5 (Data Elements and Standards for Drug Dictionaries
2.	Q and A Procedure	IWG	Creation of Q and As to assist the implementation of existing guidelines	CTD-IWG
3.	Revision procedure	EWG	Revision/Modification of existing guidelines	E2B(R3)
4.	Maintenance procedure	EWG	Adding Standards to existing guidelines and/or recommendations	Q3C(R3) M2 Recommendations

Formal ICH Procedure (Category 1)

This procedure corresponds to the original ICH process and was used for more than a decade, and it now includes some additional explanation on each activity. The Steering Committee may decide to follow an accelerated procedure for new topics, when necessary. To this end, the Steering Committee adopted the Streamlined Procedure (final version dated October 21, 2002) in Washington in September 2002.

Step 1: Consensus Building

When the Steering Committee adopts a Concept Paper as a new topic, then the process of consensus building begins.

As requested in the Concept Paper, an extended EWG or original EWG shall be established. The Rapporteur prepares an initial draft of the guideline, based on the objectives set out in the Concept Paper, and in consultation with experts designated to the EWG. The initial draft and successive revisions are circulated for comments within the EWG, giving fixed deadlines for receipt of those comments.

To the extent possible, the consultation will be carried out by correspondence, using fax and e-mail. Face-to-face meetings of the EWG will normally only take place at the time and venue of the biannual SC meetings. Additional formal meetings of the ICH EWG need to be agreed, in advance, by the Steering Committee.

Interim reports are made at each meeting of the ICH Steering Committee.

When consensus is reached among all six party EWG members, the EWG will sign the Step 2 Experts Signoff sheet.

If consensus is reached within the agreed timetable the Step 2 Experts Document with EWG signatures is submitted to the Steering Committee to request adoption under Step 2 of the ICH process.

Where complete consensus within the six ICH parties has not been reached within the agreed time frame, a report will be made to the Steering Committee indicating the extent of agreement reached and highlighting the points on which there are differences among the parties. Experts from all parties represented on the EWG will have the opportunity to explain their position to the Steering Committee. The Steering Committee may then:

- Allow an extension of the timetable, on the basis that the EWG can give assurances that consensus could be reached within a short, specified period;

- Decide to suspend or abandon the harmonisation project.

Step 2: Confirmation of Six-Party Consensus

Step 2 is reached when the Steering Committee agrees, based on the report of the EWG, that there is sufficient scientific consensus on the technical issues for the draft guideline or recommendation to proceed to the next stage of regulatory consultation. This agreement is confirmed by at least one of the SC members for each of the six ICH parties signing their assent.

Step 3: Regulatory Consultation and Discussion

(a) Regional Regulatory Consultation

At this stage, the guideline embodying the scientific consensus leaves the ICH process and becomes the subject of normal wide-ranging regulatory consultation in the three regions. In the EU it is published as a draft CHMP Guideline, in Japan it is translated and issued by MHLW for internal and external consultation and in the USA it is published as draft guidance in the Federal Register.

The difference from normal, national/regional procedures for consultation on guidelines are that the regulatory parties exchange information on the comments they have received in order to arrive at a single, harmonised guideline. Also, there is an opportunity for industry associations and regulatory authorities in non-ICH regions to comment on the draft consultation documents, which are distributed using IFPMA and WHO contact lists.

(b) Discussion of regional consultation comments

After obtaining all regulatory consultation results, the EWG who organized the discussion for consensus building will be resumed. This EWG consists of regulatory and industry parties, and Observers. If the Rapporteur was designated from an industry party until Step 2, then a new Rapporteur will be appointed from the regulatory party, preferably from the same region as the previous Rapporteur. The same procedure described in Step 1 is used to address the consultation results into the Step 2 Final Document. The draft document to be generated as a result of the Step 3 phase is called Step 4 Experts Document.

If both regulatory and industry parties of the EWG are satisfied that the consensus achieved at Step 2 is not substantially altered as a result of the consultation, or consensus is reached on any alterations, the Step 4 Experts Document is signed by the EWG regulatory experts. The Step 4 Document with regulatory EWG signatures is submitted to the Steering Committee to request adoption as Step 4 of the ICH process.

This Step 4 Document with regulatory EWG signatures is named Step 4 Experts Document, and this signoff is to be called Step 4 Experts Signoff.

Where complete consensus has not been achieved within the agreed time frame, a report will be made to the Steering Committee indicating the extent of agreement reached and highlighting the points on which differences between the parties remain. Experts from all parties represented on the EWG will have the opportunity to explain their position to the Steering Committee. The Steering Committee may then:

- Allow an extension of the time frame, if the EWG can give assurances that consensus could be reached within a short, specified period;
- Decide to abandon the current draft and resume the discussion from Step 1;
- Decide to suspend or abandon the harmonisation project.

Step 4: Adoption of an ICH Harmonised Tripartite Guideline

Step 4 is reached when the Steering Committee agrees, on the basis of the report from the regulatory Rapporteur of the EWG, that there is sufficient scientific consensus on the technical issues.

This endorsement is based on the signatures from the three regulatory parties to ICH affirming that the Guideline is recommended for adoption by the regulatory bodies of the three regions.

In the event that one or more parties representing industry have strong objections to the adoption of the guideline, on the grounds that the revised draft departs substantially from the original consensus, or introduces new issues, the regulatory parties may agree that a revised document should be submitted for further consultation. In this case, the EWG discussion may be resumed.

The Step 4 Final Document is signed off by the SC signatories for the regulatory parties of ICH as an ICH Harmonised Tripartite Guideline at Step 4 of the ICH process.

Step 5: Implementation

Having reached Step 4 the harmonised tripartite guideline moves immediately to the final step of the process that is the regulatory implementation. This step is carried out according to the same national/regional procedures that apply to other regional regulatory guidelines and requirements, in the European Union, Japan and the USA.

Information on the regulatory action taken and implementation dates are reported back to the Steering Committee and published by the ICH Secretariat on the ICH website.

Q&A Procedure (Category 2)

Additional implementation guidance/advice is usually developed in the form of Questions and Answers ("Q&As"). The development and adoption of these Q&As follows an established process described below:

The Q&A process is intended to be a mechanism by which questions received from stakeholders are collected, analyzed, reformulated and ultimately used as model questions for which standard answers are developed and posted on the ICH website.

The incoming questions will not be answered individually. They will rather serve to highlight areas that need additional clarification and will be used to develop a model question that will be answered in the Q&A document.

- Any question sent to the mailbox of the ICH website, or raised by any of the six official ICH parties, and/or by any of the official ICH Observers, will be brought to the attention of the appropriate Implementation Working Group (IWG).

- The regional questions and issues should first be handled by the regulatory party of the concerned region then shared and evaluated within the IWG, finally the proposed answer is presented to the Steering Committee for approval/endorsement before publication on the ICH website.

- The IWG Rapporteur will send the questions to the members of her / his IWG. Based on this information, the IWG will prepare model questions and their responses for presentation at the SC meeting. Based on the level of guidance given by the answers, the IWG will assess whether the Q&A document should be a Step 2 Document and published for comments or should be a Step 4 Document and published as final. The document should be Step 2 if, by the answers provided, it sets forth substantial new interpretations of the guideline(s). The document should be a Step 4 if, by the answers provided, it sets forth existing practices or minor changes in the interpretation or policy of the guideline(s).

- Each IWG presents its draft Q&A document to the SC meeting (including regional regulatory legal review process) and makes recommendations to the Steering Committee on the status of the document (Step 2 or 4).
- The Steering Committee concurs with the Q&A document and its (Step) status.
- The document will then follow the normal path of a Step 2 / Step 4 Document:
    - Step 2: the experts and the SC members will sign the Q&A document. The document will then be published for comments in the three ICH regions.
    - Step 4: the regulatory experts and the regulatory SC members will sign the Q&A document.

    Each region should develop internal procedures to deal with the case of absence of the experts at the time of signoff, which could include the possibility for the Steering Committee to signoff the Step 2/ Step 4 on behalf of the IWG experts.
- The Experts/Final Q&A document will be posted on the ICH website five working days after the SC meeting.

This procedure is intended to provide results quickly and efficiently using the minimum amount of resources consistent with the achievement of a scientifically valid result.

Conferences and Workshops

When ICH was first established, one of the objectives was to organise an International Conference on Harmonisation, and hence the name which was given to the initiative.

The name of ICH has now, perhaps, become more associated with the process of harmonisation, than the actual Conferences, although these have been extremely important for ensuring that the process of harmonisation was carried out in a transparent manner and that there was an open forum in which to present and discuss ICH recommendations. To date there have been six International Conferences on Harmonisation (see table below).

Noverber 2003 : **ICH6**	Sixth International Conference on Harmonisation, Osaka, Japan.
November 2000 : ICH5	Fifth International Conference on San Diego, USA.
July 1997 : ICH4	Fourth International Conference on Harmonisation Brussels, Belgium
November 1995 : ICH3	Third International Conference on Harmonisation Orilando, USA
November 1991 : ICH1	First International Conference on Harmonisation Brussels, Belgium.

Regional Workshops on the implementation and use of the ICH Guidelines have occasionally been organised by ICH parties, at the time of a Steering Committee meeting in the region, in order to benefit from the presence of SC Members and ICH Experts. It is envisaged that such Workshops will continue to be organised and will provide an opportunity for interaction with all "users" of the guidelines.

Revision Procedure (Category 3)

If an adopted guideline needs to be revised, then the formal ICH Step procedure should take place rather than the Q&A process. Any revision or modification to an existing ICH guideline should fall into the "Revision Procedure" category.

This procedure is almost identical to the formal ICH procedure (Category 1), i.e. 5 ICH Steps. The only difference compared to Category 1 is the final outcome: in Category 3, the final outcome will be a revised version of a current existing guideline, whereas in Category 1 the final outcome is a new guideline.

In some cases, during the process of creation of a Q&A document, the revision of the original guideline may be considered necessary. In this case, the IWG Rapporteur, when presenting the Concept Paper to the Steering Committee, may also request the setting-up of a EWG to discuss the document modifications. To increase efficiency, the same members as those forming the IWG may develop both the Q&A document and revise the guideline.

The revision of a guideline is designated by the letter R1 after the usual denomination of the guideline. When a guideline is revised more than once, the document will be named R2, R3, R4, etc at each new revision.

Maintenance Procedure (Category 4)

This procedure is currently applicable to the Q3C Guideline on Residual Solvents (see below - *Impurities: Residual Solvents*), and the M2 Recommendations.

M2 Recommendations constitute an exceptional case, because no Step 2 Document is required. However, the Steering Committee may request further clarification. In such cases, a Step 2 Document may be necessary.

Updates to the Addenda of the Q3C Guideline are considered as revisions to the Q3C Guideline and are designated by the letter R.

Each new version of the M2 Recommendations is designated by a different version number.

Impurities: Residual Solvents

Type of Maintenance: Updating Based on New Information

This has been harmonised by all six parties in Brussels on February 2002.

1. Proposal of a "permitted daily exposure" (PDE) for a new solvent or a revised PDE for an already classified solvent is submitted directly to the ICH Secretariat with supporting information through an ICH regional coordinator. This information should be based on significant toxicity data from studies such as genotoxicity studies, repeat-dose studies, reproductive toxicity studies, carcinogenicity studies and/or other relevant toxicology studies. Single-dose toxicity data alone are not sufficient. The toxicity data should be of sufficient quality to calculate a PDE.

2. Revision of an established PDE will be considered only on presentation of previously unrecognized toxicity data sufficient to result in a significant change, or because of convincing evidence that the existing data used to calculate a PDE are invalid. Minor changes in a PDE will not be considered. The Rapporteur, with the consensus of the EWG members, will assign data reviews and request subsequent recommendations to the EWG.

3. The ICH Secretariat will distribute the proposal to the Rapporteur of the ICH Ad Hoc Expert Working Group on Residual Solvents (Q3C EWG). The Rapporteur will be one of the regulatory members of the ICH who will be available for two-year terms (e.g., FDA 1999-2000, MHLW 2001-2002, EU 2003-2004, FDA 2005-2006). The ICH Secretariat will also notify the ICH Steering Committee, Coordinators, and Observers that the Q3 EWG has been called to consider the proposal. The Q3C EWG will be comprised of two members (one chemist and one toxicologist) nominated by the six sponsors of the ICH and one member nominated by IGPA, WSMI and by each pharmacopeia. As appropriate, ICH observers may be invited to join the working group.

4. The regulatory Rapporteur will ordinarily rely on correspondence or teleconferencing to avoid unnecessary travel. Based on the discussion, with requests for further information to the proposing group and/or individual as appropriate, the Rapporteur will prepare an assessment report based on committee approval with a recommendation to accept, with or without modifications, or reject the proposed PDE. Ideally, this activity would occur at the rate of 2 residual solvents per calendar year. For particular residual solvent, it is anticipated that a period of six months from receipt of the toxicological information by the Rapporteur to the recommendation of a Step 2 guideline to the Steering Committee will be necessary.

5. After endorsement by the ICH Steering Committee, either at the next formal meeting or earlier as feasible, the recommendation of the Q3C EWG will be published in each region for public comment (Step 2 ICH process). In addition, the proposal will be provided to each pharmacopeia for their publication.

6. After close of the public comment periods, the Rapporteur may convene a meeting of the Q3C EWG or will rely on correspondence or teleconferencing to consider the comments and finalize the proposal for the new/revised PDE. The

final recommendation for the new/revised PDE and implementation is then forwarded to the ICH Steering Committee for approval. Implementation will follow regional practices. With approval of the ICH Steering Committee, the change will be provided to the pharmacopoeias of the three regions for publication.

When an existing PDE is revised or a PDE for a new residual solvent is recommended by the EWG, approval by the ICH Steering Committee is required. Once approval occurs, the information should be disseminated as quickly as possible to all ICH participants and other members of the chemical and pharmaceutical communities. It is recommended that the following actions should be taken by the ICH Steering Committee to ensure rapid transmission of the new information:

- publish relevant information on the ICH web site;

- request publication of revisions by the pharmacopoeias of the three regions in their Forums or web sites;

- request that each member publish the new solvent PDE information on its respective web sites;

- request WHO to distribute this information to its non-ICH member states.

Initiation of Harmonisation Action

Suggestions for new harmonisation initiatives may arise in a number of fora, including: ICH Regional Guideline Workshops; other regional and international conferences, workshops and symposia dealing with R&D and regulatory affairs; recognised Associations, Federations and Societies which represent scientific and technical professionals concerned with the development, testing and registration of medicines. Formal proposals for ICH action must, however, be channelled through one of the six parties to ICH or one of the ICH Observers on the Steering Committee.

ICH Concept Paper

The Concept Paper is the trigger of all ICH harmonisation activities. This provides a short summary of the proposal (maximum 2 pages) and provides the information indicated below:

- **Type of Harmonisation Action Proposed:** (e.g., a new harmonised tripartite guideline/recommendation, or a revision of an existing guideline - indicating the category of procedure);

- **Statement of the Perceived Problem:** Brief description with an indication of the magnitude of the problems currently caused by a lack of harmonisation, or - in the case of new scientific developments - anticipated if harmonisation action is not taken;

- **Issues to be Resolved:** A summary of the main technical and scientific issues, which require harmonisation;

- **Background to the Proposal:** Further relevant information, e.g., the origin of the proposal, references to publications, discussions in other fora;

- **Type of Expert Working Group:** Recommendation on whether the EWG (if needed) should be a six-party group - for topics related to the R&D of new drug substances and products - or an extended EWG - for topics with implications beyond new drug research.

If necessary, further documentation and reports may be annexed to the Concept Paper.

Endorsement by the Steering Committee

A Concept Paper is normally submitted to the ICH Steering Committee by an ICH party or an Observer. The Steering Committee takes the following points into account when discussing a Concept Paper:

(a) Objectives and expected outcome of the harmonisation action;

(b) Categories of ICH process;

(c) Composition of the EWG or IWG appointed to discuss the technical issues;

(d) Setting a Timetable and Action Plan for the EWG/IWG.

The Concept Paper may need to be revised and updated to reflect the Steering Committee discussion and conclusions. The Steering Committee may also request the development of a Business Plan.

ICH Business Plan

The Business Plan, whose template was adopted at the Washington meeting in June 2004, should be submitted to the Steering Committee upon request.

Concept papers will be developed and proposed by one of the ICH parties (including Observers) for initial consideration by the Steering Committee. At this initial stage a Business Plan will not be required although one may be provided at the discretion of the proposing party. If the Steering Committee agrees that a topic may warrant further consideration and a Business Plan has not been provided and agreed, an informal EWG / IWG will be formed and the informal group will work through e-mail, teleconference and, exceptionally, face-to-face meetings. The first tasks of the informal EWG / IWG will be to finalize a Concept Paper and develop and agree a Business Plan. The revised Concept Paper and Business Plan will be sent prior to and presented at the next SC teleconference or face-to-face meeting.

Establishment of an ICH Working Group

Depending on the type of harmonisation activity proposed, the ICH Steering Committee will endorse the establishment of either an Expert Working Group (EWG) or an Implementation Working Group (IWG).

Each of the six official ICH parties shall nominate official representatives to every EWG/IWG. Unless otherwise specified by the Steering Committee, the official membership of an EWG/IWG shall be limited to two officials per party per working group, one of who shall be designated as the Topic Leader and the other as the Deputy Topic Leader. ICH Observers may nominate one representative, as may Interested Parties, where applicable.

The Steering Committee officially designates a Rapporteur among the Topic Leaders designated by the six ICH parties, and in some cases a Co-Rapporteur may be appointed.

Future of ICH

The International Conference on Harmonisation of Technical Requirements for the Registration of Pharmaceuticals for Human Use (ICH) was established in 1990 as a joint regulatory/industry project to improve, through harmonisation, the efficiency of the process for developing and registering new medicinal products in Europe, Japan and the United States, in order to make these products available to patients with a minimum of delay.

The six parties to ICH represent the regulatory bodies and research-based industry in the three regions, Europe, Japan and the USA, where the vast majority of new medicines are currently developed.

The ICH process has achieved success because it is based on scientific consensus developed between industry and regulatory experts and because of the commitment of the regulatory parties to implement the ICH tripartite, harmonised guidelines and recommendations.

The Fifth International Conference on Harmonisation (ICH 5) San Diego, November 2000, marks the end of 10 years of activity thus providing an opportunity to evaluate results and to identify future needs in the area of international harmonisation.

CHAPTER 2

FUNDAMENTAL CONCEPTS IN VOLUMETRIC ANALYSIS

Introduction

The term 'volumetric analysis' was used for quantitative determination but it has been now replaced by titrimetric analysis. It refers to quantitative chemical analysis of one reactant of known concentration (standard solution or the titrant) that is added to the solution whose concentration is to be determined. The solution of known concentration is termed as "TITRANT" and the substance being titrated is termed as "TITRAND". The weight of the substance to be determined is calculated from the volume of the standard solution used and the chemical equation, relative molecular masses of the reacting compounds. The standard solution is added from the burette to the solution of which the concentration is to be determined until a required reaction is completed. The point at which the reaction occurs is called as the equivalence point or the theoretical point (stoichiometric) end point. The completion of the reaction is detected by physical change or by addition of an auxiliary reagent known as an indicator, change in colour is noticed.

In volumetric analysis, a reaction should fulfil the following conditions.

1. It must be a simple reaction which can be expressed by a chemical equation, the substances to be determined should react completely with the reagent in stoichiometric or equivalent proportions.

2. Reaction should be relatively fast. Addition of catalyst in some cases may be necessary to increase the speed of the reaction.

3. Some alternation in physical or chemical property of the solution at the equivalence point is must.

4. An indicator should be available which by a change in physical properties should sharply define the end point of the reaction.

If no visible indicator is available the detection of the equivalence point can be achieved by measuring :

(a) The potential between an indicator electrode and a reference electrode.

(b) The change in electrical conductivity of the solution.

(c) The current which passes through the titration cell between an indicator electrode and a depolarised reference electrode at a suitable applied e.m.f.

(d) The change in absorbance of the solution.

Volumetric analysis includes the following fundamental concepts :

1. Primary Standards
2. Secondary Standards
3. Preparation of Standard Solutions
4. Standardisation
5. Ways of Expressing Concentration
6. Requirements for Reactions Used
7. Classification of Volumetric Methods
8. Steps involved in Quantitative Analysis

Primary Standard

In titrimetry, certain chemicals are used frequently in defined concentration as reference solutions.

Such substances are referred to be PRIMARY STANDARD solutions. A primary standard solution is a compound of sufficient purity from which a standard solution is prepared by direct weighting of a quantity, followed by dilution to give a defined volume.

A primary standard solution should possess the following requirements :

1. It must be easy to obtain, to purify, to dry (at 110-120 °C) and to preserve in a pure state.

2. The substance should be unaltered in air during weighing. This condition implies that it should not be hygroscopic, oxidised by air or affected by CO_2. The standard solution should maintain an unchanged composition during storage.

3. The substance should be capable of being tested for impurities by quantitative and other tests of known sensitivity i.e. the total amount of impurities should not exceed 0.01-0.02% (99.9-99.99% pure)

4. It should have high relative molecular mass so that the weighing errors may be negligible. The precision in weighing is orderinarly 0.1-0.2 mg: for an accuracy of 1 part in 1000.

5. The substance should be readily soluble under the conditions in which it is employed.

6. The reaction with the standard solution should be stoichiometric and practically instantaneous. The titration error should be negligible, or easy to determine accurately by experiment.

An ideal primary standard is difficult to obtain and compromise between the above ideal requirements is necessary.

The substances commonly employed as primary standards in the following types of titrations are:

1. Acid-Base Titrations
2. Oxidation-Reduction Titrations
3. Precipitation Titrations
4. Complexometric Titrations

Acid-Base Titrations

Basic Primary Standards

1. Sodium carbonate - Anhydrous
2. Sodium tetraborate – Borax
3. Potassium hydrogen phthalate

Acid Primary Standards

1. Oxalic acid
2. Benzoic acid
3. Sulfamic acid
4. Phenyl cinchonic acid

Oxidation-Reduction Titrations

Oxidants

1. Potassium dichromate
2. Potassium bromate
3. Potassium iodate
4. Potassium hydrogen iodate

Reductants

1. Oxalic acid
2. Sodium oxalate
3. Arsenic trioxide
4. Pure metal ion

Precipitation Titrations

1. Silver
2. Silver nitrate
3. Sodium chloride
4. Potassium chloride
5. Potassium bromide

Complexometric Titration

1. Pure metallic zinc
2. Pure metallic magnesium
3. Zinc chloride
4. Calcium chloride

Secondary Standard

A substance which is not a primary standard in nature is called a secondary standard.

Ex: Alkali hydroxides

Inorganic acids

Deliquescent substances.

Definitions

Standard Solution

The solution of accurately known strength is known as standard solution. The basic unit of quantity employed is MOLE (the amount of substance which contain as many elementary units as there are atoms in 0.012 kgs of carbon-12).

As a result standard solutions are now commonly expressed in terms of molar concentrations.

Equivalence Point

It is also called as theoretical point or stoichiometric end point. This is a oint at which the reaction gets just completed in the titration. The completion of titration is being detected by some physical change, produced by standard solution itself or more usually by the addition of an auxiliary reagent known as "indicator". The point at which this occurs is called end point of the titration.

Indicator

It is an auxiliary reagent used in all stoichiometric titrations to detect the end point of the reaction.

Titration Error

In ideal titration the visible end point will coincide with stoichiometric or theoretical end point, a very small difference usually occurs which is known as titration error.

Preparation of Standard Solution

If a reagent is available in the pure state, a solution of definite molar strength is prepared simply by weighing out a mole or a definite fraction or multiple thereof, dissolving it in an appropriate solvent, usually water, and making up the solution to a known volume. It is not essential to weigh out exactly a mole. In practice it is more convenient to prepare the solution a little more concentrated than is ultimately required and then to dilute it with distilled water until the desired molar strength is obtained. If M_1 is the required molarity, V_1 the volume after dilution, M_2 the molarity originally obtained and V_2 the original volume taken

$$M_1V_1 = M_2V_2$$

OR $$V_1 = \frac{M_2V_2}{M_1}$$

The volume of water to be added to the volume V_2 is (V_1-V_2) ml.

The standard solution is always prepared in volumetric or standard flasks.

Examples of standard solution which have state of high purity are Na_2CO_3, potassium hydrogen phthalate, benzoic acid, sodium tetraborate, sulphamic acid, sodium oxalate, silver, $AgNO_3$, $NaCl$, KCl, l_2, KBr_2, Kl, $K_2Cr_2O_7$ $PbNO_3$, AS_2O_3.

Standardisation

When the reagent is not available in a pure form, solution of approximately known normality is first prepared. These are then titrated against a standard solution. This process is called standardisation.

In general normal acids like HCl and sulphuric acid can be standardised by using anhydrous sodium carbonate. Similarly alkali hydroxides like $NaOH$ and KOH can be standardised against a standard solution of Benzoic acid or oxalic acid.

Ways of Expressing Concentration of Standard Solution

Concentration is the amount of solute present in a given amount of solution.

It is generally expressed as the quantity of solute in a unit volume of solution.

$$\text{Concentration} = \frac{\text{quantity of solute}}{\text{volume of solution}}$$

Some forms of expression of concentration are:

1. Percent by Weight
2. Mole Fraction
3. Molarity
4. Normality
5. Equivalent Weight

Percent by Weight

It is defined as the weight of the solute as a percent of the total weight of the solution

$$\%\text{ by weight of solute} = \frac{\text{weight of solute}}{\text{weight of solution}} \times 100$$

Ex: HCl contain 36% by weight for 100 gm of solution.

Mole Fraction

It is the ratio of the number of moles of solute and the total number of moles of solute and solvent.

It is expressed as

$$X_{\text{solute}} = \frac{\text{moles of solute}}{\text{moles of solute} + \text{moles of solvent}}$$

If moles of solute is represented as 'n' and moles of solvent as N then the equation can be written as

$$X_{\text{solute}} = \frac{n}{n+N}$$

Since mole fraction is "unitless"

$$X_{\text{soulte}} + X_{\text{solvent}} = 1$$

Molarity

Molarity is defined as the number of moles of the solute per litre solution. Molarity is nothing but the concentration of the solution. It is being denoted by the symbol (M). It is defined in terms of mass of solvent.

$$\text{Molarity} = \frac{\text{moles of solute}}{\text{volume in litres}}$$

If moles of solute = n

Volume in litres = V

then $\qquad M = \dfrac{n}{V}$

Molarity has a unit of Mol litre^{-1}

Formal Concentration

Some substances do not exist in molecular form, they remain in ionic form in solid states as well as in solution. In such cases instead of molecular weight, formula weight is used and it is expressed as "formality". It is defined as number of formula weight of a solute per litre of solution. It is represented by "F".

$$F = \frac{\text{weight of solute in grams}}{\text{volume of solution in litres}} \times \text{formula weight.}$$

Molarity

It is the number of moles of solute per/kg of solvent. It is represented by symbol "m". It is defined in terms of volume of solution.

$$\text{Molarity} = \frac{\text{moles of solute}}{\text{moles of solvent in kilograms}}$$

Normality

It is the number of equivalents of solute per litre of solution. It is denoted by "N".

$$\text{Normality} = \frac{\text{equivalents of solute}}{\text{volume of solution in litres}}$$

Equivalent Weight

The equivalent weight of an acid or base is weight that contains 1.008 g of replaceable hydrogen. In redox titrations the equivalent weight is that weight which yields or combines with 1.008 g of "available" hydrogen or 8.00 g of "available" oxygen, available being defined as available for use in the oxidation or reduction reaction. The equivalent weight in precipitation reactions is defined as that weight of substance which contains or combines with 1g atom of a univalent metal.

Parts Per Million and Parts Per Billion

Parts per million is frequently employed to express the concentration of very dilute solution and is expressed as PPM

$$\text{Concentration in PPM} = \frac{\text{mass of solute}}{\text{mass of solution}} \times 10^6 \text{ PPM}$$

Requirements for Reaction used in Volumetric Analysis

For the uses of chemical reaction in volumetric analysis methods, the reaction should fulfil some of the requirements.

1. In titration, the reagent is used not in excess, but in a quantity which exactly corresponds to the reaction equation and is chemical equivalent to the substance being determined.
2. To determine the equivalence point with sufficient accuracy.
3. The reaction should be simple and expressed by well defined chemical equation.
4. There should not be any side reactions, so that from the reaction stoichiometry, calculation of amount of the reacting substance can be done.
5. The reaction should be rapid.
6. The reaction must proceed to completion when an equivalent amount of standard solution has been added. This gives satisfactory end-point detection.
7. Reaction should have some simple methods for the detection of end-point or equivalence point of titration.

Classification of Volumetric Methods

Volumetric determination can be subdivided into following principal methods:

1. Neutralisation Reactions
2. Complex Formation Reactions
3. Precipitation Reactions
4. Oxidation-Reduction Reactions
5. Non-Aqueous Titrations

    Neutralisation reactions, complex formation reactions, precipitation reactions do not involve any change in oxidation state as they are dependent on combination of ions. But oxidation reduction reaction involves a change of oxidation state i.e. transfer of electrons.

Neutralisation Reaction [Acidimetry and Alkalimetry]

A hydrogen electrode or a glass electrode is immersed in solution of the acid, whose strength is to be determined. The gas electrode is coupled with a standard calomel electrode. The cell thus formed is connected to the potentiometric or electronic voltameter. The pH and emf changes when an alkali is added to the solution (Fig. 2.1).

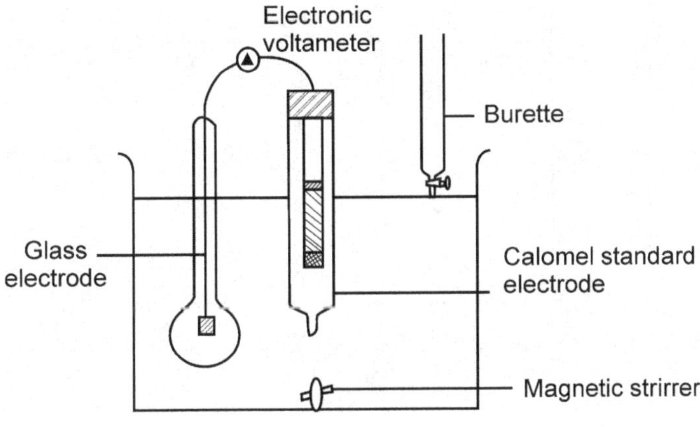

Fig. 2.1

The standard alkali solution is then added from the burette in small volumes. After each addition the emf of the cell is recorded. The emf is then plotted against the volume of alkali added. The shape of the curve for the titration of a strong acid against strong alkali is given below in Fig. 2.2. The steepest point of the curve indicates the equivalence point.

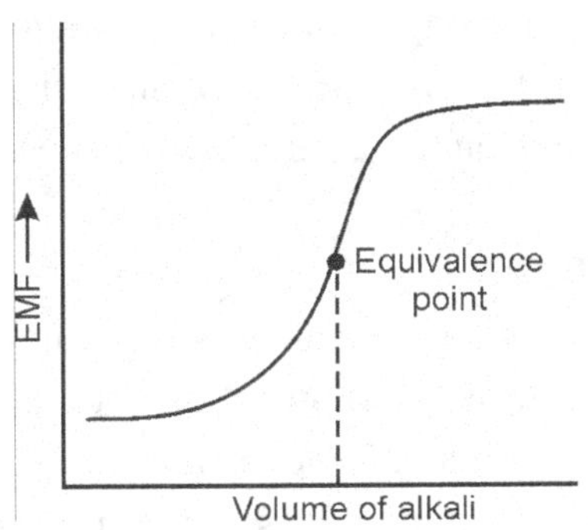

Fig. 2.2

However when the solutions are dilute or weak acids or bases are involved the steepness of the curve is less marked and it is difficult to judge the end-point. In such cases we plot the slope of the curve against the volume of alkali used. The maximum of the curve indicates the end point (Fig. 2.3).

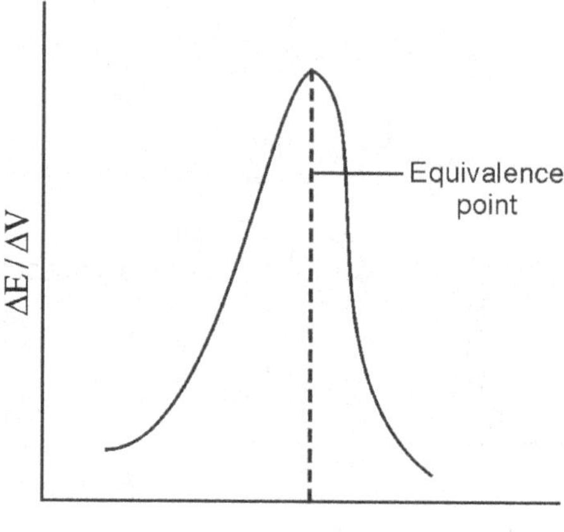

Fig. 2.3

Complex Formation Reactions

These depend on the combinations, other than hydrogen or hydroxide ions, to form a soluble slightly dissociated ion or compound, as in the titration of a solution of a cyanide with silver nitrate $[2CN^- + Ag^+ \rightleftharpoons [Ag(CN)_2]^-]$ or of chloride ion with mercury nitrate solution $(2Cl^+ + Hg^{2+} \rightleftharpoons HgCl_2)$.

Ethylenediaminetetra-acetic acid, largely as the disodium salt of EDTA is a very important reagent for complex formation titration and has become one of the most important reagents used in titrametric analysis. Equivalence point detection by the use of metal-ion indicators has greatly enhanced its value in titrimetry.

Precipitation Reaction

A typical precipitation titration is that of NaCl solution against silver solution. A silver electrode dipping in the unknown NaCl solution is coupled with a calomel electrode through a salt bridge. However if the calomel electrode were in direct contact with a solution containing excess silver ions, chloride would seep through the sintered base and react to form an insoluble layer of NaCl (Fig. 2.4).

Any change in the cell potential is due to change in concentration of Ag^+ ion around silver electrode

$$Ag^+ + e \rightarrow Ag$$

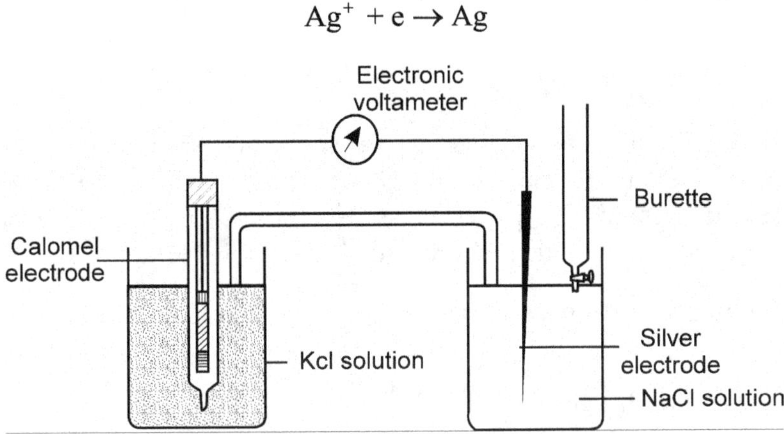

Fig. 2.4

Initially the concentration of Ag^+ ion will be zero. But as silver nitrate is added from the burette silver chloride is precipitated. Now the solution will contain a small concentration of Ag^+ ions formed by the slightly dissociation of silver chloride. This concentration will increase slightly as Cl^- ions are removed in order to maintain solubility product $KSP = [Ag^+][Cl^-]$. After the equivalence point the concentration of Ag^+ ions and therefore the silver electrode potential will rise very sharply (Fig. 2.5).

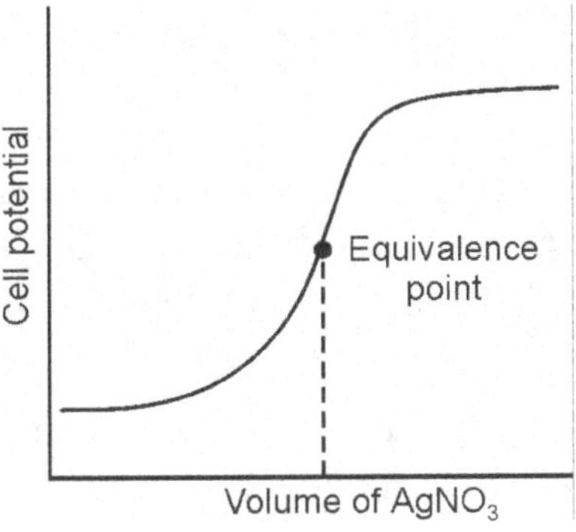

Fig. 2.5

Oxidation-Reduction Titrations

The titration of Fe^{2+} with cerricc ions (Ce^{4+}) is an example of Oxidation Reduction or Redox titrations. Fe^{2+} ion is oxidised to Fe^{3+} ion while Ce^{4+} is reduced to Ce^{3+} ion.

$$Fe^{2+} + Ce^{4+} \rightarrow Fe^{3+} + Ce^{3+}$$

This titration can be carried in the apparatus given below. The indicator electrode is a shiny platinum strip dipping in the solution of Fe^{2+} ions and it is connected to a standard calomel electrode. The Ce^{4+} solution is added from the burette and the cell potential, E is recorded after each addition. The potential of the platinum electrode depends on the ratio $\dfrac{[Fe^{3+}]}{[Fe^{2+}]}$. The potential of the cell E_1 also changes with the change of the ratio $\dfrac{[Fe^{3+}]}{[Fe^{2+}]}$.

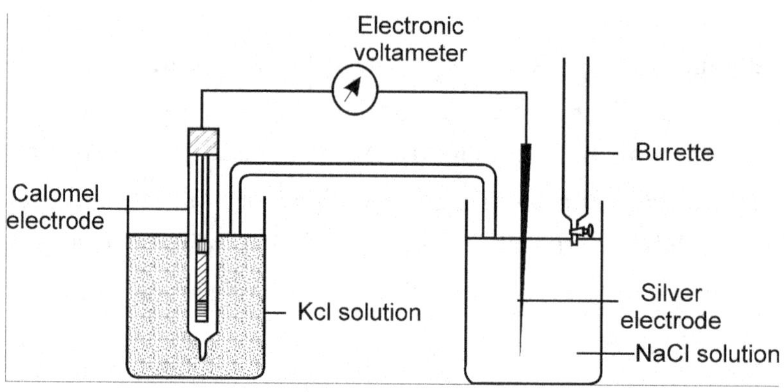

Fig. 2.6

Therefore the cell potential changes with the addition of Ce^{4+} ion from the burette. It shows how the potential of the cell changes during the titration. At the equivalence point there is a sharp rise of potential which indicates the end point (Fig. 2.7).

Potentiometric titrations of this type are particularly useful for coloured solution in which an indicator cannot be employed.

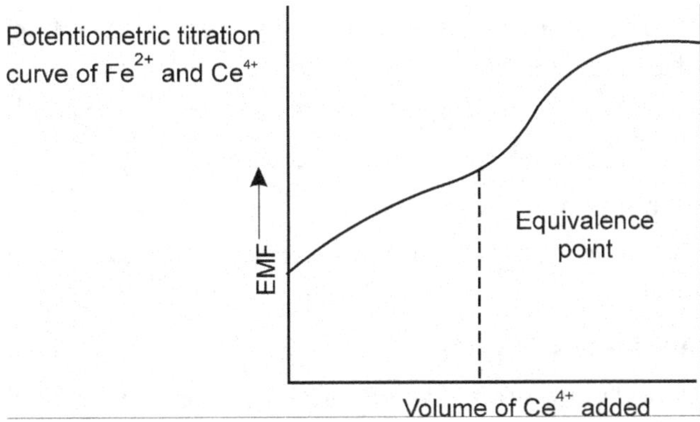

Fig. 2.7

Non Aqueous Titrations

The reactions occurring in non-aqueous titrations are of the ordinary neutralisation type and can be explained by the Lowry-Bronsted and Lewis concepts.

There are 3 common reasons why titration in non-aqueous solvents is preferred.

1. The reactants or products might be insoluble in H_2O.
2. The reactants or products might react with water.
3. The analyte is too weak, an acid or a base to be titrated in water.

Steps Involved in Quantitative Analysis

1. Selection of method of analysis.
2. Sampling.
3. Preparation of sample solution.
4. Elimination of interferences.
5. Calibration and measurement.
6. Calculation of results.
7. Evaluation of results and their reliability.

1. Selection of Methods of Analysis

Selection requires experience as well as scientific knowledge. It should be accurate, simple, precise and economic.

2. Sampling

This is a very important operation. It is the process of extracting from a large quantity of material, a small portion which is truly representative of the composition of material. Sampling techniques are quite different in different cases such as each type of material has its own special sampling instructions. The principle is that the average sample must be compared of the largest possible number of portions of the substances. There are 3 types of sampling methods.

1. Those in which the whole material is examined.
2. Casual sampling on adhoc basis.
3. Methods where portions of material are selected based upon statistical probabilities.

3. Preparation of Sample Solution

The samples (solids) are ground to decrease their particle size and mixed to ensure homogeneity. Required amount of sample is weighed and dissolved in the solvent in the mild conditions.

4. Elimination of Interferences

The reaction used and properties measured are characteristic of group of compounds. The analyst has to design a scheme which effectively isolates the species of interest from all others in the sample that can influence the measurement.

5. Calibration and Measurement

All analytical result depend on a final measurement of a physical property of the analyte. The physical property measured is often directly proportional to the concentration.

$$C = KX$$

The method of determining K is a vital step and is termed as calibration.

6. Calculation of Results

Until the results have been expressed in such a way that the person can understand the significance of it, the analysis is not complete. Computation of analyte from data is simple and easy with the help of calculators.

7. Evaluation of Results and their Reliability

Any analytical result is incomplete without an estimate of their reliability. Now-a-days, more attention is given to statistical methods to confirm the reliability and accuracy of the results.

Chapter **3**

ACIDIMETRY AND ALKALIMETRY

"Aqueous Acid base Titrations"

> **OR**

Acid Base Titrations

Neutralization or aqueous acid–base titrations are usually a reaction in which H_3O in solution is titrated by OH^-.

E.g.

$$HCl + NaOH \rightleftharpoons NaCl + H_2O$$

$$CH_3COOH + NaOH \rightleftharpoons NaOOCH_3C + H_2O$$

$$HCl + NH_4OH \rightleftharpoons NH_4Cl + H_2O$$

$$HClO_4 + CH_3COONa \rightleftharpoons CH_3COOH + NaClO_4$$

Basically,

$$H_3O^+ + OH^- \rightleftharpoons 2H_2O$$

Such type of Titration are carried out under standard volumetric conditions using internal indicator to detect the end point of titration.

Acid Base Theory

Arrhenius Theory

Acid $\rightarrow$ releases H^+.

Base $\rightarrow$ releases OH^-.

E.g. $HA \rightleftharpoons H^+ + A^-$
Acid

$H^+ + H_2O \rightleftharpoons H_3O^+$

Acid is a substance that when dissolved in water gives rise to hydrogen ions which on association with solvent form hydronium ions. A base is defined as the substance that when dissolved in water ions to give hydroxyl ions

$$BOH \rightleftharpoons B^+ + OH^-$$

Limitations

It does not give any explanation for these substances which don't contain the hydroxyl ions

Eg.   Amines

$$NH_3 + H_2O \rightleftharpoons NH_4^+ + OH^-$$

- The behaviour of these substances is explained on the basis of hydrolysis or their reaction with water and are referred to as "pseudo bases."

$$B + H_2O \rightleftharpoons BH^+ + OH^-$$

- This theory explains the quantitative acid base behaviour in aqueous solution but doesn't account for acid-base behaviour in non-aqueous solvents.

  1. Can't mention any idea about solvent.

  2. Basic compound in H_2O – dissolve $\rightarrow$ concentration of OH^- ions.

Lowry - Bronsted Theory

According to this theory, an acid donate protons and a base accepts proton.

$$HA \rightleftharpoons H^+ + A^-$$

$$B + H^+ \rightleftharpoons BH^+$$

In the theory, an acid donates proton. It is independent of solvent.

$$HA \rightleftharpoons H^+ + A^-$$

The anion $\bar{A}$ acts as a base as it accepts proton.

$$B + H^+ \rightleftharpoons BH^+ \text{ conjugate acid of base B}$$

The cation BH^+ acts as an acid as it donates proton.

The acid and base pairs in the above reactions are called as conjugate acid base pair i.e. the base is the conjugate base of the acid and the acid is the conjugate acid of the base.

$$\text{Acid} \rightleftharpoons \text{Base} + H^+$$

For the acid-base reaction, it is necessary to have two conjugate acid-base systems as it involves proton transfer from one system to other.

Limitations

- Charge on acid is greater than its conjugate part by 1 unit. But practically, individual H^+ ion is not possible. $\therefore$ Protons is soluble.

- This theory explains the acid-base reactions in various solvents.

- The conjugate acid-base system is essential in order to observe a reaction. The reaction can be considered as proton transfer from one system to another.

Acid   **Base**

$$CH_3COOH \rightleftharpoons CH_3COO^- + H^+$$

$$CH_3NH_3^+ \rightleftharpoons CH_3NH_2^- + H^+$$

$$H_2PO_4^- \rightleftharpoons HPO_4^{-2} + H^+$$

In general,

$$HA \rightleftharpoons H^+ + A^- \rightarrow \text{conjugate of acid HA}$$
$$H^+ + B^- \rightleftharpoons BH^+$$
$$HA + B^- \rightleftharpoons A^- + BH$$

Water

- Water can act as acid-base pair as they have acid-base properties.

- Water can act as both acid and base i.e. its amphoteric in nature.

$$H^+ + H_2O \rightleftharpoons H_3O^+$$

$$\text{Base} \rightleftharpoons \text{Acid}$$

The dual behaviour of water allows it to act as second conjugate acid-base system with solutes that are either acids or bases.

Lewis Theory

- An acid as a species that can accept an electron pair and a base as a species that can donate an electron pair.

- Every proton acceptor is an electron pair donor.

- This theory is useful to describe the indicator colour change in non-protonic systems exhibiting acid-base reaction.

E.g.   1. $H^+ + \ddot{N}H_3 \rightarrow NH_4^+$ $[NH_3 \rightarrow H^+]$ co–ordinate covalent bond

$\downarrow$

2. $BF_3 + \ddot{N}H_3 \rightarrow BF_3 \leftarrow NH_3$

	Acid	**Base**
Arrhenius theory	$\overset{+}{H}$ donor	$\overset{-}{OH}$ donor
Lewry Bronsted theory	Proton donor	Proton acceptor
Lewis theory	electron pair acceptor	electron pair donor

Strength of Acid and Base

Depends on :

Nature of solvent

E.g.: Acts as acid

1. $HCl + H_2O \rightarrow H_3O^+ + Cl^-$

$HCl + CH_3COOH \rightarrow CH_3COOH_2^+ + Cl^-$

$\downarrow$ $\downarrow$

Acts as weak acid   S.A.

2. $CH_3COOH + H_2O \rightarrow CH_3COO^- + H_3O^+$

$CH_3COOH + NH_3 \rightarrow CH_3COO^- + NH_4^+$

$\downarrow$ $\downarrow$

S.A   S.B

Ability of solvent to donate or accept proton/electron

Stability of structure after donation of proton

E.g.
$$HCl \rightarrow H^+ + Cl^-$$
$$HBr \rightarrow H^+ + Br^-$$
$$HF \rightarrow H^+ + F^-$$

acidity inc.

S. A.

$$\underrightarrow{C, O, N, F}$$

EN ⇑ as atomic no.

As EN ⇑ it becomes WB and SA.

Acid–Base Equilibrium

Dissociation of WA in Aq. solution

$$HAC + H_2O \rightarrow H_3O^+ + AC^-$$

Ka = acid dissociation constant.

$$Ka = \frac{[H_3O^+][AC^-]}{[HAC][H_2O]}$$ (H_2O Negligible so avoided)

$$Ka = \frac{[H_3O^+][AC^-]}{[HAC]}$$

.....(3.1)   Now, $2H_2O \rightarrow H_3O^+ + OH^-$

Kw = ionic product or water dissociation constant.

$$K_w = [H_3O^+][OH^-]$$

$$= [H^+][OH^-]$$

$$[OH^-] = \frac{Kw}{[H^+]}$$ .....(3.2)

Similarly, $AC^- + H_2O \rightarrow HAC + OH^-$

Kb = base dissociation constant.

$$Kb = \frac{[HAC][OH]}{[AC^-]}$$

$$Kb = \frac{[HAC]\,KW}{[AC^-][H^+]}$$

$$Kb = \frac{KW}{\dfrac{[AC^-][H^+]}{[HAC]}}$$

$$Kb = \frac{Kw}{Ka} \qquad\qquad .....(3.3)$$

$$PKw = PKa + PKb \qquad\qquad .....(3.4)$$

$$PKw = 14 \text{ at } 25\ ^\circ C$$

Ionization or Dissociation

Ionization (In)

Separation of ions from pairs.

Dissociation (Ds)

Formation of ions

Eer,   S.A & S.B – direct dissociation of ions

For,   S.A & S.B – No formation of ion pair

$$AB \xrightarrow{\ IN\ } A^+\,B^- \xrightarrow{\ DS\ } A^+ + B^-$$

Ion pair

Degree of Dissociation of A & B

Depends on

- Nature of acid/Base.

  SA & SB – completely dissociated into ions

   WA & WB – forms pairs and then separation of ions
- Nature of solvent

  Acidity of solvent varies from solvent to solvent.
- Dielectric constant

  ⇑ Dielectric const. ⇑ ionization

- Concentration

  Degree of dissociation α 1/concentration

  Dilute solution $\rightarrow$ degree of dissociation more

- Temperature

  $\Uparrow$ Temp, more molecular velocity

  $\therefore$ degree of Ds $\Uparrow$

Dissociation of Strong Acid (SA)

C = Analytical cont. of SA

$$HA \rightarrow H^+ + A^-$$
$$H_2O \rightarrow H^+ + OH^-$$

- According to electro-neutrality rule

  $$H^+ = A^- + OH^-$$

- $\therefore$ +ve ions counter balanced by –ve ions

- For S.A. concentration $> 10^{-6}$

  Concentration of [OH$^-$] value is less

  $$\therefore [H^+] = [A^-] = C \qquad \qquad .....(3.5)$$

  Here, momentary acidity = Total acidity = C (for S.A)

Dissociation of Strong Base (SB)

C = Analytical cont. for S.B.

$$MOH \rightarrow M^+ + OH^-$$

$$H_2O \rightarrow H^+ + OH^-$$

According to electroneutrality rule,

$$O\bar{H} = M^+ + H^+$$

Similarly if concentration of S.B $> 10^{-6}$ Then, **[H$^+$]** value is less.

$$\therefore [OH^-] = [M^+] = C$$

Here, momentary basicity = Total basicity = C (for S.B.)

Ionization of Weak Acid (WA)

C = Analytical const of W.A

X = concentration of ionic electrolytes

$$HAC \rightarrow H^+ + AC^-$$

$$H_2O \rightarrow H^+ + OH^-$$

According to electroneutrality rule

$$H^+ = AC^- + OH^-$$

$$[H^+] = [AC^-] = X$$

$$Ka = \frac{[H^+][AC^-]}{[HAC]}$$

$$Ka = \frac{[H^+][H^+]}{HAC} = \frac{[H^+]^2}{C-[H^+]} = \left[\frac{X^2}{[HAC]}\right]$$

[HAC] = Reversed acidity = Total acidity − Momentary acidity = C − [H$^+$]

$$\therefore Ka = \frac{[H^+]^2}{C}$$

$$[H^+] = \sqrt{Ka \times C}$$

$$\text{Log } [H^+] = \frac{1}{2}\log Ka + \frac{1}{2}\log C$$

$$-\log [H^+] = -\frac{1}{2}\log Ka - \frac{1}{2}\log C$$

$$pH = \frac{1}{2}pKa - \frac{1}{2}\log C$$

$$pH = \frac{1}{2}\left(pKa - \frac{1}{2}\log C\right) \qquad \dots\dots(3.6)$$

Ionization of Weak Base (WB)

C = Analytical const of W.B.

X = concentration of ionic electrolytes

$$NH_4OH \rightarrow NH_4^+ + OH^-$$

$$H_2O \rightarrow OH^- + H^+$$

According to electro neutrality rule

$$OH^- = NH_4^+ + H_4 + H^+$$

$$[OH^-] = [NH_4^+] = X$$

$$\therefore \ Kb = \frac{[NH_4^+][OH^-]}{[NH_4OH]}$$

$$Kb = \frac{[OH^-][OH^-]}{[NH_4OH]} = \frac{[OH^-]^2}{[NH_4OH]}$$

Here, [NH$_4$OH] = Reversed basicity = Total   Momentary basicity $= C - [OH^-]$

$$Kb = \frac{[OH^-]^2}{C - [OH^-]}$$

$$Kb = \frac{[OH^-]^2}{C}$$

$$[OH^-] = \sqrt{Kb.C}$$

$$Log \ [OH^-] = \frac{1}{2}\log Kb + \frac{1}{2}\log C$$

$$-\frac{1}{2}\log[OH^-] = -\frac{1}{2}\log Kb - \frac{1}{2}\log C$$

$$pOH = \frac{1}{2}pKb - \frac{1}{2}\log C$$

$$pOH = \frac{1}{2}\left(pKb - \log C\right) \qquad\qquad .....(3.7)$$

$$pH = pKw - POH$$

$$pH = pKw - \frac{1}{2}\left(pKb - \log C\right)$$

$$pH = 14 - \frac{1}{2}\left(pKb - \log C\right) \qquad\qquad .....(3.8)$$

Common Ion Effect

Common ion presence, decrease in solubility of salt.

Also, acidity & basicity decreases

$$NaOH \rightarrow Na^+ + OH^-$$

$$HAC \rightarrow H^+ + AC^-$$

$$\downarrow$$

Formation water

$$HAC + NaOH \rightarrow NaAC + H_2O$$

$$\left. \begin{array}{l} HAC \rightarrow H^+ + AC^- \\ NaAC \rightarrow Na^+ + AC^- \end{array} \right\} \text{High Concentration}$$

$$\downarrow \qquad \downarrow$$

$$\text{S.B} \qquad \text{W.A}$$

Concentration of H^+ decreases

$\therefore$ acidity decreases and we have to add sodium acetate.

$$\Rightarrow \quad HAC \rightarrow H^+ +$$

$$HCl \rightarrow H^+ + Cl^-$$

High concentration

$\therefore$ Basicity decreases. (H^+ concentration $\Uparrow$)

Hydrolysis

- Change in pH when reacted with water
- For S.A & S.B no hydrolysis, occurs as no change in pH occurs.

$$E.g. \qquad NaCl \rightarrow Na^+ + Cl^-$$

$$H_2O \rightarrow H^+ + OH^-$$

- As strong acid-base salt as complete dissociation occurs.

  $\therefore$ No change in pH

  $\therefore$ No hydrolysis

- Hydrolysis occurs in salts of
    - (i)   SA & WB
    - (ii) WA & SB
    - (iii) WA & WB

    If any cation or anion which can be reacted with H^+ and OH^- of water so that change in pH occurs is hydrolysis. It is reversible or irreversible.

- SA & WB eg. HCl & NH_4OH

    $$Salt \rightarrow NH_4HCl$$

- SB & WA eg. NaOH & CH_3COOH

    $$Salt \rightarrow CH_3COONa$$

- WA & WB e.g HAC & NH_4OH

    $$Salt \rightarrow CH_3COONH_4$$

    $$i.e\ NH_4AC$$

Weak Acid & Strong Base (WA & SB)

e.g. $NaOH \rightarrow$ (SB)

$CH_3COOH \rightarrow$ (WA)

$CH_3COONa \rightarrow$ Salt

$CH_3COONa \rightarrow CH_3COO^- + Na^+$

$CH_3COO^- + H_2O \rightarrow OH^- + CH_3COOH$

Due to formation of unionized acetic acid, concentration of OH^- increases and acidity decreases.

- pH > 7 $\therefore$ alkaline in nature

    according to law of mass action

$$Kh = \frac{[HAC][OH^-]}{[AC^-]}$$

$$Kh = \frac{[HAC]Kw}{[AC^-][H^+]}$$

$$Kh = \frac{Kw}{Ka} \qquad \qquad \qquad .....(3.9)$$

Now, $Kh = \dfrac{[HAC][OH^-]}{[AC^-]}$

$[HAC] = x = [OH^-]$

And, $[AC^-] = C - x \approx C$ ($\because$ x is negligible)

$Kh = \dfrac{x^2}{C} = \dfrac{Kw}{Ka}$

$x = [OH^-] = \sqrt{\dfrac{Kw \times C}{Ka}}$

Applying log,

$$Log\ [OH^-] = \frac{1}{2}\log Kw + \frac{1}{2}\log C - \frac{1}{2}\log Ka$$

$$-\log\ [OH^-] = -\frac{1}{2}\log Kw - \frac{1}{2}\log C + \frac{1}{2}\log Ka$$

$$pOH = +\frac{1}{2}pKw - \frac{1}{2}\log C - \frac{1}{2}pKa$$

$$pOH = \frac{1}{2}\left[pKw - \log C - pKa\right]$$

now, $pH = pKw - pOH$

$$pH = pKw - \frac{1}{2}pKw + \frac{1}{2}\log C + \frac{1}{2}pKa$$

$$pH = \frac{1}{2}\left(pKw + \log C + pKa\right) \qquad .....(3.10)$$

Degree of Hydrolysis

Degree of hydrolysis,

$$\lambda = \frac{x}{C}$$

E.g. $KCN \rightarrow K^+ + CN^-$

W.A (more weak acid than HAC and HCl)

$$Ka = \frac{[K^+][CN^-]}{[KCN]}$$

$$CN^- + H_2O \rightarrow HCN + OH^-$$

$$Kh = \frac{[HCN][OH^-]}{[CN^-]}$$

Eg.
$$HAC \rightarrow H^+ + AC^-$$

$$Ka = \frac{[H^+][AC^-]}{[HAC]}$$

$$AC^- + H_2O \rightarrow HAC + OH^-$$

$$Kh = \frac{[HAC][OH^-]}{[AC^-]}$$

$$\therefore Kh = \frac{\lambda C . \lambda C}{C - \lambda C}$$

$$Kh = \frac{\lambda^2 C^2}{C(1-\lambda)}$$

$$Kh = \frac{\lambda^2 C}{(1-\lambda)}$$

$$Kh = \lambda^2 C \times Ka \qquad \text{Where, } Kh = \text{hydrolysis constant}$$

$$\frac{Kw}{Ka} = \lambda^2 C$$

$$\lambda = \sqrt{\frac{Kw}{Ka \times C}} \qquad \qquad .....(3.11)$$

Strong Acid & Weak Base (SA & WB)

E.g. $NH_4OH \rightarrow WB$

$HCl \rightarrow$ Strong acid

$NH_4Cl \rightarrow$ Salt

$NH_4Cl \rightarrow NH_4^- + Cl^-$

$H_2O \rightarrow H^+ + OH^-$

$NH_4^+ + H_2O \rightarrow NH_3 + H_3O^-$

$$Kh = \frac{[NH_3][H_3O^+]}{[NH_4^+]}$$

$$Kh = \frac{Kw\,[NH_3]}{[OH^-][NH_4^+]}$$

$$Kh = \frac{Kw}{Kb}$$

$$\text{Now, } Kh = \frac{[H^+][NH_3]}{[NH_4^+]} = \frac{x^2}{C}$$

$$Kh = \frac{Kw}{Kb} = \frac{x^2}{C}$$

$$[H^+] = x = \sqrt{\frac{Kw}{Kb}.C}$$

Applying log,

$$\text{Log }[H^+] = \frac{1}{2}\log Kw + \frac{1}{2}\log C - \frac{1}{2}\log Kb$$

$$-\log[H^+] = -\frac{1}{2}\log Kw - \frac{1}{2}\log C + \frac{1}{2}\log Kb$$

$$pH = \frac{1}{2}pKw - \frac{1}{2}\log C - \frac{1}{2}pKb$$

$$pH = \frac{1}{2}(pKw - \log C - pKb) \qquad\qquad .....(3.12)$$

Degree of Hydrolysis

$$\lambda = \frac{x}{C}$$

$$\lambda = \sqrt{\frac{Kw}{Kb.C}}$$

$$\therefore Kh = \frac{[NH_3][H^+]}{[NH_4^+]} = \frac{x^2}{C-x}$$

$$Kh = \frac{Kw}{Kb} = \frac{\lambda C.\lambda C}{C(1-\lambda)} \qquad (\because x = \lambda C)$$

$$\frac{Kw}{Kb} = \frac{\lambda^2 C}{(1-\lambda)}$$

$$\frac{Kw}{Kb} = \lambda^2 C$$

$$\lambda = \sqrt{\frac{Kw}{Kb.C}} \qquad\qquad \ldots..(3.13)$$

Weak Acid & Weak Base (WA & WB)

$$CH_3COONH_4 \rightarrow CH_3COO^- + NH_4^-$$

$$H_2O \rightarrow H^+ + OH^-$$

$$CH_3COO^- + NH_4^+ + H_2O \rightarrow CH_3COOH + NH_3 + H^+ + OH^-$$

$$Kh = \frac{[HAC][NH_3]}{[NH_4^+][AC^-]} \quad \text{i.e.} \quad \frac{x.x}{(C-x)(C-x)} = \frac{x^2}{(c-x)^2}$$

$$Kh = \frac{[HAC][NH_3]}{[NH_4^-][AC^-]} \times \frac{[H^+][OH^-]}{[H^+][OH^-]}$$

$$Kh = \frac{[HAC]}{[AC][H^+]} \times \frac{[NH_3]}{[NH_4][OH^-]} \times [H^+][OH^-]$$

$$Kh = \frac{1}{Ka} \times \frac{1}{Kb} \times Kw$$

$$Kh = \frac{Kw}{Ka.Kb} = \frac{x^2}{C^2}$$

$$X = C\sqrt{\frac{Kw}{Ka.Kb}}$$

$$X = [H^+] = C\sqrt{\frac{Kw}{Ka.Kb}}$$

$$\log [H^+] = \log C + \frac{1}{2}\log Kw - \frac{1}{2}\log Ka - \frac{1}{2}\log Kb$$

$$- \log [H^+] = - \log C - \frac{1}{2} \log Kw + \frac{1}{2} \log Ka + \frac{1}{2} \log Kb$$

$$pH = - \log C + \frac{1}{2} pKw - \frac{1}{2} pKa - \frac{1}{2} pKb$$

$$pH = \frac{1}{2} pKw - \log C - \frac{1}{2} pKa - \frac{1}{2} pKb \qquad .....(3.14)$$

Degree of Hydrolysis

$$\frac{x}{C} = \sqrt{\frac{Kw}{Ka.Kb}}$$

$$\lambda = \sqrt{\frac{Kw}{Ka.Kb}}$$

$$Kh = \frac{x^2}{(C-x)^2} = \frac{\lambda^2 C^2}{C^2(1-\lambda)^2} = \frac{\lambda^2}{(1-\lambda)^2}$$

$$\sqrt{Kh} = \frac{\lambda}{(1-\lambda)} \qquad .....(3.15)$$

Now, $\qquad Ka = \dfrac{[H^+][AC^-]}{[HAC]}$

$$[\overset{+}{H}] = \frac{Ka.[HAC]}{[AC^-]}$$

$$= Ka.\frac{x}{C-x}$$

$$= Ka.\frac{\lambda}{(1-\lambda)}$$

$$[H^+] = Ka . \sqrt{Kh}$$

$$[H^+] = Ka . \sqrt{\frac{Kw}{Ka.Kb}} \qquad (\because Kh = \frac{Kw}{Ka.Kb})$$

Applying log, $Log [H^+] = \log Ka + \dfrac{1}{2} \log Kw - \dfrac{1}{2} \log Ka - \dfrac{1}{2} \log Kb$

$$- \log [H^+] = - \log Ka - \frac{1}{2} \log Kw + \frac{1}{2} \log Ka + \frac{1}{2} \log Kb$$

$$pH = + pKa + \frac{1}{2} pKw - \frac{1}{2} pKa - \frac{1}{2} pKb$$

$$pH = \frac{1}{2} pKa + \frac{1}{2} pKw - \frac{1}{2} pKb$$

$$pH = \frac{1}{2} (pKa + pKw - pKb) \qquad\qquad .....(3.16)$$

"End Point Detection"

- The point at which complete neutralisation is achieved is called as the 'end point' or the 'equivalence point'.

- If both acid and base are strong electrolytes, the resulting solution will be neutral having pH = 7.

- But if either of the two is a weak electrolyte, the resulting salt formed will hydrolyse to some extent and solution will possess some acidic or alkaline properties.

Indicator

- It is a substance which exhibits colour change at a particular stage of a chemical reaction.

Neutralisation Indicator

- These are substances which exhibit different colours at various values of pH.

- Indicators are weak acids/WB which have different colours in their conjugate base and acid forms.

- Most indicators are used in dilute solution form.

- For an acid–base titration, we select an indicator which will show a distinct colour change at pH close to equivalence point.

Two Theories

(A)   Ostwald Theory

According to this theory the undissociated indicator acid [HIn] or base [InOH] has a colour difference than its ions.

For such an acid Indicator equivalence $\rightarrow$

$$\text{HIn} \rightleftharpoons \text{H}^+ + \text{In}^-$$

Unionized colour   Ionized colour

- In acid solution, there is depression of ionization of indicator due to common ion effect.

- Hence initially concentration of In^- is greater than that of In^- and the colour exhibited will be that of unionized form.

- As titration proceeds, the alkali medium will promote removal of H^+ and there is gradual increase in concentration of ionized form In^- and the solution requires colour of ionized form.

- Low concentration of In^- but on addition of alkali, In^- concentration increases and H^+ decreases. Therefore gives different colour in ionized form.

By applying law of mass action,

$$\text{KIna} = \frac{[\text{H}^+][\text{In}^-]}{[\text{HIn}]}$$

$$[\text{H}^+] = \frac{\text{KIna}[\text{HIn}]}{[\text{In}^-]}$$

Applying log,

$$\text{Log}\,[\text{H}^+] = \log \text{KIna} + \log [\text{HIn}] - \log [\text{In}^-]$$

$$-\log [\text{H}^+] = -\log \text{KIna} - \log [\text{HIn}] + \log [\text{In}^-]$$

$$\text{pH} = -\log \text{KIna} + \log \frac{[\text{In}^-]}{[\text{HIn}]}$$

$$\text{pH} = \text{pKIna} + \log \frac{[\text{In}^-]}{[\text{HIn}]} \qquad .....(3.17)$$

$$\text{pH}\,\alpha\,\frac{[\text{In}^-]}{[\text{HIn}]}$$

$$\text{pH}\,\alpha\,\frac{\text{ionized form}}{\text{unionized form}}$$

- The change in colour is affected by H^+ concentration and as this change is gradual the colour change of indicator is also a gradual one.

- In order to detect the colour change the ratio $\dfrac{[In^-]}{[HIn]}$ must be at least $\dfrac{1}{10}$.

- The pH values at which these limits of observable colour change occur are

$$pH = pKIna + \log \dfrac{[In^-]}{[HIn]}$$

- For limit on acid side,

$$\dfrac{[In^-]}{[HIn]} = 0.1$$

$$\therefore pH = pKIn - 1 \qquad\qquad .....(3.18)$$

- KIna is dissociation constant of indicator.

- The colour of indicator depends upon the ratio of concentration of ionized and unionized form and hence directly proportional to pH. Ratio is $\dfrac{1}{10} \Rightarrow 0.1$.

For Base Indicator

$$InOH \rightleftharpoons In^+ + OH^-$$

$$KInb = \dfrac{[In^+][OH^-]}{[InOH]}$$

$$[OH^-] = KInb \dfrac{[InOH]}{[In^+]}$$

Now, $Kw = [H^+]\,[OH^-]$

$$[OH^-] = \dfrac{Kw}{[H^+]}$$

$$\dfrac{Kw}{[H^+]} = KInb \dfrac{[InOH]}{[In^+]}$$

$$[H^+] = \dfrac{Kw\,[In^+]}{KInb\,[InOH]}$$

Taking log,

$$\text{Log } [H^+] = \log Kw + \log [In^+] - \log KInb - \log [InOH]$$

$$-\log [H^+] = -\log Kw - \log [In^+] + \log KInb + \log [InOH]$$

$$pH = pKw - \log [In^+] - pKInb + \log InOH.$$

$$pH = pKw - pKInb + \log \frac{[InOH]}{[In^+]}$$

For limit on base side,

$$pH = pKIn + 1$$

In general, the pH range in colour change is observed is,

$$pH = pKIn \pm 1$$

This is called "Transition Interval" of the indicator.

The indicator should be such that the pH at equivalence point falls within the transition interval of the indicator.

Titration between	pH at End Point	Indicator
WA AND SB	Alkaline range	Thymel blue Phenolphthalein Thymol phthalein
WB and SA	Acid range	Methyl orange Methyl red Bromocresol green

Examples

1. *Phenolphthalein*

   Acidic – colourless

   Alkaline – pink

   pH range – 8.3 to 11

2. *Methyl orange*

   Acidic – red

   Alkaline – orange

   pH range – 3.1 to 4.1

3. *Methyl red*

   Acidic – red

   Alkaline – yellow

   pH range – 4.2 to 6.3

4. *Phenol red*

   Acidic – yellow

   Alkaline – red

   pH range – 6.8 to 8.4

Resonance Theory

- All the acid–base indicators which are commonly used are organic compounds.
- The difference in colour of same compound is associated with the capability of the compound discribe visible light and this capability is related to the electronic structure.
- Change in the electronic features will result in absorption of different colour components of light with resultant colour change.
- Acid base titration give different colour in different media and colour depends on capability of compounds to absorb UV light and related to electronic structures.

  E.g.   1. Phenophthalein

  2. Azodye

Phenolphthalein

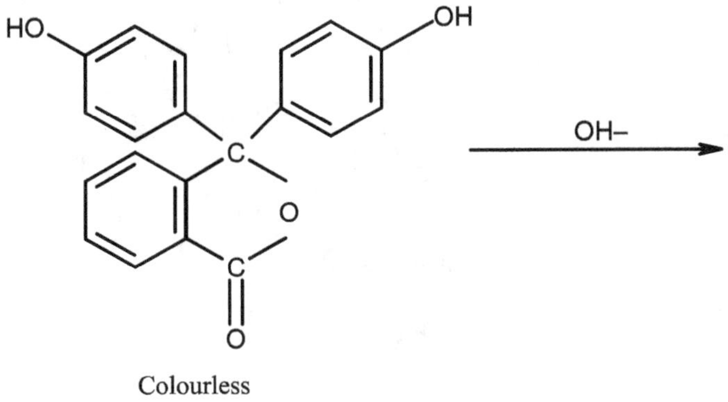

HO

OH

C

O

C

O

OH–

Colourless

Fig. 3.1

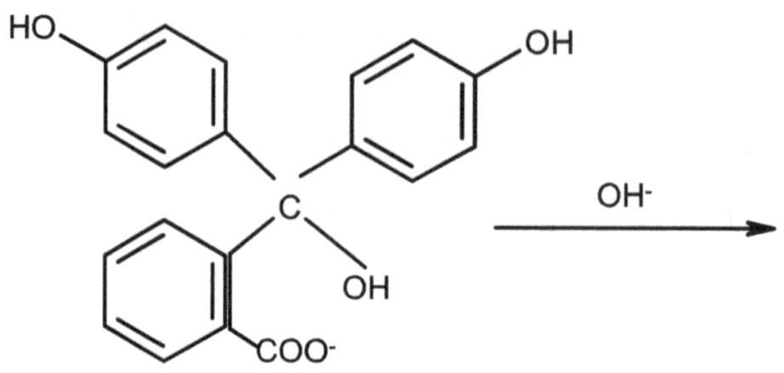

Triphenyl carbonyl structure

Fig. 3.2

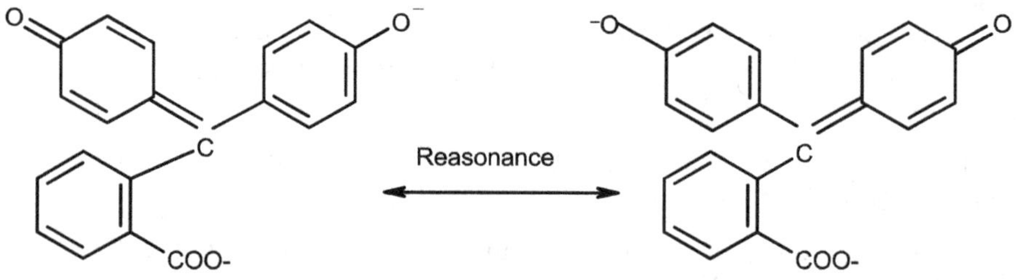

Red colour

Fig. 3.3

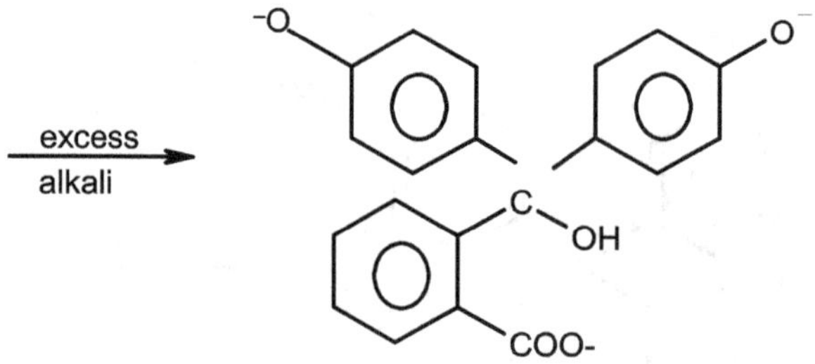

Colour Disaapears

Fig. 3.4

The red colour in alkaline solution is due to the quinatioid structure $\bar{c}$ resulting increased possibilities for resonance between various ionic forms.

Azodye:

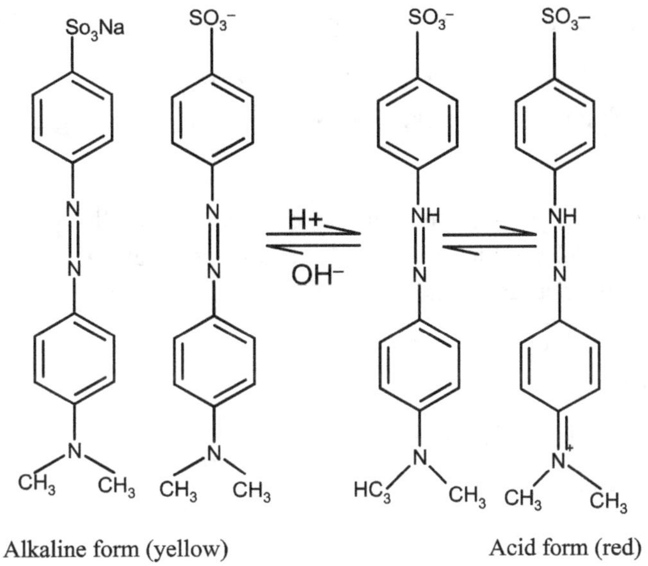

Alkaline form (yellow)   Acid form (red)

Fig. 3.5

Methyl orange is red in acid and yellow in alkaline solution. This colour change is associated with a rearrangement involving the azo link.

Mixed Indicators

- In some cases, the pH range is narrow and the colour change cover this range must be very sharp.

- This is not easily possible with ordinary acid–base indicators.

- The result may be achieved by the use of suitable mixture of indicators.

- These are generally selected so that their pKIn values are close together and overlapping colours are complementary at an intermediate pH value

  Eg. A mixture of equal parts of neutral red (0.1 % solution in alcohol) and methylene blue (0.1% solution in alcohol) gives a sharp colour change from violet–blue to green in passing from acid to alkaline solution at pH 7.

- A mixture of phenolphthalein (3 parts of 0.1%) and α–naphtholphthalein (1 part 0.1%) passes from pale rose to violet at pH 8.9. Titration of phosphoric acid to dibasic stage)

- The colour change of single indicator may also be improved by addition of pH sensitive dyestuff to produce the complement of the indicator colour.

  Eg. Addition of xylene cyanol to methyl orange.

  Here, colour changes from alkaline to acid side is green $\rightarrow$ grey $\rightarrow$ magenta.

When used?

They are used where sharp colour change is required for smaller pH interval. These are selected so that their pKIn value are close together and overlapping colour and they are complementary as intermediate value.

E.g.　Bromocresol green and methyl red

　　　　pH $\rightarrow$ 5.1

　　　　colour $\rightarrow$ Red $\rightarrow$ acidic and

　　　　　　　green $\rightarrow$ Basic

Universal Indicator

Multiple Range Indicator

- By mixing certain indicators the colour change may be made to an extent over the considerable portion of pH range.

- Such mixtures are called UNIVERSAL indicator. Not suitable for quantitative titration but for determination of approximate pH by colorimetric titration.

  E.g.　Dissolve 0.1 gm of phenolphthalein

　　　　+ 0.2 gm of methyl red

　　　　+ 0.3 gm of methyl yellow

　　　　+ 0.4 gm of bromo thymol blue

　　　　+ 0.5 gm thymol blue

　　In 500 ml absolute alcohol

Add sufficient sodium hydroxide solution until colour is yellow.

Colour changes are

　　　　pH $\rightarrow$ 2　　　–　　　red

　　　　pH $\rightarrow$ 4　　　–　　　orange

$$pH \rightarrow 6 \quad - \quad \text{yellow}$$
$$pH \rightarrow 8 \quad - \quad \text{green}$$
$$pH \rightarrow 10 \quad - \quad \text{blue}$$

Several indicators are available commercially as solution and as the test papers and are used in colorimetric determination of pH.

Titration Curves

- If we study the changes in hydrogen ion concentration during the course of titration we get a clear idea about the mechanism of neutralization process.

- The pH value of greatest important is the ore near the equivalence point as it gives us help in selecting an indicator which will give the smallest titration error.

- The curve obtained by plotting pH as ordinate against the percent of acid neutralised for the number of ml of alkali (titrant) added as abscissa during titration is known as "Neutralisation" or more generally "Titration curve"

$$pH \xrightarrow{\text{Vs}} \text{ml of titrant}$$

Factors Affecting Titration Curves

1. Strength of acid and base

2. Concentration

3. Influence of Buffer condition

4. Neutralization or Hydrolysis

1. SA – SB Titration

- When strong acid and strong base are mixed together as in titration of one by other the reaction can be represented as:

$$H^+ + OH^- \rightleftharpoons H_2O$$

- Since it is reverse of ionization of water its equilibrium concentration is very large.

- This requirement for a reaction to form the basis of a good titration

$$Eg. \quad HCl + NaOH \xrightarrow{\text{Neutralisation}} NaCl + H_2O$$

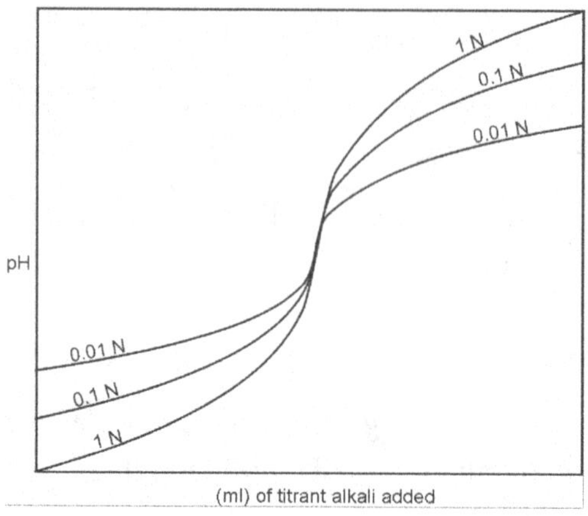

Titration curve $\forall$ SA – SB

Fig. 3.6

2. WA – SB Titration

- It is possible to derive exact equation that describes the entire course of titration the calculation is just as convenient with the approximate equation above.

- Titration considered in four stages.

$$pH = \frac{1}{2} pKw + \frac{1}{2} pKa + \frac{1}{2} \log C$$

(a) Before titration begins

at this point sample solution contains only the acid and pH is calculated.

$$[H^+] = \sqrt{Ka.C} \qquad\qquad .....(3.19)$$

(b) During titration

- After some SB has been added, its reaction with the WA will produce an equivalent amount of conjugate WB. The solution now is a mix of WA and its conjugate base, it is a buffer solution and we apply Handerson – Hasselbalch equation.

$$pKa = pH - \log \frac{b}{a}$$

(c) At end point

Now, an amount of SB has been added that is exactly to amount of WA initially added.

- The solution now contains only the conjugate base of WA and pH can be calculated.

$$Kb = \frac{[OH^-]^2}{C - [OH^-]}$$

$$[OH^-] = \sqrt{Kb.C}$$

(d) After the end point

- An excess of titrant has been now added, and pH determined essentially by this excess, the appropriate dilution within the solution being taken into account.

- It is true that the conjugate WB produced also contributes to the solution pOH, but its contribution is small relative to effect of excess titrant. After equivalence point, the solution contains excess of OH^- which will represent the hydrolysis of salt.

  Eg. $HAC + NaOH \rightleftharpoons NaAC + H_2O$

  $HAC + H_2O \xrightarrow{H} AC^- + H_3O^+$

  $H_2O + H_2O \xrightarrow{H} H_3O^+ + OH^-$

- For 0.1 N acetic acid and 0.1 N NaOH

- Indicator used $\rightarrow$ alkaline range

  E.g. Phenolphthalein, thymolphthalein or Thymol blue

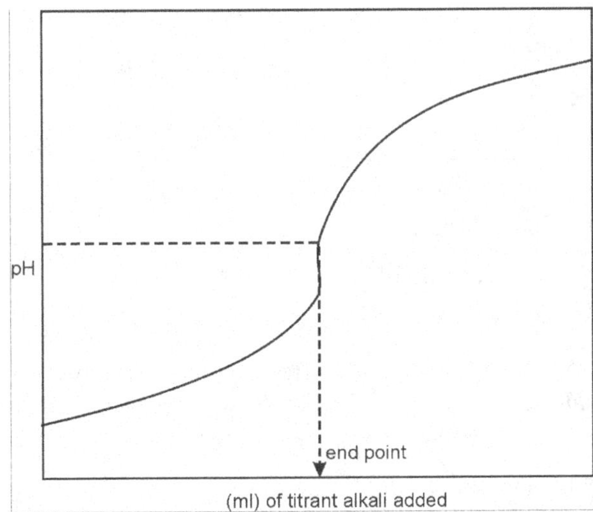

Titration curve for WA – SB

Fig. 3.7

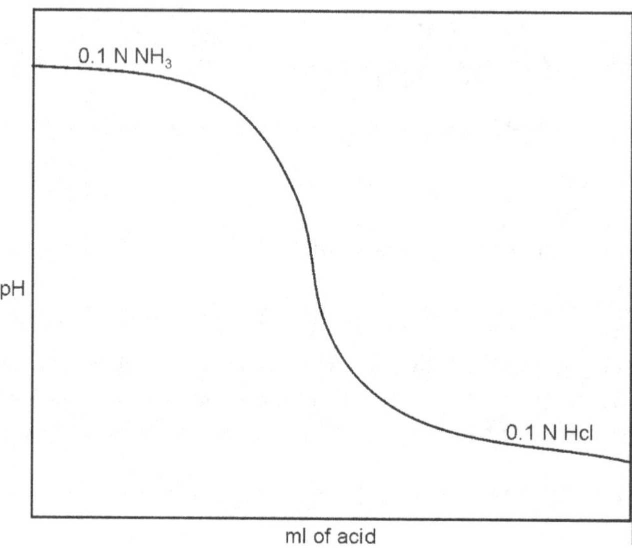

Fig. 3.8

3. WB – SA Titration

Eg. Titration of 100 ml of 0.1 N Aq. ammonia

$Kb = 1.8 \times 10^{-5}$ $\overline{C}$

100 ml of 0.1N HCl

pH – at equivalence point

$$pH = \frac{1}{2} pKw - \frac{1}{2} pKb - \frac{1}{2} \log C$$

and also, for other calculations,

$$pH = pKw - \frac{1}{2} pKb - \log \frac{[salt]}{[base]}$$

- After equivalence point has been reached the solution contains excess of H^+ ions, hydrolysis of salt be repressed and subsequent change of pH will be due to excess of acid present.
- The indicator must be acidic range

    Eg. Methyl orange

    Methyl red

    Bromophenol blue

    Bromocresol green

Titration curve $\forall$ WB – SA

Eg. $HCl + NH_4OH \xrightarrow{\text{N}} NH_4Cl + H_2O$

$NH_4OH + H_2O \xrightarrow{\text{H}} NH_4^+ + OH^-$

$H_2O + H_2O \rightarrow H_3O^+ + OH^-$

4. WA – WB Titration

Eg. 100 ml 0.1 N acetic acid with 0.1 N NH_3

pH at equivalence point is,

$$pH = pKw + \frac{1}{2}(pKa - pKb)$$

- The chief feature of curve is that the change of pH near equivalence point and during whole neutralization is very gradual.
- Hence, the end point can't be detected by ordinary indicator.
- Hence, mixed indicator is use.

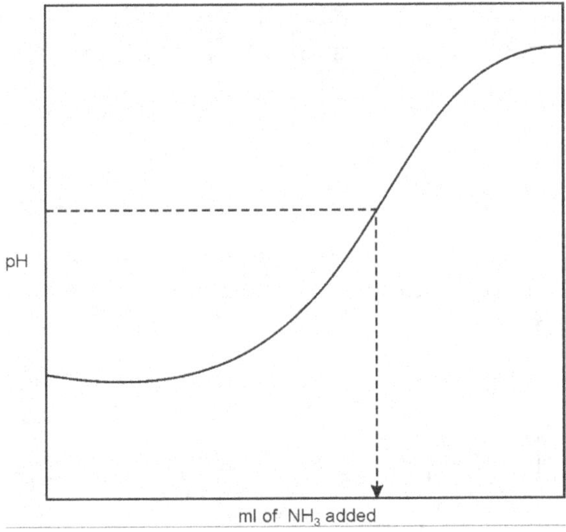

Fig. 3.9

Titration Curve for WA – WB

Eg. $HAC + NH_4OH \xrightarrow{\text{N}} NH_4AC + H_2O$

$NH_4OH + H_2O \xrightarrow{\text{H}} NH_4^+ + OH^-$

$$H_2O + H_2O \xrightarrow{\text{H}} OH^- + H_3O^+$$

$$HAC + H_2O \xrightarrow{\text{H}} H_3O^+ + AC^-$$

5. Titration Curves of Polybasic Acids

- A polybasic acid is considered as a mixtured acids i.e. it furnishes more than 1 proton on dissociation.

Eg.   Carbonic acid gives two protons.

Phosphoric acid gives three protons

Hence are called polybasic or polyprotic acid

Each stage of dissociation gives a separate monobasic acid

Dissociation Constant

$$H_3A \rightleftharpoons H_2A^- + H^+ \qquad \rightarrow \qquad K_1$$

$$H_2A \rightleftharpoons HA^- + H^+ \qquad \rightarrow \qquad K_2$$

$$HA^- \rightleftharpoons H^+ + A^- \qquad \rightarrow \qquad K_3$$

$$K_1 > K_2 > K_3$$

- Neutralization curve can be constructed by treatment of tribasic acid as a mixture of three monobasic acids.

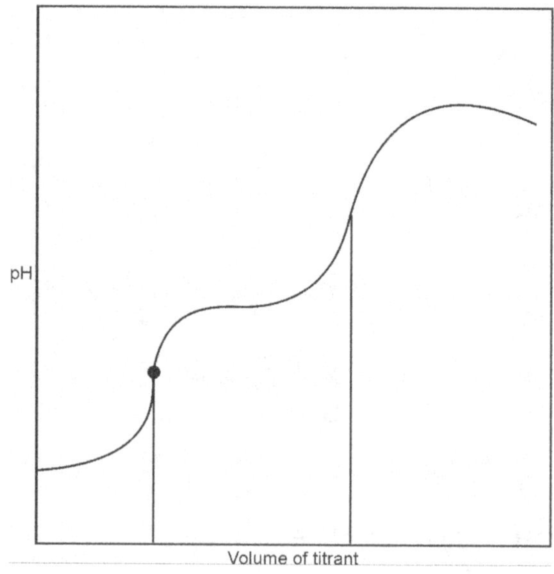

Fig. 3.10

Importance of (Acid Aqueous Base Titration)

- In aqueous acid base titration various drugs can be analysed easily
  Titration can be performed using direct titration.

  Eg :

Drug	Type	Titrant
HCl	Direct titration	NaOH
Benzoic acid	Direct titration	NaOH
Tartaric acid	Direct titration	NaOH
Thiopentone sodium	Direct titration	H_2SO_4
NaOH	Direct titration	H_2SO_4

- If the acidic or basic solute have a sufficient strength, they can be titrated with SB or SA respectively to give quantitative results.

- In case of insoluble substances, substances which are volatile, reactions requiring bcating and substanccs for which reaction proceeds rapidly only in presence of excess of reagent, direct titration will not be possible. These substances are determined by back titration.

- The determination involves addition of excess but known quantity of standard solution to the weighed sample of analyte and after the complete reaction, the excess of solution, not required by the analyte is back titrated with standard solution.

- Similarly, blank reading is performed by omitting the sample.

- The difference in these two titration gives the quantity of solution required for the reaction with the analyte and quantitative analysis is carried out.

- Neutralization titration are used in assay of various drugs and formulations.

Drug	Type	Titrant
Asprin	Back titration	H_2SO_4
Dientestrol	Back titration	NaOH
Urea	Back titration	HCl
Methyl saliaylate	Back titration	HCl
Indomethacin	Back titration	NaOH
Benzyl alcohol	Back titration	NaOH

CHAPTER 4

GRAVIMETRIC ANALYSIS

- Gravimetric analysis involves the separation of the constituents to be estimated in the form of an insoluble compound of known composition.
- The insoluble compound is then washed to free it from impurities, dried and weighed either as such or ignited that leaves a residue of some other compound which is then weighed as pure form as possible.
- It involves transformation of the element, ion or radial to be determined into a pure stable compound which is then weighed.
- The separation of element or the compound containing it, may be possible by following ways:

  (i) Precipitation method.

  (ii) Volatilisation or evolution method.

  (iii) Electro-analytical method.

  (iv) Chromatography.

Advantages of Gravimetric Analysis

- It is accurate and precise when using modern analytical balance.
- Possible sources of errors can readily be checked, since filterates can be tested for completeness of precipitation and precipitates may be examined for the presence of impurities.
- It is an absolute method i.e. it involves direct measurement without any form of calibration being required.

- Determination can be carried out with relatively inexpensive apparatus. The most expensive items are a muffle furnace and sometimes platinum crucible.
- A very high level of accuracy can be achieved.

Disadvantages

- It is slow.
- It is time consuming.
- It is tedious.
- Gravimetric analysis is a macroscopic method and it involves large samples.

Advantages

- Analysis of standards to be used for the testing and calibration of instrumental techniques.
- Analysis requiring high accuracy, although the time consuming nature of gravimetry limits this application to small number of determination.

The Factors which Determine a Successful Analysis by Precipitation

- The precipitates must be insoluble so that no applicable loss occurs, the quantity remaining in solution does not exceed 0.1 mg.
- The physical nature of precipitates must be such that it can be readily separated from the solution by filtration and can be washed free of soluble impurities. These conditions require that the particles does not pass through the filtering medium that the particle size is unaffected.
- The precipitates must be convertible into a pure substance by definite chemical operation such as evaporation.

The Rules for Precipitation

- The precipitating agent should be mixed slowly and with constant agitation. This will keep that degree of supersaturation small and will help in the formation of crystalline precipitate.
- The precipitation should be carried out in dilute solution.
- The precipitation should be carried out in hot solution so the precipitates produced can be stable at higher temperature.
- Crystalline precipitates should be digested for a longer time.
- Precipitates should be preferably washed with dilute solution of appropriate electrolyte. Washing with water is avoided as it leads to peptization.
- Precipitates that are contaminated by co-precipitation or others are dissolved in a suitable solvent and then reprecipitated from the solution.

Colloid State

- Colloidal suspensions are not suitable in gravimetric analysis because of its particle size.

- The size ranges in between 10^{-7} to 10^{-4} cm.

- This cannot be readily filtrated.

- The stability of this suspensions can be decreased by stirring, heating and by adding an electrolyte. This causes individual particles to bind together to give colloidal mass and is filterable.

- The process of converting colloidal suspensions into a filterable mass is called coagulation or agglomeration.

Lyophobic Colloids	Lyophilic Colloids
These are only slightly viscous.	They are very viscous almost jelly like, known as gels.
Addition of water has no effect on these colloids.	Addition of water or solvents has effect on these colloids.
Comparatively small concentration of electrolyte results in flocculation of these colloids.	Comparatively large concentration of electrolytes can result in flocculation of these colloids.
They possess electrical charge of definite sign which can be changed only by specific methods.	They change their charge easily
Ultramicroscopy reveals the particles in vigorous motion known as 'Brownian movement ' e.g. Gold solution	Under ultramicroscope only a diffused light concentration is exhibited.

Stability of Colloidal Suspensions is due to following reasons

- All particles are either positively charged or negatively charged so they repel one-another.

- The primarily adsorbed ions and secondarily adsorbed negative counter ions constitute a classical double layer that stabilises a colloidal suspension by preventing individual particles coming close enough to one another to agglomerate.

- Coagulation of colloidal suspension can be brought about by heating accompanied by stirring and even more effective way to coagulate colloid is to increase the concentration of electrolyte.

- If we add a suitable ionic compound to the suspension the concentration of counter ions increases as a result the volume of solution that contains sufficient counter ion to balance the charge of the primary adsorption layer decreases.
- This leads to shrinkage of counter 1M layer and then the particles can approach more closely to one-another and agglomerate.
- By increasing the particle's size, solubility is decreased.

Peptization of Colloids

- Peptization refers to the process by which a coagulation reverts to its original dispersed state.
- When a coagulated colloid is washed, some of the electrolytes responsible for its coagulation is reached from the internal liquid in contact with the solid particles.
- Removal of the electrolytes has the effect of increasing the volume of the counter ion layer.
- The repulsive forces responsible for the original colloid state are then re-established and particles detach themselves from the coagulated mass.
- The washing becomes cloudy as the freshly dispersed particles pass through the filter.
- Washing is needed to minimize contamination, on the other hand there is risk of losses resulting from peptization if pure water is used.
- The problem is resolved by washing the precipitates with a solution containing an electrolyte that volatilizes during the subsequent drying or ignition.

Factors

Post Precipitation: Sometimes when a precipitate is allowed to stand in presence of the mother liquor the second substance will form the precipitate with peptizing reagent, called post precipitation.

- It occurs with sparingly soluble substance which form supersaturated solution. They usually have an ion in common with that precipitate.

   E.g. when calcium oxalate is precipitated in presence of Mg^{+2} ions, Magnesium Oxalate does not precipitate out immediately because it tends to form supersaturated solution but if this precipitate is allowed to stand for a longer time before filtration, Magnesium Oxalate separates out on precipitates of solution, greater will be the error due to post precipitation.

Post Precipitation	Co-Precipitation
Extent of contamination increases with time of contact with mother liquor in case of post precipitation.	Extent of contamination decreases with time of contact with mother liquor in case of co-precipitation.
Extent of contamination increases with faster agitation by mechanical or thermal means.	Extent of contamination decreases with faster agitation by mechanical or thermal means.
Magnitude of contamination by post precipitation is greater.	Magnitude of contamination by co-precipitation is lesser.

Digestion: It is a process in which a precipitate is heated for an hour or more in the solution from which it was formed (mother liquor).

- In this, small particles tend to dissolve and reprecipitate on the surface of larger crystals in addition individual particles agglomerate to share a common counter ion layer and finally cement together to form large crystals.
- Digestion is carried out at elevated temperature.
- It is also possible sometimes at room temperature.
- It improves filterability of precipitates and its purity.
- Smaller particles which have greater solubility and surface area will after precipitation tend to pass the solution and will ultimately redeposit on larger particles resulting into elimination of co-precipitation by surface adsoption.
- In addition the rapidly formed precipitates are irregular and have more surface area.
- On digestion the precipitates tend to become more regular, dense, crystalline particle resulting in decrease of surface area, thus digestion results in decrease of adsorption of co-precipitation and increase size of crystals of precipitate, Thus facilitating filtration.

Drying of Precipitates: There are three different ways of drying of precipitates.

(i)   Air drying at room temperature (Ambient)
(ii) Air drying at low temperature
(iii) Ignition

(i) **Ambient Temperature**: If precipitates are obtained from solvents like ether or ethanol then they can be dried at ambient temperature,
e.g. precipitates of $MgNH_4PO_4$ [Magnesium Ammonium Phosphate].

(ii) **Low Temperature**: AgCl precipitates can be dried at 100 at 130°C because water is not bound to precipitate.

(iii) *Ignition*: Water is bound to $Fe_2O_3 \cdot 6H_2O$. Here conversion takes place from one compound to another.

$$CuSO_4.5H_2O \xrightarrow{\text{Ignition}} CH_2O + \frac{1}{2}O_2$$

Reprecipitation

A drastic but effective way to minimize the effects of absorption is reprecipitation or double precipitation.

Here the filtrated solid is redissolved and reprecipitated.

The first precipitates ordinarily carries down only a fraction of the contaminant present in the original solvent. Thus, the solution containing the redissolved precipitates has a significantly lower contaminant concentration than the original and even less adsorption occurs during the second precipitation.

Reprecipitation adds substantially to the time required for an analysis but is often necessary for such precipitates as the hydrous excide of iron (III) and aluminium which have extra ordinary tendencies to adsorb the hydroxides of heavy metal cations such as Zn, cd and Mn.

Thermogravimetry

A technique in which a change in the weight of a substance is recorded as a function of temperature or time using the balance and furnace.

Two types of graphs are obtained here

(i)   TG curve (the thermogravimetric curve).

(ii) Derivative of the thermogravimetric curve (DTG curve).

(i) *TG Curve*: The basic instrument requirement for thermogravimetry is a precision balance with a furnace programmed for a linear rise of temperature with time.

The results may be presented as a thermogravimetric (TG) curve, in which weight is recorded as the function of temperature or time.

(ii) *DTG Curve (derivative thermogravimetric curve)*: The first derivative of the thermogravimetric curve (TG) is plotted with respect to either temperature or time.

(i)   *TG Curve*: Here the figure shows a typical thermogravimetric curve for copper sulphate pentahydrate $CuSO_4.5H_2O$.

It can be divided into horizontal portions (plateau) and curved portions.

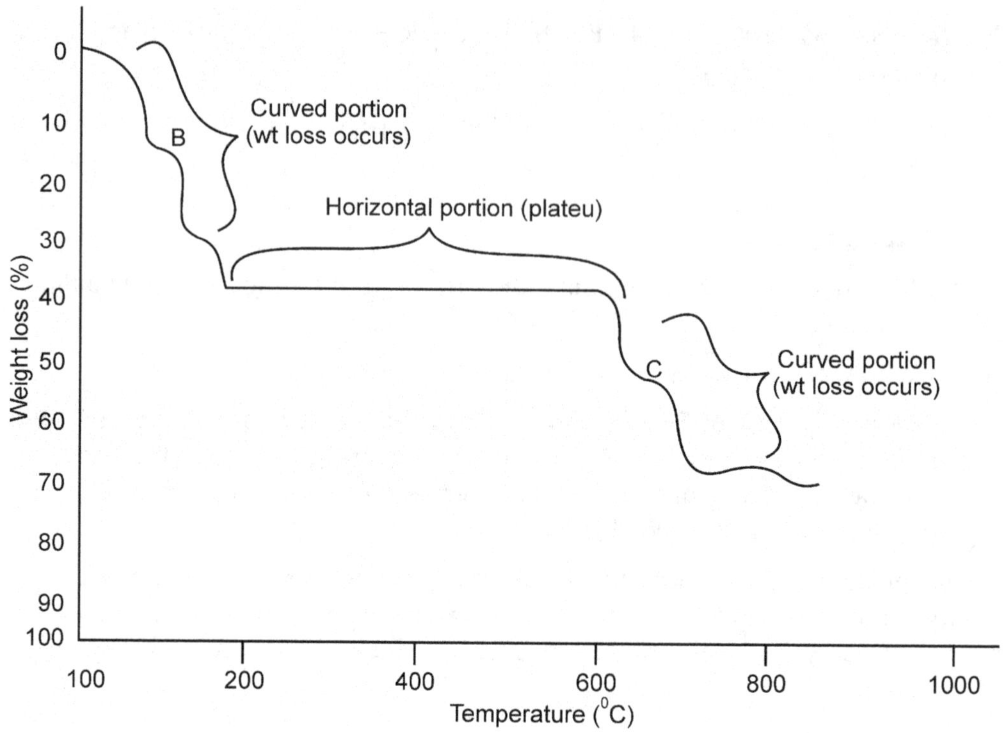

Fig. 4.1 $CuSO_4$, SH_2O : Typical TG curve.

***Horizontal Portion (Plateau)*:** It indicates the region where there is no weight loss.

***Curved Portion*:** It indicates the region of weight loss.

Since the TG curve is quantitative, calculation on compound stoichiometry can be made at any given temperature.

Copper sulphate pentahydrate has four distinct regions of decomposition.

They are listed here along with the approximate temperature ranges :

$$CuSO_4.\, 5H_2O \longrightarrow CuSO_4.\, H_2O \qquad \text{90 to 150 °C}$$

$$CuSO_4.\, H_2O \longrightarrow CuSO_4 \qquad \text{200 to 275 °C}$$

$$CuSO_4 \longrightarrow CuO + SO_2 + \frac{1}{2}\,O_2 \qquad \text{700 to 900 °C}$$

$$2CuO \longrightarrow Cu_2O + \frac{1}{2}\,O_2 \qquad \text{1000 to 1100 °C}$$

***Extra*:** The precise temperature regions for each of the reactions depend up on the experimental conditions. Although in the figure the co-ordinate is shown as the percentage weight loss, the scale on this axis may take other forms like :

   (i)   True weight.

   (ii) Percentage of the total weight.

   (iii) Relative molecular mass units.

  (ii) DTG curve (Derivative thermogravimetric curve)

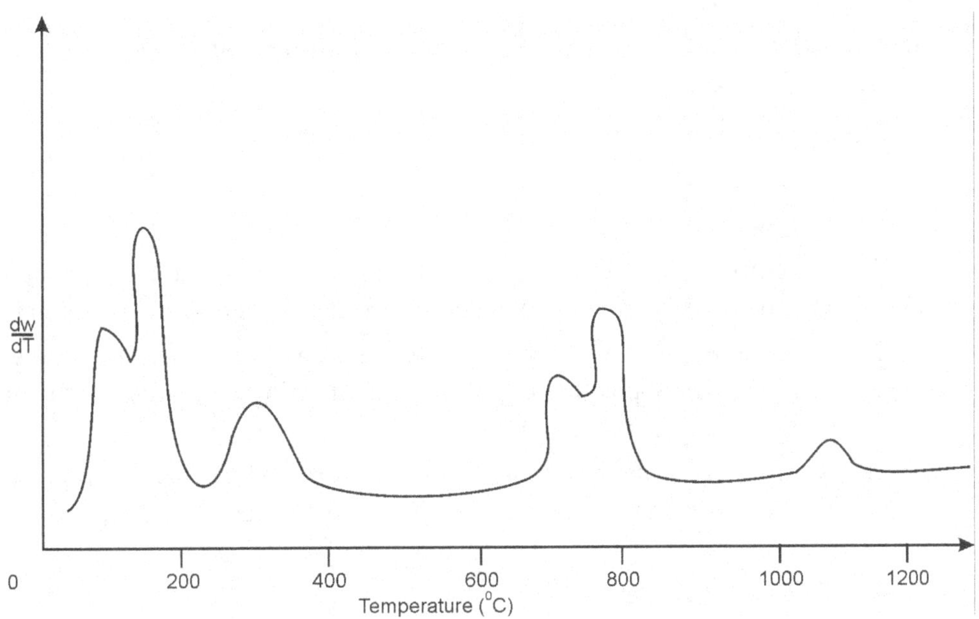

Fig. 4.2 Typical DTG Curve.

If the rate of change of weight with time dW/dT is plotted against temperature, a derivative thermogravimetric (DTG) curve is obtained.

In the DTG curve when there is no weight loss then $dW/dT = 0$

The peak on the derivative curve corresponds to a maximum slope on the TG curve

When dW/dT is a maximum but not zero there is an inflexion i.e. a change of slope on the TG curve.

Inflexions B and C on Fig. 4.1 may imply the formation of the trihydrate $CuSO_4 . 3H_2O$ and at point C it is reported by Duval as due to formation of a golden yellow basic sulphate composition $2CuO.SO_3$.

Derivative thermogravimetry is useful for many complicated determinations and any change in the rate of weight loss may be readily identified as a trough indicating consecutive reactions hence weight loss changes occurring at close temperature may be ascertained.

Factors Affecting these Curves

Factors affecting the gravimetry curve are mainly classified into two classes:

(i)   Instrumental effects.

(ii) Sample characteristics.

(i)   ***Instrumental Effects*** : There are three types of instrumental factors which affect these curves. They are

(a) Heating rate.

(b) Furnace atmosphere.

(c) Crucible geometry.

(a) **Heating Rate:** When a substance is heated at a fast rate, the temperature of decomposition will be higher than that obtained at a slower rate of heating.

Extra: The effect is shown for single step reaction in Fig. 4.3. The curve AB represents the decomposition curve at a slow heating rate, whereas the curve CD is due to the faster heating rate.

If T_A and T_C are the decomposition temperatures at the start of the reaction and the final temperatures on the completion of the decomposition are T_B and T_D, then

$$T_A < T_C$$

$$T_B < T_D$$

$$T_B - T_A < T_D - T_C$$

The heating rate has only a small effect when a fast reversible reaction is considered.

The points of inflexion B and C obtained on the thermogravimetric curve for copper sulphate pentahydrate may be resolved into a plateus if a slower heating rate is used.

Hence the detection of intermediate compounds by thermogravimetry is very dependent upon the heating rate employed.

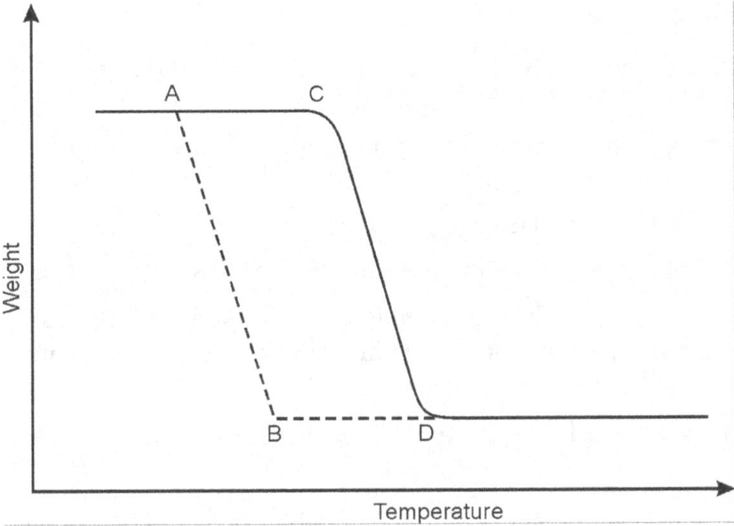

Fig. 4.3 Faster heating rates lead to higher decomposition temperatures.

(b) Furnace Atmosphere: Normally the function of the furnace atmosphere is to remove the gaseous products evolved during thermogravimetry, in order to ensure the nature of surrounding gas remains as constant as possible throughout the experiment.

There are three atmospheres most commonly employed in thermogravimetry.

(i) *Static Air* : Air form the surroundings flows through the furnace.

(ii) *Dynamic Air* : Compressed air from a cylinder is passed through the furnace at a measured rate flow.

(iii) *Nitrogen Gas*: Oxygen-free nitrogen gas provides an inert environment

(c) Crucible Geometry: The geometry of the crucible can alter the slope of the thermogracimetric curve. A flate shaped crucible is generally preferred to a 'high-form' cone shape because the diffusion of any evolved gases is easier with a flat shape.

(d) Sample Characteristic

- The weight
- The particle size
- The mode of preparation of a sample all govern the thermogravimetric results.
- The smaller sample size and less amount of sample is desirable.

Applications of Thermogravimetry

- Determining the purity and thermal stability of both primary and secondary standards.

- Investigating the correct drying temperatures and the suitability of various weighing forms for gravimetric analysis.

- Direct application to analytical problems

- Determining the composition of alloys and mixtures.

Thermogravimetry is a valuable technique for assessing the purity of materials. Analytical reagents, especially those used in titrimetric analysis as primary standards, e.g. Na_2CO_3, KHP have been examined.

Many primary standards absorb appreciable amounts of water when exposed to moist atmospheres.

TG data can show the extent of this absorption, hence the most suitable drying temperature for a given reagent may be determined.

The thermal stability of EDTA as the free acid and also as the more widely used disodium salt Na_2 EDTA $2H_2O$ has been reported. According to that the dehydration of the disodium salt commences at between 110 and 125 °C, which confirmed the view that Na_2 EDTA $2H_2O$ could be safely heated to constant weight at 80 °C.

Initially the widespread application of thermogravimetry in analytical chemistry has been in the study of the recommended drying temperatures of gravimetric precipitates.

Thermogravimetry may be used to determine the composition of binary mixtures. e.g. for Ca (calcium) and strontium binary mixture. Here the decomposition temperature for $CaCO_3$ is 650 to 850°C.

- where for strontium carbonate the decomposition temperature is 950 to 1150 °C.

- Both carbonates decompose to their oxides with the evolution of carbon dioxide.

- Hence the amount of calcium and strontium present in a mixture may be calculated from the weight losses due to the evolution of carbon dioxide at the lower and higher temperature ranges respectively.

- This method can also be extended to the analysis of a three-component mixtures.

- The most important applications of thermogravimetry is in examining the thermal stability of polymers.

CHAPTER 5

NON-AQUEOUS TITRATIONS

Introduction

- Non-aqueous titrations are those in which the titration of weakly acidic or weakly basic substances are carried out using non-aqueous solvents so as to get a sharp end-point.

- They replaced aqueous titrations for many substances which are either too weakly acidic or too weakly basic for the problem of quality control and as they do not give sharp end-point because of poor solubility and weak reactivity.

- In short, non-aqueous titrations have replaced the aqueous titrations for many substances which are either too weakly acidic or too weakly basic.

Principle of Non-Aqueous Titrations: These titrations are based upon Bronsted-Lowry and Lewis theory of acids and bases and the nature and influence of levelling effects of non-aqueous solvents on substances.

- An additional advantage is that many substances which are insoluble in water are sufficiently soluble in organic solvents to permit their titrations in the non-aqueous media.

- Speed, precision and accuracy of non-aqueous methods are close to that of classical acidimetric and alkalimetric titrations.

- The apparatus is also same but moisture and CO_2 are to be avoided because water which is a weak base can compete with a weak nitrogen base and end-point would not be sharp at all.

- Moisture content should not be more than 0.05%. Temperature during standardisation should not vary.

- In aqueous titrations the neutralization is between proton donor and acceptor, i.e. acid and a base.

- But in non-aqueous titrations, the neutralization is between a weakly protophyllic substance which tends to accept a pair of electrons and a highly protophyllic substance which tends to provide a pair of electrons in the formation of covalent bonds by co-ordination.

- The chemical reaction of acid with base in aqueous solution is different from the reaction that take place in non-aqueous solution.

- The chemical reaction of acid HA with base B in aqueous solution is represented by

$$HA + H_2O \rightarrow H_3^+O + A^- \qquad \text{Conjugate base of acid HA.}$$

$$H_3^+O + B \rightarrow BH^+ + H_2P$$

- A very weak base B may be a weak proton acceptor as compared to H_2O in aqueous medium. However, in non-aqueous solvents like glacial acetic acid, it can accept proton readily when acetous perchloric acid is used as titrant.

$$HClO_4 + CH_3COOH \rightleftharpoons CH_3COO\,H_2^+ \quad \text{(Acetous perchloric acid)}$$
$$\text{Titrant}$$
$$CH_3COO\,H_2^+ + B \rightleftharpoons BH^+ + CH_3COOH$$

Reasons for Non-Aqueous Titrations

- The reactants or products might be insoluble in water.
- The reactants or products might react with water.
- The analyte to be titrated is too weak acid or too weak base.

Solvents for a Weak Base in Non-Aqueous Titrations

- Glacial acetic acid + acetic anhydride
- Dioxane
- Benzene
- Acetonitrile
- Carbon tetrachloride
- Chlorobenzene

Solvents for a Weak Acid in Non-Aqueous Titration

- Ethylene diamine
- n-Butyl amine
- Pyridine

- Dimethyl formamide
- Ethyl-methyl ketone
- Acetone
- Methanol
- Ethanol

Titrants for a Weak Base

- Perchloric acid
- Alkyl sulfonic acid
- O – fluoro sulfonic acid
- 2, 4 dinitro benzene sulfonic acid
- 2, 4, 6 trinitro benzene sulfonic acid

Titrants for a Weak Acid

- Alkali methoxide
- Tetra butyl NH_4OH
- Li-methoxide

Indicators for Weak Bases

- α-napthol benzene
- Oracet blue
- Crystal violet
- Quinaldine red

Indicators for Weak Acids

- Quinaline red in alcohol
- Thymol blue in DMF
- Azoviolet in benzene

Types of Solvents

There are four classes.

(i) Aprotic Solvents

- These are chemically neutral and unreactive in nature or we can say they are inert in nature.
- They have low dielectric constant.

    They are useful in dissolving substances, thus act as solvents and are useful for diluting solutions.

    e.g.   Chloroform

    Benzene

(ii)   Proto acidic solvents

- These are acidic in nature
- They donate protons

  e.g., H_2SO_4

  HCl

  Formic acid

  HNO_3

(iii)   Photophobic solvents

- These are basic in nature
- They abstract protons from acids to give soluated protons

  $$HB + Sol \rightleftharpoons Sol.\ H^+ + B^-$$

  e.g.   Pyridine

  n-butyl amine

  ethylene diamine

(iv)   Amphiprotic solvents

- These solvents behave as an acid or as a base depending upon the substances dissolved in it.
- They have both protogenic and protophyllic properties in being able to donate and accept protons.

  e.g.   Glacial acetic acid

  Dioxan

  H_2O

Classification of Non-Aqueous Titrants

Non-aqueous titrants are categorised as follows:

- Substances which behave as bases under appropriate conditions of titrations
- Substances which behave as acids under appropriate conditions of titration
- Substances which have both acidic and basic functional groups, can be titrated as acid or base under appropriate conditions of titrations.
- For determination of basic substances a solution of perchloric acid in glacial acetic acid is most commonly used as a titrant.

Selection of Solvents

While selecting the solvents, the following factors must be considered :

(i)   Solubility and nature of sample under investigation, for example, if the sample is a weak acid then basic solvents like DMF or pyridine are used.

(ii)   There should not be any side-reaction of the sample or titrant with the solvent.

(iii) The solvent choosen should not affect the sharpness of the end-point during titration.

(iv)   The titrant and solute should be readily miscible with solvents.

(v)   The solvent should have a reasonably high dielectric constant.

(vi)   The solvent should be readily available, of low toxicity, easily purified and inexpensive.

While selecting the solvents, the following must also be considered.

(a)   Titrimetric determinations of weak acids require basic solvents such as ethylene diamine or formamide as media.

(b)   Weak bases are titrated in acidic solvents such as anhydrous acetic acid, glycols and their mixtures with other solvents.

(c)   Amphoteric solvents in determining acids, bases, salts and various mixtures. Examples are alcohols, ketones and their derivatives.

(d)   Inert solvents are generally employed for preparing mixed solvents. These are benzene and its derivatives and also chlorine derivatives of saturated hydrocarbons.

Interference due to Water

- When a weakly basic drug is present, water (OH^-) acts as stronger base and preferentially accepts protons from an acid. Thus there is interference in the reaction of weak base with an acid.

- When a weakly acidic drug is present, water (H^+) behaves like a strong acid and preferentially donates proton to the base. Thus, there is interference in the reaction of weak acid with a base.

- Hence in the presence of water, titration of either weakly acidic substances with stronger base or weakly basic substances with stronger acid is not possible.

Solvents used for Non-Aqueous Titrations

A very large number of both inorganic and organic solvents have been used but few are more frequently used.

e.g.   (i)   Glacial acetic acid

(ii) Acetonitrile

(iii) Dioxan Alcohol

(iv)   Dimethyl formamide (DMF)

(v)   Benzoic acid and phenyl cinchonic acid

(i)   Solute   Titrant   Solvent   Indicator

       WA compund $\rightarrow$ SB $\rightarrow$ Basic/ no acidic $\rightarrow$ WA

(ii)   Solute   Titrant   Solvent   Indicator

       WB compound $\rightarrow$ SA $\rightarrow$ non Basic/ acidic $\rightarrow$ WB

Solvents may be :

(i)   SA : less capacity to accept H^+ ions

(ii)   WA : less capacity to donate H^+ ions

(iii)   SB : more capacity to accept H^+ ions

(iv)   WB : less capacity to accept H^+ ions

Dissociation of Solute

In dissociation, solute gives either +ve or –ve ions

   +ve ions are called *Lionium ions*

   –ve ions are called *Liate ions*

Non-Aqueous Titration of Weak bases with Perchloric Acid

- *Principle* : Weak bases are dissolved in acetic acid and are titrated with acetous perchloric acid.

- Acetic acid behaves as a weak acid because of poor dissociation into H^+.

$$CH_3COOH \rightleftharpoons CH_3CO\bar{O} + \overset{+}{H}$$

- But when a strong acid (perchloric acid) is added to acetic acid, there is formation of *onium ions* which have more tendency to donate protons.

$$HClO_4 \rightleftharpoons H^+ + ClO_4^-$$

$$\therefore\ CH_3COOH + H^+ \rightleftharpoons CH_3COO\,H_2^+$$

$$\text{(onium ion)}$$

- When weak bases like pyridine are dissolved in acetic acid, equivalent amount of acetate ions are produced which have more tendency to accept protons.

$$\therefore\ C_3H_5N + CH_3\,COOH \rightleftharpoons C_2H_5NH^+ + CH_3COO^-$$

- Ultimately the titration of weakly basic drug in acetic acid against acetous perchloric acid yields accurate end-point.

- The series of reactions is given as follows :

$$HClO_4 + CH_3COOH \rightarrow CH_3COO\,H_2^+ + ClO_4^-$$
$$\text{(onium ions)}$$

$$C_5H_5N + CH_3COOH \rightarrow C_5H_5NH^+ + CH_3COO^-$$
$$\text{(acetate ion)}$$

$$CH_3COO\,H_2^+ + CH_3COO^- \rightarrow 2CH_3COOH$$
$$\text{(Burette)} \qquad \text{(Conical flask)}$$

- The net reaction is given as

$$HClO_4 + C_5H_5N \rightarrow C_5H_5NH^+ + ClO_4$$

On one hand, the tendency of acid to donate proton is increased and on the other hand, the tendency of base to accept proton is increased. These lead to sharp end-point in non-aqueous titrations.

- **Preparation of 0.1 N Perchloric Acid**

  - 8.5 ml perchloric acid + 500 ml of glacial acetic acid + 21 ml of acetic anhydride

$$\downarrow$$

  Cool + glacial acetic acid to make 1000 ml

- **Standardization**

  Weight 0.7 g potassium hydrogen pthalate (KHP) + 50 ml glacial acetic acid + 2 ml drops of crystal violet solution and titrate with perchloric acid solution until violet colour changes to dark green.

  KHP 0.7 g + 50 ml glacial acetic acid + 2 ml drops of crystal violet

$$\downarrow\ \text{Titrate with } HClO_4$$

  Violet colour changes to dark green

Important Terminology

Lyonium/Lionium Ion: (Positive (+ve) ion)

On dissociation of acid and bases in non-aqueous solvents, the positive radical or most probably cation is termed as lionium ion.

Lyate/Liate Ion: (Negative (–ve) ion)

On dissociation of acid and bases in non-aqueous solvents, the negative radical or most probably anion is called as liate ion.

- If lyonium ion concentration increases, the compound is called acidic in nature.
- If lyate ion concentration increases, the compound is called basic in nature.

0.1 N Lithium Methoxide

- Titrant is prepared as follows : (Lithium Methoxide)
- 0.7 g freshly cut lithium metal + 150 ml of methyl alcohol

↓ Cool flask during addition of metal.

When reaction is completed add toluene

Standardisation

Weight 0.25 g benzoic acid

↓

Dissolve in 25 ml of dimethyl formamide

Add quinaldine red as indicator

↓

Titrate with lithium methoxide

- Protect during titration solution from O_2.
- Perform blank titration using dimethyl formamide (DMF)

Drug Assayed : Amylo barbiturate

0.1 N Tetra Butyl Ammonium Hydroxide

- Dissolve 40 g of tetra butyl ammonium iodide in 90 ml of dehydrated methyl alcohol in stoppered glass flask + place in ice bath add 20 g of silver oxide.
- Shake vigorously for one hour.

Comment : HAC is differentiating solvent for $HClO_4$ and HCL

- when $HClO_4$ is dissolved in the solvent HAC

$$\underset{\text{SA}}{HClO_4} + \underset{\text{WA}}{CH_3COOH} \rightarrow \underset{\text{(onium ion)}}{CH_3COOH_2^+} + ClO_4^- \qquad \text{.....(i)}$$

Whereas when HCl is dissolved in the solvent HAC

$$\underset{\text{WA}\downarrow}{HCl} + \underset{\text{SA}}{CH_3COOH} \rightleftharpoons \underset{\text{(onium ion)}}{CH_3COOH_2^+} + \bar{Cl} \qquad \text{.....(ii)}$$

- Here in eq. (i) $HClO_4$ in acetic acid gives $CH_3COO\,H_2^+$ (onium ion) which is weaker acid than $HClO_4$. So, here the reaction will go in only one direction.

- Whereas HCl in e.q. (ii) gives onium ion but onium ions are stronger acid than HCl. So, reaction will be possible in reverse also. So, here reaction goes in both the direction.

- Therefore we can say that the CH_3COOH is the differentiating for HCl and $HClO_4$.

H_2O is Differentiating Solvent for HCl and CH_3COOH

- When HCl reacts with H_2O,

$$\underset{\text{SA}}{HCl} + \underset{\text{WB}}{H_2O} \rightarrow \underset{\text{WB}}{H_3O^+} + Cl^-$$

- It gives H_3O^+ ions which are weaker than HCl, so HCl here being stronger acid reaction will go in only forward direction.

- Whereas when H_2O reacts with acetic acid,

$$\underset{\text{WA}}{CH_3COOH} + H_2O \rightleftharpoons \underset{\text{SA}}{H_3O^+} + CH_3COO^-$$

it gives H_3O^+ which is stronger acid than CH_3COOH

- So, reaction will go backward also

- Therefore we can say that H_2O is differentiating solvent for CH_3COOH and HCl.

Applications of Non-Aqueous Titrations

Official drugs analysed by this method are:

S.NO.	Name of the drug	Medium	Titration
1.	Caffeine	Glacial acetic acid	Perchloric acid
2.	Phenobarbitane	Pyridine	Perchloric acid
3.	Atropine Sulphate	Glacial acetic acid	Perchloric acid
4.	Ephedrine HCl	Glacial acetic acid + mercuric acetate solution	Perchloric acid

CHAPTER 6

COMPLEXOMETRIC TITRATIONS

Ligand

- Complexometric titrations are those reactions in which simple metal ion is transformed into complex ion by addition of reagent which is known as ligand.

- Ligand donates electron. Thus in a ligand molecule there is presence of at least one lone pair of electrons through which co-ordinate linkage with metal ion takes place.

- The ligand molecule usually possess oxygen, nitrogen or sulphur in one or more number in their structure.

- There is a particular number of ligand molecules associated with metal ion (like 2, 4, 6 etc) which is called as co-ordinate linkage with metal ion takes place.

- Ligand may be a neutral molecule with ion pair of $\bar{e}$, $\bar{e}$ donating groups are S, N, O, H.

Complexation

- The Process of complex ion formation can be termed as complexation.

- A complexation reaction with a metal ion involves the replacement of one or more of the co-ordinated solvent molecules by other nucleophilic groups.

- The group bound to the central ion are called ligands.

Ligands are Classified as

(i) Unidentate with- Ligand bound to metal ion only at 1 point by donation of lone pair of $\bar{e}$, e.g. Cl^-

(ii) Bidentate- Ligand bound to metal ion by 2 points, eg : oxalate ion

(iii) Tridentate - 3 points, eg : Glycerin

(iv) Tetradentate - 4 points, eg : $NH_2\ CH_2\ CH_2\ NH_2$

(v)   Multidentate-   Ligand contains more than 2 co-ordinating atoms.

e.g.   EDTA has 2 donor N group and 4 donor 0 atoms (hexadentate)

Binuclear Complexes

- It is possible to form a binuclear complex. i.e., containing two metal ions.
- Ever a poly nuclear complex, which contains more than two metal ions is formed. : eg : $(Zn_2Cl_6)^{-2}$ complex

Chelate

- The process of ring formation is called chelation and a complex having ring like structure with the metal ion is called 'Chelate'.

  Thus,   Titrant   +   Sample   →   complex

↓	↓
Ligand	M. ion
↓	↓
Levis	Lewis
Base	Acid
Donates $\bar{e}$	accepts $\bar{e}$

Complexing Agent

- Complexing agent is one which donates $\bar{e}$ and is capable of forming 1 or more co-ordinate covalent bond with metal ion.
- The properties of complex metal ion differ.
- If complexing agent forms single bond and is unidentate and forms a co-ordination compound, is refered to as ligand. If forms more than 1 bond and form is polydentate is called chelating agent.
- If complexing agent is soluble in H_2O, it is called a sequestering agent.
- Sequestering agents have groups like $-COOH$, SO_3H, NH_2, OH, eg : EDTA

Eg : $\ddot{N}H_3$ + Cu^{+2} →

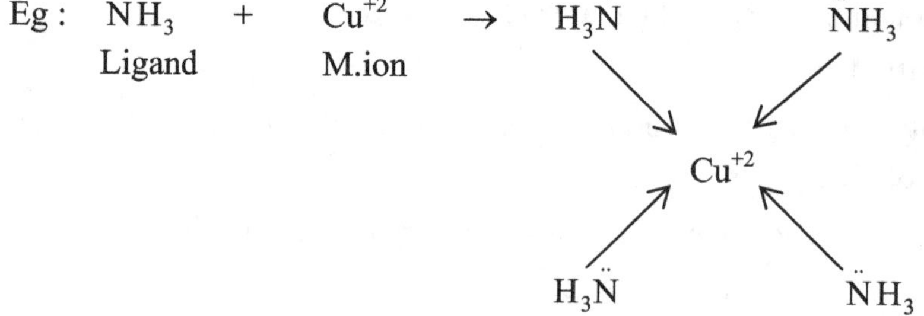

Stability of Complex

- Stability of complex is governed by law of mass action.
- Consider a metal ion M with monodentate ligand L.

$$M + L \rightleftharpoons ML$$

$$K_1 = \frac{[ML]}{[M][L]}$$

$$ML + L \rightleftharpoons ML_2$$

$$K_2 = \frac{[ML_2]}{[ML][L]}$$

Similarly, $$ML_{(n-1)} + L = ML_n$$

$$K_n = [ML_n]$$

$$[ML_{n-1}]\,[L]$$

This equi constant are called K_1, K_2, …. K_n

Step-wise Stability Constant

Verner's Co-ordination no: It is a small group attached to central atom in complex n't depending upon valency and depends on space available.

E.g. : Elements of 2nd period can accomodate 4 groups.

Thus, consider,

$$M + L \rightleftharpoons ML$$

$$K = \frac{[ML]}{[M][L]}$$

$$\therefore [M] = \frac{[ML]}{K[L]}$$

Now, take –ve log on both sides,

$$- \log [M] = - \log \frac{[ML]}{[L]} - (- \log K)$$

$$\therefore - \log [M] = \frac{[L]}{[ML]} - PK$$

$$\therefore PM = \frac{\log [L]}{[ML]} - PK$$

- Thus, value of PM is fixed by value of K and ratio of concentration of Ligand to complex.

- Stability of [ML] is always less than M – EDTA complex.

- The value of PM doesn't change if concentration of Metal ion is changed. So, this system of complex Ligand can act as buffer solution and can be referred as metal ion buffer.

- Also, as value of K increases, stability of complex increases.

- Values of K

    - decrease in acidic PH

    - increase with temperature

    - increase in presence of ethanol

    - increase in presence of electrolyte which causes common ion effect.

        e.g.: Cu^{+2} – metal ion

        NH_3 – Ligand

    Since Cu^{+2} has co-ordination no.4, therefore reacts with 4 NH_3 molecule.

$$Cu^{+2} + NH_3 = Cu\,(NH_3)^{+2} \qquad K_1 = 2 \times 10^4$$

$$Cu^{+2} + (NH_3) + NH_3 = Cu\,(NH_3)_2^{+2} \qquad K_2 = 47 \times 10^4$$

$$Cu\,(NH_3)_2^{+2} + NH_3 = Cu\,(NH_3)_3^{+2} \qquad K_3 = 1.1 \times 10^4$$

$$Cu\,(NH_3)_3^{+2} + NH_3 = Cu\,(NH_3)_4^{+2} \qquad K_4 = 2 \times 10^2$$

$$Cu^{+2} + 4NH_3 = Cu\,(NH_3)_4^{+2} \qquad K_f = K_1 + K_2 + K_3$$

$$(K_s)\,K_4$$

$$= 2.1 \times 10^{13}$$

For a successful titration the value of $\log k_f$ should be above 8

e.g. : Ba complex $\log k_f = 7.8$

Na $\rightarrow \log k_f = 1.7$

Can't be titrated successfully.

Comment

1.   Why disodium EDTA is used ?

Ans. As it is more soluble in water than EDTA. Disodium EDTA stable in alkaline solution.

2. We use buffer solution for complexometric titration with pH 10.5 i.e. Ammonia Ammonium chloride.

Ans. We use this Buffer solution as at this pH, complex is more stable and sharp end point is obtained.

3. Why it is essential to maintain pH ?

Ans. 1. Because of complex, stability is changed with change in pH.

2. formation of complex with metal ion.

3. Colour of indicator – metal complex depends on PM which depends on pH.

Detection of End Point

- There are various methods for detection of end point.
- Few of the methods are :
    1. Potentiometry
    2. Conductometry
    3. Amperometry
    4. Spectrophotometry
    5. PM indicator

1. Potentiometry

- In this method Platinum electrode is generally used, with a standard reference electrode like calomel electrode.
- Platinum electrode measures redox potential associated with metal EDTA complex.
- Potential of electrode is a function of ratio of two oxidation states of metal given by equation,

$$E = E_0 \log_e \frac{[ox]}{[Red]}$$

Where,

E = The potential of the electrode

E_0 = The standard electrode potential

$[Ox]$ = concentration of ions in the oxidised state

$[Red]$ = concentration of Ions in the reduced state.

- Another indicator electrode used in potentiometric titration is mercury electrode.

- It measures potential changes accompanying the replacement reaction between metal ion Mn+ and Hg(ion) present in Hg-EDTA complex in titration.
- Electrode is immersed in solution to be titrated and small quantity of Hg-EDTA (0.01 M) is added.
- Hg(II) is displaced from Hg-EDTA by metal ion and equilibrium is reset.

    E.g. : with divalent Metal ion,

$$M^{2+} + Hg - EDTA^{2+} \rightarrow Hg^{2+} + M - EDTA^{2+}$$

- The potential of mercury electrode depends upon the ratio of $M^{2+}/(M\text{-}EDTA)^{2+}$ and it changes abruptly (drastic) at the end point.

    Graph $\rightarrow$ ml titrant vs mv $\rightarrow$ sigmoidal graph

2. Conductometric Titration

- The Principle is based upon the substitution of ions of one mobility by the ions of another mobility.
- The conductance increases or decreases depending upon mobility of ion which can be greater or lesser.
- To measure conductance of solution, conductance cell is dipped into and terminals are connected to test terminals of conductivity bridge. The selector switch is set in appropriate range and recording is done from galvanometer.
- As conductance is reciprocal of resistance, its unit is expressed as, Mho's or $ohm's^{-1}$, siemens, millisiemens.

3. Amperometric Titrations

- Metal ions give diffusion current at adjusted half wave potential.
- During titration with EDTA, metal ion concentration decreases and so also the diffusion current.
- This forms the basis of amperometric titration.

4. Spectrophotometric Titration

- There is always a change in absorption spectrum when complexes are formed and this forms the basis of photometric titration.
- The change in absorption spectrum occurs more prominently in dilute (0.001 to 0.005 M) solutions.
- Some metals form complexes which are colorless in nature and these can be estimated in uv region.
- Metal like Fe (III), Cu (II) etc form coloured complexes which are intense than the colour of metal ions. For such metals, colorimetric analysis is carried out.

5. PM Indicators (metal ion indicators)

General Properties

- For visual consideration of end points, a metal ion indicator should satisfy the following criteria :

    1. The colour reaction must be such that before the end point, when nearly all the metal ion is complexed with EDTA, the solution is strongly coloured.

    2. The colour reaction should be specific or at least selective.

    3. The metal indicator complex must possess sufficient stability else, because of disassociation a sharp colour change is not obtained.

- But the metal indicator complex must be stable than the metal - EDTA complex.

- This change in equilibrium from the metal indicator complex to metal-EDTA complex should be sharp and rapid.

    4. The colour contrast between the free indicator and metal indicator complex should be readily observable.

Name	pH range	Titratable Metal Ions	Colour Change + Extra
1. Calcon (Mordant Black, Solochrome dark blue)	12 - 14	$Na+$, $Ca+$, $CaCl_2$, Ca-Gluconate CaNa-lactate $CaCO_3$, NaCl	With $ca^{+2} \rightarrow$ Purple red with excess EDTA $\rightarrow$ blue
2. Catechol Violet	4 - 7	Th^{+4}, Bi, Mg, Mn, Co, Zn, Ca, Cd	Acid $\rightarrow$ blue ($Th^{+3} \rightarrow$ pH 3) (Bi $\rightarrow$ pH 1.5)
3. Mordant Black II – (Solochrome black) (Eriochrome black T)	10	Mg, Ca, Cd, Zn, Mn, Hg, Pb. (Not used for Sr, Sn, Ti, Fe, Ce,Vn)	Red $\rightarrow$ blue (Below – 6.3 pH and above 11.5 $\rightarrow$ Reddish brown)
4. Mordant Blue 3 (Solochrome Cyanne R)	-	Al	Al present $\rightarrow$ purple Al absence $\rightarrow$ pink
5. Murexide (Amm. purpurate	10 -11	Cu, Ni, Co, Ca	Yellow – blue violet (Ni Co) orange $\rightarrow$ blue V (Cu) Red $\rightarrow$ blue violet (Ca)
6. Xylenol orange	1-2 (Bi $\rightarrow$1.3) (Pb $\rightarrow$ 4-5) (Zn – 8-9) (Hg, cd – 5-6)	Bi, Th, Zn, Co, Cd, Pb, Sn, Ni, Mn,	Red $\rightarrow$ lemon yellow
7. Methyl thymol blue	0 - 2	Th, Hg, Zn, Co, Cd, Al, Ni etc.	Blue $\rightarrow$ yellow

Other example are:

- Variamine blue
- Diphenyl Carbazone
- Zincon
- Alizarine
- Alizarine Flourine blue
- Na – Alizarine sulphonate
- Calcichrome

  Why we use $MgSO_4$ Titrant – EDTA

  PH 10.5, Buffer – NH_3 – NH_4Cl

  Indicator – murexide

- Why we use $MgSO_4$ in the estimation of ca^+ ? Concentrated EDTA abstracts Ca^{+2} slowly but at end point this EDTA abstracts Mg^{+2} suddenly, so the clear transaction of colour and sharp end point is obtained and also the stability of Mg^- oxide complex is less than Ca muroxide complex.

- Why mordant black can't be used for Cu, Ni, Pt $\Rightarrow$ $\because$ forms more stable complex with M ion than EDTA.

  The indicator must be very sensitive to metal ions (i.e. PM) so that the colour change occurs as near to the equivalence point as possible.

  The PH range should be maintained.

  These metal ion indicators are chelating agents.

  E.g : EDTA

  - The use of metal ion indicator or PM indicator with EDTA can be represented as,

$$M - In + EDTA \rightarrow M–EDTA + In$$

The stability of metal ion-indicator complex can be represent as K_{In},

$$M + In \rightarrow M - In$$

$$K_{In} = \frac{[M - In]}{[M][In]}$$

- The indicator colour change is affected by the H^+ ion concentration of the solution.

  For PH range $\rightarrow$ 7-11

  Dye – exhibits – Blue colour

  Metal ion – red colour

- These colours are extremly sensitive as $10^{-4} - 10^{-7}$ M solution of M_g ions give red colour with indicator.

- Now, defining apparent indicator concentration

$$K'_{In} = \frac{[M\ In]}{[M^{n+}][In]}$$

$$\therefore \ \log(k'\ In) = PM + \log \frac{[MIn]}{[In]}$$

$$\therefore \ PM = -\log \frac{[MIn]}{[In]} + \log K'In$$

- Stability of M^{in} is always less than M–EDTA complex

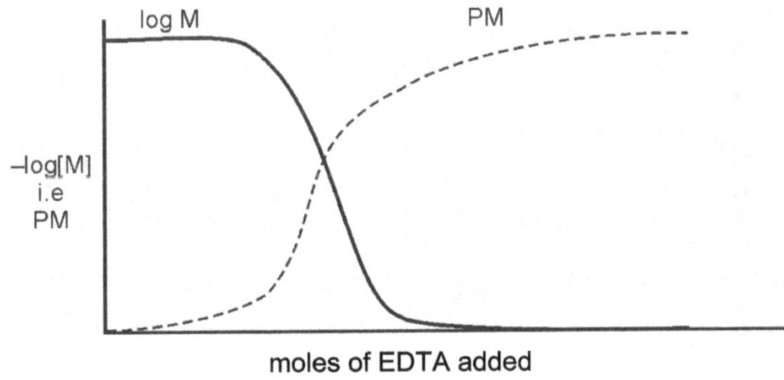

Fig. 6.1

$\Rightarrow$ after addition of more titrant more indicator is liberated

$\therefore$ If $In = M'In$

$\therefore$ $PM = -Pk'$ or pk''

Different Types of Titrations in Complexometry

1. Direct titration
2. Back (Residual) Titration
3. Replacement titration
4. Alkalimetric titration

1. Direct Titration

- The solution containing metal ion to be determined is buffered to the desired pH.

  E.g. : pH = 10 with $NH_3 - NH_4Cl$ (aq) and titrated directly with standard EDTA solution.

- It may be necessary to prevent precipitation of hydroxide of metal by the addition of some auxillary complexing agent such as lactate or citrate or triethanolamine.

- At the equivalence point, the magnitude of the concentration of the metal ion being determined decreases abruptly.

- This is generally determined by the change in colour of a metal indicator or by amperometric, spectrometric or potentiometric methods.

- Mainly used for estimation of :

  CaCl

  Ca – Gluconate

  Ca – Lactate

  $MgSO_4$

  $ZnSO_4$

Assay of $MgSO_4$

Formula = $MgSO_4\ 7H_2O$

Mol. Wt = 246.47

Indicator used = Mordant black or Murexide

Buffer used = Ammonia – Ammonium Chloride

Factor = 0.00602 G of $MgSO_4$

  $\cong$ 1 m*l* of 0.85 M disodium EDTA

pH = 10.5,

colour change = Pink to Blue

Titrant – Disodium EDTA

$$Mg + In \xrightarrow[\text{NH}_4\text{Cl}]{\text{NH}_3^-} Mg - In$$

  complex

$$Mg - In\ +\ EDTA\ \rightarrow\ Mg - EDTA\ +\ In$$

  Complex   (liberated)

2. Back Titration

- Many metals cannot be titrated directly, they may precipitate from the solution in the pH range necessary for the titration, or they may form inert complexes.

- Or if a suitable metal indicator is not available, then an excess of standard EDTA solution is added. The resulting solution is buffered to the desired PH, and the excess of the EDTA is back titrated with a standard metal Ion solution of $ZnCl_2$ or sulphate or $MgCl_2$ or sulphate is often used for this purpose.

- The end point is detected with the aid of the metal indicator which responds to the zinc or Mg ions introduced in back titration.

Why we use Back Titration?

- Metal which can precipitate as hydroxide in alkaline solution of buffer.
- Metals insoluble in nature Cal. oxalate and cal sulfate)
- Compounds which do not react with EDTA titrant.
- When metal forms complex with EDTA rather than In.
- Used for – Ca – Phosphate

$$Al\,(OH)_3 - gel$$

$$Al\,(OH)_3$$

$$Al - Sulphate$$

Assay of Calcium Phosphate

Dibasic Calcium phosphate

Formula $\rightarrow$ $CaHPO_4$

M.W 136.2

Indicator used $\rightarrow$ Mordant black

Buffer $\rightarrow$ $NH_3 - NH_4Cl$

Sample + Buffer + In + Titrant (Disodium EDTA) $\rightarrow$ unreacted EDTA (excess) + Titrated with zinc

$$Ca^{+2} + EDTA \rightarrow Ca^{+2}\,EDTA + In + unreacted \rightarrow$$
$$\qquad\qquad Complex \quad EDTA$$

$$+Zncl_2 \rightarrow Zn^{+2}\,EDTA\;complex \xrightarrow{\;+In\;} Zn^{+2} - In$$
$$\qquad\qquad\qquad\qquad Complex$$

Assay of Alluminium Hydroxide gel

Wt to be taken – 5g

Indicator : xylenol orange

Buffer – Hexamine

Factor – 0.00254 g $\cong$ 1 ml 0.85M disodium EDTA

Assay of Al. Sulphate

$Al_2(SO_4)_3$ $(342.15 \rightarrow M.w)$

Wt to be taken $\rightarrow 0.6g$

In $\rightarrow$ xylenol orange, Buffer $\rightarrow$ Hexamine

Factor: 0.008554 g $\cong$ 1ml 0.85 disodium. EDTA

3. Replacement Titration

- Substitution may be used for metal ions that don't react (or react unsatisfactorily) with a metal indicator, or for metal ions with form EDTA complexes that are more stable than those of other metals such as Mg or Ca.

- The metal cation M^{n+} to be determined may be treated with the Mg complex of EDTA, when the following reaction occurs

$$M^{n+} + Mg^{y-2} \rightleftharpoons (My)^{(n-4)+} + Mg + 2$$

- The amount of Mg ion set free is equivalent to cation present and can be titrated with a standard solution of EDTA and suitable metal indicator.

- In direct titration of Ca ions, solochrome black gives poor end point, if Mg is present, it is displaced from its EDTA complex by Ca and an improved end point results.

    Used for estimation of

    - Ca – lactate
    - Ca – Gluconate
    - Ca – Levulinate

Assay of Calcium gluconate

Formula : $C_{12}H_{22}CaO_{14}.H_2O$

M.W : 448.4

Wt to be taken in gram – 0.5

Indicator : Mordant black

Buffer Factor: Ammonium – Ammonium Chloride,

Titrant $\rightarrow$ Disodium EDTA + $MgSO_4$

Factor – 0.00224 g $\cong$ 1 ml 0.85 M Disodium EDTA

Colour Changes ; Red to Blue

$$Ca^{+2} + Mg^{+2}\ EDTA \rightarrow Ca^{+2}\ EDTA + Mg^{+2}$$

(more stable)

Assay of Ca- Lactate

Formula : $C_6H_{10}\ CaO_6.\ H_2O$

M.W : 218.22 (Anhydrous)

Wt to be taken : 0.3 g

Indicator : Mordant balck II

Buffer : Ammonia – Ammonia Chloride

Titrant $\rightarrow$ Disodium EDTA + Mg So$_4$

Factor : 0.01090 g $\cong$ 1 ml 0.85 M disodium. EDTA

4. Alkalimetric Titration

- Protons from disodium EDTA are liberated resulting in formation of acid. (2H atoms)

- The liberated acid is titrated with standard alkali.

- Either visual pH indicator or potentiometric method is adopted for detecting end point.

- No buffer solution is used as pH change is evolved.

  e.g.: Assay of $BaSO_4$

- Suitable control of the pH of the solution

  E.g.: Assay of $BaSO_4$

- Control of pH makes use of different stabilities of metal – EDTA complexes.

  E.g.: Bismuth and thorium can be titrated in an acidic medium (PH = 2) with xylenol orange or methylthymol blue as indicator, and most divalent cations don't interfere.

- A mixture of bismuth and lead ions can successfully titrated by first titrating the bismuth at pH-2 with xylenol orange as indicator, then adding hexamine to raise the pH to about 5, and titrating the lead.

Masking Agents

- Masking may be defined as the process in which a substance without physical separation of it or its reaction products, is so transformed that it does not enter into a particular reaction.

- Demasking is the process in which the masked substance regains its ability to enter into a particular reaction.

- By using masking agents, some of the cations in a mixture can often be masked so they can no longer react with EDTA, or with the indicator.

- An effective demasking agent is the cyanide ion, this forms stable cyanide complexes with the cations of Cd, Zn, Hg (II), Cu, CO, Ni, Ag and the platinum metals, but not with the alkaline earths, manganese and lead.

$$M^{2+} + 4CN^- \rightarrow [M(CN)_4]^{2-}$$

- It is therefore possible to determine cations such as Ca^{+2}, Mg^{+2}, Pb^{+2} and Mn^{+2} in the presence of these metals by masking with an excess of K or Na cyanide.

Demasking

- The Cyanide complexes of zinc and cadmium may be demasked with methanol ethanoic acid solution or better with chloral hydrate.

$$[Zn (CN)_4]^{2-} + 4H^+ + 4HCHO \rightarrow Zn^{+2} + 4HO - CH_2 - CN$$

- The use of masking and selective demasking agent permits the successive titration of many metals.

  Thus, a solution containing Mg, Zn and Cu can be titrated as follows :

1. Add excess of standard EDTA and back titrate with standard Mg solution using solochrome black as indicator. This gives the sum of all the metals present.

2. Treat an appropriate portion with excess KCN and titrate as before. This gives Mg only.

3. Add excess of chloral hydrate to titrated solution to liberate Zn from cyanide complex, and titrate until the indicator turns blue, this gives Zn only. Cu content can be found by difference.

- Demasking and masking agents are required.

   (i)   If EDTA or Disodium EDTA forms complex with metal ion during estimation of ion and other impurities are also estimated which give false result.

   (ii) Two or more metal ions estimated in mixture and each ion selectively titrated.

Demasking carried out by Three Methods.

   (i)   Addition of precipitate.

   (ii) Addition of complexing agent

   (iii) pH control

(i)   Addition of precipitate

- to remove the interference precipitants are added to collect the precipitate and estimation is carried out.

  E.g.: Ferrocynaide as precipitate for copper as an interfering agent. Similarly sulfate used for Li, Ba as interfering agent.

(ii)   Addition of Complexing Agent

- Ferrus complex with interfering ion. This complex is more stable than EDTA complex and thus impurities are removed.

  E.g.: NH_4Cl used as complexing agent for Fe and Al and KCN for Ag, Cu, Mg, Fe, Zn, Co, Ni, Ca as interfering agent.

(iii) By pH Control

- In EDTA complex the alkaline earth matter are not stable with pH 3.7.
- They form complex with Fe^{+3}, Co^{+3}, Th^{+4}, Ti^{+4}, Sn^{+4} and they are stable and titrated by varying the pH.

Disodium Ethylene Diamine Tetra Acetate

(0.05 M) standard

Preparation

- Dissolve 18.6 g of Disodium EDTA in sufficient water to produce 100 ml.

Slandardization

- Weigh 0.8 g of granulated zinc, dissolve by gently warming in 12 ml diluted HCl,

- Add 5 drops of bromine water.

- Boil to remove excess of bromine

Cool

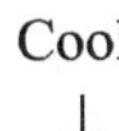

Add water upto 200 ml

Pipette out 20 ml of solution into flask and neutralize by 2N NaOH.

Dilute to about 150 ml with water

Add Ammonia buffer of pH 10 to dissolve ppt and 5 ml in excess

Add 50 mg of mordant black II mixture and titrate with the disodium EDTA until solution turns green.

Factor

0.003269 g of granulated zinc $\cong$ 1 ml of 0.05 M Disodium EDTA.

$$Zn^{+2} + [H_2y] \rightarrow [zny]^2 + 2H^+$$

2nd Method

PSC $\rightarrow$ CaO$_3$ + HCl (to dissolve CaCO$_3$)

Heat and cool + 250 ml solution with H_2O

20 ml solution of sample + Buffer + Indicator

Indicator $\rightarrow$ Calcon

Titrate with Disodium EDTA

CHAPTER 7

DIAZOTISATION TITRATIONS
(Sodium Nitrite Titrations)

Introduction

Many simple primary aromatic amino compounds can be estimated quantitatively by determining the volume of a standard sodium nitrite solution which is required to bring about their conversion into diazonium salt. Hence this type of titrations are also called as Sodium Nitrite Titrations. All the drugs containing primary aromatic amino groups (NH_2) can be estimated by diazotisation titrations. In some cases, drugs containing other functional groups like Nitro (NO_2), acetyl, succinyl and phthanlyl groups, by subjecting to Hydrolysis and reduction, are converted to amino groups, and then they are estimated.

Principle

Aromatic primary amines react with Sodium Nitrite in acid solutions (Nitrous acid) to form diazonium slats.

$$C_6H_5\,NH_2\,NaNO_2 + HCl \rightarrow C_6H_5\,N_2Cl + NaCl + 2H_2O$$

Under controlled experimental conditions, the reaction is quantitative and can be used for the determination of substances containing a free primary amino group. Simple chemical reactions like Hydrolysis and Reduction can be used in case of drugs having groups like Nitro etc. For conversion into amino groups and then this primary amino group can be diazotised.

The addition of Sodium Nitrite to Hydrochloric acid causes the formation of nitrous acid. This nitrous acid diazotises the aromatic amino group. After the end point, excess nitrous acid formed is shown by immediate formation of deep blue colour with starch iodide paper.

$$NaNO_2 + HCl \rightarrow HNO_2 + NaCl$$

End Point Detection

Observation of the end point depends on the detection of the small excess of nitrous acid which is then present. This can be demonstrated visually using starch-iodide paper or paste. This method is called as 'External Indicator Method'.

Starch iodide paper is prepared by immersing a filter paper in starch mucilage and potassium iodide solution. The Iodine formed reacts with starch mucilage to give the blue colour.

$$kl + HCl \rightarrow KCl + Hl$$

$$2HI + 2HNO_2 \rightarrow l_2 + 2NO + 2H_2O$$

Amperometric End Point Detection Method

Using external indicator method, some times it is difficult to locate the end point. In such cases the end point can be determined amperometrically. In this method a pair of platinum electrodes are immersed in the titration liquid. Electrode polarization occurs when a small voltage (30-50 mV) is applied across the electrodes and no current flows through the sensitive galvanometer included in the circuit. Liberation of excess nitrous acid at the end point de-polarizes the electrodes and current flows in the galvanometer. This is known as the dead stop end point. The electrodes must be clean, otherwise the end point is delayed.

Preparation and Standardization of 0.1 m Na NO₂

7.5 g of sodium nitrite is dissolved in sufficient water to produce 1000 ml which gives 0.1 M (M/10) sodium nitrite solution. Standardization of this solution is done by running into warm, acidified potassium permanganate solution and determining the volume of permanganate required for oxidation of sodium nitrite. Alternately sodium nitrite solution is standardized (M/10 or M/20) against pure sulphanilic acid.

First Method

In the analysis, a weighed amount of the substance is dissolved in dilute hydrochloric acid and the solution is cooled below 15°C. A standard solution of sodium nitrite is added into the solution slowly and the end point is determined by withdrawing drops of a titrated solutions and spotting on starch iodide paper. The end point is shown by a blue colour on the paper.

$$Na\,NO_2 + HCl \rightarrow NaCl + HNO_2$$

$$ArNH_2.HCl + HONO \rightarrow ArN2 + Cl^- + 2H_2O$$

Second Method

About 0.5 g of sulphanilamide previously dried at 105 °C for three hours is transferred to a suitable beaker. 50 ml of water and 20 ml of hydrochloric acid is added, stirred until it dissolves and cooled to 15 °C. The contents of the beaker are titrated against 0.1 M Sodium Nitrite solution.

Each ml of 0.1 M Sodium Nitrate solution $\equiv$ 0.01722 g of sulphanilamide.

Assay Procedure for Diazotisation Titration

Specified amount of the drug is dissolved in about 50 ml of water and 20 ml of Hydrochloric acid. The solution is stirred and cooled to about 15°C. The mixture is titrated against 0.1 M Sodium nitrite solution. The end point is determined by using any one of the techniques either by external indicator method or using amperometric dead stop end point technique by using platinum electrodes.

Types of Diazotisation Titrations

Commonly employed titration techniques in case of diazotisation are three types.

1. Direct titration

2. Reverse method and

3. Special methods

1. Direct Titration

- One mole of the drug + three moles of concentrated Hydrochloric acid
- Temperature lowered to 4°C by using ice or ice cold solution externally to the reaction mixture.
- 0.1 N $NaNO_2$ is the titrant
- End point by external starch iodide paper or by potentiometric end point method.

2. Reverse Method

This method is used when the resulting diazonium salt is insoluble like napthylamine sulphonic acid. In such cases, witter ions are formed which are difficult to solubilise. Hence first the solution of amine is treated with sodium nitrite and the resulting solution is run into a solution of Hydrochloric acid.

3. Special Methods

For aminophenols, direct method cannot be used because when treated with sodium nitrite they form quinines which are highly unstable and hence titration cannot be carried out. In such a case the reaction is carried out in the presence of copper sulphate which forms stable diazo oxide and diazo coupling reaction can be carried out.

Applications

Direct Titration with Nitrite Solution

1. Benzocaine
2. Dapsone
3. Primaquine phosphate and its tablets
4. Procainamide hydrochloride and its injection
5. Procaine hydrochloride
6. Sodium amino salicylate, tablets and granules
7. Suramin
8. All sulpha drugs containing free aromatic amino group like, sulphacetamide sodium, sulphadimethoxine, sulphdoxine, sulphadimidine, sulphadiazine, sulphaguanidine, sulphapyridine, sulphamethizole, sulphalene, sulphamethoxazole, sulphaphenazole, sulphamethoxydiazine and sulphamethoxypyridazine.

Conversion to Amino Group by Chemical Reactions

(a) By reduction

1. Metronidazole
2. Secnidazole
3. Chloramphenicol

These drugs contain aromatic nitro group, which can be reduced by using reducing agent to get aromatic amino group. This primary aromatic amino group can be diazotised by using nitrite solution.

(b) Hydrolysis

1. Paracetamol (Acetyl derivative)
2. Phthalyl sulphathiazole (Pthalyl derivative)
3. Succinyl sulphathiazole (Succinyl derivative)

These drugs are derivatives of amino groups like acetyl or phthalyl or succinyl derivative. After hydrolysis to free amino group, these drugs can be titrated with nitrite solution.

CHAPTER 8

OXIDATION–REDUCTION TITRATION

Oxidation Reduction

Oxidation reduction reaction is a process involving the transfer of electrons from one elements or ion to another resulting in the change of the valency of reacting atoms or ions.

When an atom or ion is oxidised, it loses electrons resulting in the increase in the positive valency or decrease in the negative valency of an element.

While in reduction, the electrons are added to it resulting in the increase in negative valency or decrease in the positive valency of the element.

e.g. Conversion of $FeCl_3$ to $FeCl_2$

$$Fe^{+3} + \bar{e} \rightarrow Fe^{+2}$$

$\left.\right\}$ Reduction

Undergo Reduction

Oxidising Agents

Oxidising agents are the substances containing an atom or ion capable of taking an $\bar{e}$ resulting in decrease in +ve valency and increase in –ve valency.

e.g. $KMnO_4$, $K_2Cr_2O_7$, Malogens, H_2O_2

Reducing Agents

Reducing agents are the substances containing an atom or ion capable of losing electrons resulting in the increase of their +ve valency and decrease of their –ve valency.

e.g. Metals, $FeCl_2$, H_2S, H_2O_2

e.g.   (i) $Zn \rightarrow Zn^{+2} + 2\bar{e}$

  (ii) $Fe^{+2} \rightarrow Fe^{+3} + 2\bar{e}$

Hence, increase in +ve charge, decrease in –ve charge.

e.g.   (i) $Ce^{+4} + \bar{e} \rightarrow Ce^{+3}$

Decrease in +ve charge, increase in –ve charge

Oxidation – Reduction Cell

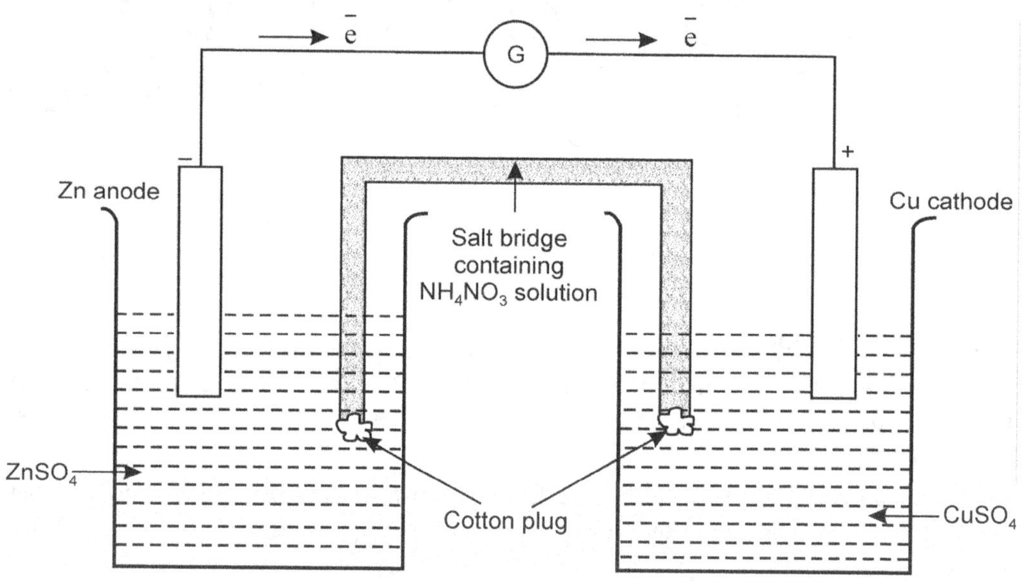

Fig. 8.1 Electro chemical cell.

Zinc strip is dipped into solution of $CuSO_4$

$$Zn(s) + Cu^{+2}_{(aq)} \rightleftharpoons Zn^{+2}_{(aq)} + Cu(s)$$

Half Reactions are,

$$Zn(s) + \rightleftharpoons Zn^{+2}_{(aq)} + 2\bar{e} \quad \text{(Oxidation)}$$

$$Cu^{+2}_{(aq)} + 2\bar{e} \rightleftharpoons Cu(s) \quad \text{(Reduction)}$$

In one vessel solution of zinc sulphate is taken and zinc strip is dipped. In other vessel, a solution of $CuSO_4$ is taken and in that a copper strip of definite weight is dipped.

These two vessels are connected by U-shaped glass tube filled with solution of ammonium nitrate. This U tube is called salt bridge.

Zinc and copper strips with a thin wire connected to a galvanometer (G).

When both strips are carefully washed with water and then dried, are weighed, it is found that the weight of zinc strip decreases and weight of copper strip increases.

When both the electrodes are connected by a copper wire, the flow of $\bar{e}$ is from anode to cathode in the external circuit.

The U-shaped tube filled with a solution of ammonium nitrate is called salt bridge. The flow of electricity in the solution is through ions.

Zn^{+2} ions produced by oxidation in the vessel on left hand side enter solution and so solution $ZnSO_4$ becomes +vely charged.

On Right hand side, cu formed by reduction of Cu^{+2} ions.

Hence concentration of Cu^{+2} decreases and due to SO_4^{-2} ions, the solution of $CuSO_4$ becomes -vely charged.

For the reaction to occur continuously, solution should be without electric charge. The salt bridge: connected between both vessels, contains liquid of appropriate salt, the SO_4^{2-} ions from $CuSO_4$ are diffused to the solution on the left hand side.
The salt bridge functions to maintain electrical charge neutrality.

LHS – anode $\rightarrow$ oxidation $\bar{e}$ flow

RHS – cathode $\rightarrow$ reduction
$$\downarrow$$
$ZnSO_4$ solution $\rightarrow$ +ve charged

$CuSO_4$ solution $\rightarrow$ –ve charged

SO_4^{1-} or RHS $\rightarrow$ LHS

Half Cell

- The electrode and the solution in which it is dipped is collectively known a Half-cell

- It is represented by putting a single vertical line between an electrode and active ions.
  e.g. $Zn \,|Zn^{+2}$ and $Cu|\,Cu^{+2}$

- The representation of gas electrode is shown by inert electrode and active ions.
  e.g. $Pt\,|H_2\,(1atm)|\,H^+$

- Salt bridge represented by two vertical lines.
  e.g. $Zn\,|Zn^{+2}(1M)\,||\,Cu^{+2}(1M)|Cu$

- Anode(O) is on left hand side and cathode on RHS.

  e.g. $Ag\,|Ag^+(1M)\,\|\,Cl^-(1M)|Cl_2(1atm)|pt$

- Concentration is expressed in molarity in bracket and pressure $\forall$ gas in atmosphere.

  e.g. $pt\,|H_2(1\ atm)/H^+(1m)\,\|\,Ag^+(1M)|Ag$

- If the concentration of the solution of a half cell is 1M for pressure of gas is 1 atm and temperature is 25 °C, the cell of such type is called standard half cell. By connecting 2 standard half cells, standard cell is formed.

Nernst Equation

- Potential of electrochemical cell depends on,

  - Temperature of cell

  - Concentration of solution

  - Nature of electrode

- Equation showing relation between potential of a non-standard electro-chemical cell and concentration of solution is known as Nernst Equation.

$$E = E^\circ + \frac{0.0592}{n}\ \log\ \frac{[Oxi]}{[Red]}$$

where, $\dfrac{Rt}{F}$ at 25°C temp is constant,   R = gas const

$$F = Faraday$$

OR

$$E_N = E^\circ - \frac{0.0592}{n}\ \log\ \frac{[Red]}{[Oxi]}$$

Also,

$E\ cell = E^\circ_{Oxi} - E^\circ_{Red}$ (if oxidation potential given)

$E\ cell = +ve$ (Spontaneous Reaction)

$E\ cell = -ve$ (Non-spontaneous reaction)

Oxidation-Reduction Titration Curves

- In Oxidimetric titrations the concentration of the substances or ions involved in the reaction are changing continuously.

- The oxidation potential of the solution (E) must therefore also change, just as the solution pH changes continuously during titration by neutralization method.

- By plotting the oxidation potentials corresponding to different points in the titration we obtain a titration curve.

  e.g. Plot the curve for titration of a ferrous ion salt with permanganate in acid solution.

Reaction

$$MNO_4^- + 5\,Fe^{+2} + 8H+ \rightleftharpoons M_n^{+2} + 5\,Fe^{+3} + 4H_2O$$

- The reaction is reversible, at any stage the solution always contains two redox systems, Fe^{+3}/Fe^{+2} and MnO_4^-/M^{+2}

$$E = 0.77 + \frac{0.058}{1}\,\log\frac{[Fe^{+3}]}{[Fe^{+2}]} \qquad \text{.....(i)}$$

$$E = 1.51 + \frac{0.058}{5}\,\log\frac{[MnO_4^-][H^+]^8}{[Mn^{+2}]} \qquad \text{.....(ii)}$$

- With excess permanganate it is easy to calculate concentration of MnO_4^- and Mn^{+2} ions in solution and much more difficult to calculate the concentration of the remain Fe^{+2} ions, therefore equation 2 is used.

  At the paint when half $KMnO_4$ is added to $FeSO_4$, then only 50% of Fe^{+2} ions contained in original solution has been converted to Fe^{+3} ions.

$$E = 0.77 + \frac{0.058}{1}\,\log 1.$$

  The change in potential occurs when there is a break of potential at equivalence point.

  At this point only 0.1 ml of $KMnO_4$ is reqd, by reaction.

  $\therefore$ only 0.1 ml Fe^{+2} remains unchanged and rest is converted to Fe^{+3}

$$E = 0.77 + \frac{0.058}{1}\,\log\frac{[Fe^{+3}]}{[Fe^{+2}]}\ \text{(unchanged) (Here, 0.1 ml)}$$

- The amount of permanganate ion added in excess (0.1 ml) remains in form of MnO_4^- rest is converted to Mn^{+2} by reaction with Fe^{+2}.

$$\therefore E = 1.51 + \frac{0.058}{5}\,\log\frac{[MnO_4^-][H^+]^8}{[Mn^{+2}]}\ \text{excess here (0.1 ml)}$$

- Multiply equation (ii) by 5 and (i) by 1

$$E = 0.77 + 0.058 \log \frac{[Fe^{+3}]}{[Fe^{+2}]}$$

$$5E = 5 \times 1.51 + 0.058 \log \frac{[MnO_4^-]}{[Mn^{+2}]}$$

$$6E = 0.77 + 5 \times 1.51 + 0.058 \log \frac{[Fe^{+3}][MnO_4^-]}{[Fe^{+2}][Mn^{+2}]} \qquad .....(iii)$$

(H^+ concentration is taken as 1. In both equations E represents oxidation potential of given solution, therefore has same value).

At equivalence point the amount of MnO_4^- ions added corresponds to the reaction equation,

$$5\, Fe^{+2} + MnO_4^- + 8H^+ \rightleftharpoons 5\, Fe^{+3} + Mn^{+2} + 4H_2O$$

$\therefore$ at equilibrium there must be 5 Fe^{+2} ions for each MnO_4^- ion remaining in Solution.

$\therefore$ at equivalence point, the molar curve of Fe^{+2} is 5 times the concentration of MnO_4^- i.e.

$$[Fe^{+2}] = 5\,[MnO_4^-]$$

Similarly, $$[Fe^{+3}] = 5\,[Mn^{+2}]$$

Thus, $\dfrac{[Fe^{+3}]}{[Fe^{+2}]} = \dfrac{[Mn^{+2}]}{[MnO_4^-]}$

$\therefore \dfrac{[Fe^{+3}][MnO_4^-]}{[Fe^{+2}][Mn^{+2}]} = 1$

So, From eqn. (iii)

$$6\,E = 0.77 + 5 \times 1.51$$

$$E = 1.38711$$

If the standard potential of the system corresponding to oxi-red are taken as, E_o' and E_o''

Their stoichiometric co-efficients are a and b, then the oxidation potential of solution at equivalence point is,

$$E = \frac{b\,E_o' + a\,E_o''}{a + b}$$

$\therefore$ Eqn. of Reaction

$$a\ Oxi_1 + b\ Red_2 \rightleftharpoons a\ Red_1 + b\ Oxi_2$$

$\therefore$ Concentration at equivalence point

$$\frac{[Red_1]}{[Oxi_1]} = \frac{[oxi_2]}{[Red_2]} = a + b\sqrt{K}$$

K = equi-const.

- The magnitude of potential change depends on.

  (i) difference between standard oxidation potentials of two system.

  Greater the difference, greater the change in potential

- The oximetric curves are independent of dilutions, as Nernst equation contains the ratio of the concentration of oxidised form and reduced form which doesn't alter in dilution.

- The titration curve terms is independent of dilution and thus is advantage of oxidimetric method over neutralization method.

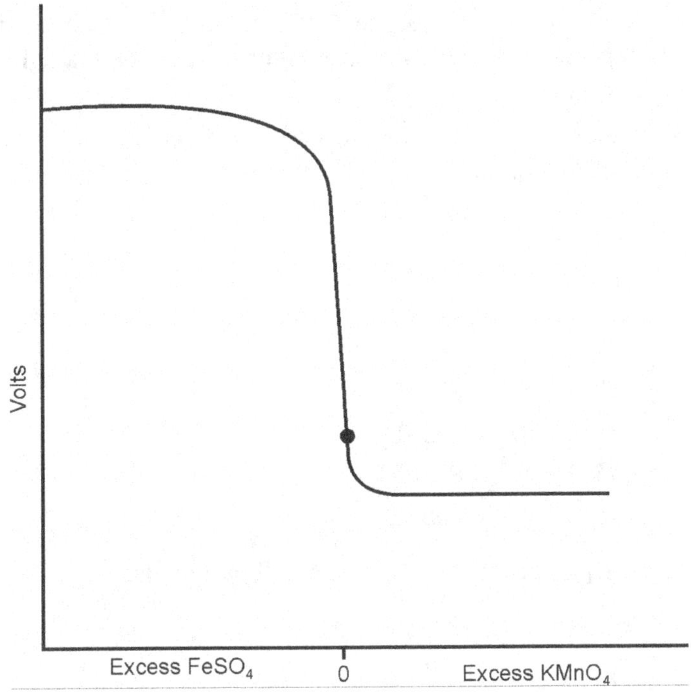

Fig 8.2 Titration curve of FeSO$_4$ with permagnate.

Redox Potential

- The direction of a redox potential can be predicated provided some quantitative characteristic of the relative force involved is known. This characteristic is Redox Potential.

- It is possible to measure the potential difference between two systems by connecting them into a galvanic cell.

- The more powerful the oxidant of the pair of Oxi. Red couple the weaker is the reductant.

  Eg. $Cl_2 \rightarrow$ powerful oxidising agent $Cl_2 + 2\bar{e} \rightarrow 2\,Cl^-$

  $\therefore$ it has ability to accept $\bar{e}$ and change to Cl^-, $\therefore$ Cl^- is weak reducing agent.

- No absolutely pure oxidising or reducing agent. Their solution always contain the products of their red or oxi respectively.

  Eg. Fe^{+2} always contains some Fe^{+3} possessing oxidising properties.

- The oxidants Cl_2, MnO_4^- always contain Cl^-, Mn^{+2}, therefore they act as reducing agents.

- Redox potentials of various couples are determined by taking into account that their values depend on strengths of oxidising and reducing agents and also ratio of their concentration.

- All oxidising reducing agents differ in strength i.e. chemical activity.

  Prove that equivalent point

  $$E_{cell} = \frac{n_1 E_1^0 + n_2 E_2^0}{n_1 + n_2}$$

Proof

$$E_R = E_R^0 - \frac{0.0592}{n} \times \log \frac{[Red\,R]}{[oxi\,R]} \qquad \qquad .....(i)$$

$$E_O = E_O^0 - \frac{0.0592}{n} \times \log \frac{[Red\,L]}{[oxi\,L]} \qquad \qquad .....(ii)$$

- Now, consider E_1 and E_2 as two different cell potentials.

- $E_1 \times n_1$ and $E_2 \times n_2$

$$E_1 = n_1 E_1^0 - 0.0592 \times \log \frac{Red_1}{Oxi_1}$$

$$n_2 E_2 = n_2 E_2^0 - 0.0592 \times \log \frac{Red_2}{Oxi_2}$$

Now, $n_1 E_1 + n_2 E_2 = n_1 E_1^0 + n_2 E_2^0 - 0.0592$

$$\log \left[\frac{Red_1}{Oxi_1} \times \frac{Red_2}{Oxi_2} \right]$$

- An equivalence point, the amount of concentration of reduction equals concentration of oxidation.

$$\therefore \ Red_1 = Oxi_2$$

$$Red_2 = Oxi_1$$

$$\therefore \ n_1 E_1 + n_2 E_2 = n_1 E_1^o + n_2 E_2^o - 0.0592 \log 1.$$

$$n_1 E_1 + n_2 E_2 = n_1 E_1^o + n_2 E_2^o$$

Also, $E_1 = E_2 = $ Equivalent point $= E.$

$$E (n_1 + n_2) = n_1 E_1^o + n_2 E_2^o$$

$$E = \frac{n_1 E_1^o + n_2 E_2^o}{n_1 + n_2} \ \text{(proved)}$$

Equivalent Weights and Oxidation Number

Equivalent weight of an oxidising or reducing agent is defined as that weight of the agent which reacts with or contains 1.008 g of H or 8 g of available oxygen.

Eg. $2 \, KMnO_4 \rightarrow K_2O + 2 \, MnO + 50$

in acid solution

$$\text{Equi. wt} = \frac{\text{Mol.wt}}{5}$$

$KMnO_4$

in acidic medium,

$$MnO_4^- + 8H^+ + 5\bar{e} \rightarrow Mn^{+2} + 4H_2O$$

Thus, $KMnO_4 \xrightarrow[\text{medium}]{\text{acidic}} MnSO_4$

$\qquad\qquad \downarrow \qquad\qquad\qquad \downarrow$

$\qquad\qquad +1 \qquad\qquad\quad +2$

Change in O.N = 5

$$\text{Equi. wt} = \frac{\text{Mol.wt}}{5}$$

In Basic Medium

$$MnO_4^- + 4H+ + 3\bar{e} \rightarrow MnO_2 + 2H_2O$$

$$\therefore KMnO_4 \xrightarrow{\text{basic medium}} MnO_2$$

$$\downarrow \qquad\qquad\qquad \downarrow$$

$$+7 \qquad\qquad\qquad +4$$

Change in O.N. = 3

$$\text{Equi. Wt.} = \frac{\text{Mol.wt}}{3}$$

In neutral medium

Mol. Wt = equi. wt.

$K_2\,Cr_2\,O_7$

in acid medium,

$$K_2Cr_2O_7 \rightarrow K_2O + Cr_2O_3 + 30$$

$$\downarrow \qquad\qquad\qquad \downarrow$$

$$+12 \qquad\qquad\qquad +6$$

Change in O.N = 6

$$\text{Equi. Wt.} = \frac{\text{Mol.wt}}{6}$$

$$Cl_2, Br_2, I_2 \rightarrow Cl^-, Br^-, I^-$$

$$0 \qquad\qquad\qquad -1$$

Change in O.N = 1

$$\therefore \text{Mol. Wt} = \text{equi. wt}$$

$KClO_3$

$$KClO_3 \rightarrow Cl^-$$

$$\downarrow \qquad\qquad\qquad \downarrow$$

$$+5 \qquad\qquad\qquad -1$$

Change in O.N = 6

$$\text{Equi. wt} = \frac{\text{Mol.wt}}{6}$$

$$FeCl_3 \quad \rightarrow \quad FeCl_2$$
$$\downarrow \qquad\qquad \downarrow$$
$$+3 \qquad\qquad +2$$

Change in O.N = 1

Mol. Wt = equi. wt

$Na_2S_2O_3$

$$Na_2S_2O_3 \quad \rightarrow \quad Na_2S_4O_6$$
$$\downarrow \qquad\qquad\quad \downarrow$$
$$+4 \qquad\qquad\quad +10$$
$$\qquad\qquad\qquad\quad \downarrow$$
$$\qquad\qquad\qquad\quad +5$$

Change in O.N = 1

M.W = EW

$C_2O_4^-$ (oxalic Acid)

$$\downarrow \qquad\qquad \downarrow$$
$$C_2O_4^{-2} \longrightarrow CO_2$$
$$\downarrow \qquad\qquad \downarrow$$
$$+6 \qquad\qquad +4$$
$$\downarrow$$
$$+3$$

Change in O.N $\rightarrow$ 1

Equi. wt = M.W.

Zinc

$$Zn \rightarrow Zn^{+2}$$
$$\downarrow \qquad \downarrow$$
$$0 \qquad +2$$

Change in O.N = 2

$$\therefore \text{Equi. wt} = \frac{M.W}{2}$$

Cerium

$$Ce^{+4} \rightarrow Ce^{+3}$$

$$\downarrow \qquad\qquad \downarrow$$

$$+4 \qquad\qquad +3$$

change in O.N = 1

eq.wt = Mol. Wt

KB_rO_3

$$KBrO_3 \rightarrow Br^-$$

$$\downarrow \qquad \downarrow$$

$$+5 \qquad -1$$

change in O.N = 6

$$Equi.\ wt = \frac{Mol.Wt}{6}$$

Balancing of Reaction Equations

(A) Electron Balance Method

- Electrons are transferred

- No. of $\bar{e}$ lost must be no. of $\bar{e}$ gained. This is done by multiplying reaction by suitable coefficient required to balance the no. of $\bar{e}$.

  Eg. Ferrous sulphate is oxidised by $KMnO_4$ in acidic medium.

  $$KMnO_4 + H_2SO_4 + FeSO_4 \rightarrow Fe_2(SO_4)_3 + K_2SO_4 + MnSO_4 + H_2O$$

  Here, $Fe^{+2} \rightarrow Fe^{+3} + \bar{e}$ \qquad (Oxidation)

  $$Mn^{+7} + 5\bar{e} \rightarrow Mn^{+2} \qquad \text{(Reduction)}$$

- Thus, to balance,

  $$[Fe^{+2} \rightarrow Fe^{+3} + \bar{e}\,] \times 5 \times 2$$

  $$[Mn^{+7} + 5\bar{e} \rightarrow Mn^{+2}] \times 2$$

  $\therefore$ Overall reaction,

  $$2KMnO_4 + 10\ FeSO_4 + 8H_2SO_4 \rightarrow 5Fe_2(SO_4)_3 + K_2SO_4 + 2MnSO_4 + 8H_2O$$

(B) Ion-Electron Balance Method

- The $\bar{e}$ are transferred as well as, no. of ions are balanced.

  Eg. Reduction of $KMnO_4$ by $FeSO_4$ in presence of dil H_2SO_4

  (In dilute solution, H^+, OH^-, H_2O also take part)

$$KMnO_4 + FeSO_4 + H_2SO_4 \rightarrow Fe_2(SO_4)_3 + K_2SO_4 + 2MnSO_4 + H_2O$$

$$MnO_4^- \rightarrow Mn^{+2} \qquad \text{(Reduction)}$$

To balance no. of atoms, we require $8H^+$

$$MnO_4^- + 8H^+ \rightarrow Mn^{+2} + 4H_2O$$

To balance, no. of $\bar{e}$, $5\bar{e}$ required,

$$MnO_4^- + 8H^+ + 5\bar{e} \rightarrow Mn^{+2} + H_2O$$

$$Fe^{+2} \rightarrow Fe^{+3} \qquad \text{(Oxidation)}$$

To balance electrically, $1\bar{e}$ required

$$Fe^{+2} \rightarrow Fe^{+3} + \bar{e}$$

Balance no. of $\bar{e}$,

$$[MnO_4^- + 8H^+ + 5\bar{e} \rightarrow Mn^{+2} + 4H_2O] \times 1$$

$$[Fe^{+2} \rightarrow Fe^{+3} + \bar{e}] \times 5$$

To balance molecules of $FeSO_4$ multiply both eqns. by 2.

$$2[MnO_4^- + 8H^+ + 5\bar{e} \rightarrow Mn^{+2} + 4H_2O]$$

$$10[Fe^{+2} \rightarrow Fe^{+3} + \bar{e}]$$

$\therefore$ Final eqn,

$$2KMnO_4 + 8H_2SO_4 + 10FeSO_4 \rightarrow 5Fe(SO_4)_3 + 2MnSO_4 + K_2SO_4 + 8H_2O$$

Eg : Reduction of H_2O_2 with $KMnO_4$ in acid medium

Reaction $KMnO_4 \rightarrow$ Oxidizing agent

$$2kMnO_4 + 3H_2SO_4 \rightleftharpoons K_2SO_4 + 2MnSO_4 + 3H_2O + 5[0]$$

$$5H_2O_2 + 5[0] \rightleftharpoons 5H_2O + 5O_2$$

$$2KMnO_4 + 3H_2SO_4 + 5H_2O_2 \rightleftharpoons K_2SO_4 + 2MnSO_4 + 8H_2O + 5[0]$$

Redox Reaction

$$MnO_4^- + 8H^+ \rightarrow Mn^{+2} + 4H_2O$$

$$\downarrow \qquad\qquad\qquad \downarrow$$

$$+7 \qquad\qquad\qquad +2$$

Change in O.N = +5

We have to add $7 - 2 = 5\bar{e}$

$$MnO_4^- + 8H^+ + 5\bar{e} \rightarrow Mn^{+2} + 4H_2O \qquad \text{.....(i)}$$

$$2H_2O_2 \rightarrow 2H_2O + O_2$$

$$MnO_4^- + 2H_2O_2 + 8H^+ + 5\bar{e} \rightarrow Mn^{+2} + 6H_2O + O_2$$

$$H_2O_2 \rightarrow 2H^+ + O_2$$

$$\downarrow \qquad\qquad \downarrow$$

$$+4 \qquad\qquad +2$$

$$H_2O_2 \rightarrow 2H^+ + O_2 + 2\bar{e} \qquad \text{.....(ii)}$$

$\therefore$ Balancing, Multiply (ii) by 5/2

$$\frac{5}{2}H_2O_2 \rightarrow 5H^+ + \frac{5}{2}O_2 + \frac{5}{2}\bar{e}$$

$$MnO_4^- + 8H^+ + 5\bar{e} \rightarrow Mn^{+2} + 4H_2O$$

$$\overline{\frac{5}{2}H_2O_2 + MnO_4^- + 8H^+ \rightarrow 5H^+ + \frac{5}{2}O_2 + Mn^{+2} + 4H_2O}$$

1. $Cr_2O_7^{-2} + Fe^{+2} \rightarrow Cr^{+3} + Fe^{+3}$

First convert it into Half cell-reaction

$\therefore$ Separate the equation into oxi-half cell and Red. Half cell.

Balance: then combine and balance again by addition with $\bar{e}$ or H^+ or H_2O

$$Cr_2O_7^{-2} \rightarrow 2Cr^{+3} + 7H_2O$$

$$\downarrow \qquad\qquad \downarrow$$

$$+2 \qquad\qquad +6$$

$$Cr_2O_7^{-2} + 6\bar{e} \rightarrow 2Cr^{+3} + 7H_2O$$

$$\text{Now, } Fe^{+2} \rightarrow Fe^{+3} + \bar{e}$$

$$6Fe^{+2} \rightarrow 6Fe^{+3} + 6\bar{e}$$

$$\text{Now, } \frac{Cr_2O_7^{-2} + 6\bar{e} + 14H^+ \rightarrow 2Cr^{+3} + 7H_2O}{Cr_2O_7^{-2} + 6Fe^{+2} + 14H^+ \rightarrow 6Fe^{+3} + 2Cr^{+3} + 7H_2O} \Big] \text{Balanced}$$

2. $AS_2S_3 + ClO_3^- \rightarrow H_3ASO_4 + SO_4^{-2} + Cl^-$

$$\downarrow$$

Arsenic sulfide

$$AS_2S_3 \rightarrow H_3ASO_4 + SO_4^{-2}$$

$$AS_2S_3 + 20H_2O \rightarrow 2H_3ASO_4 + 3SO_4^{-2} + 34H^+$$

Here, we have to balance the whole charge on both sides of equation's since there are two different atoms AS and S, as change in O.N. of both.

So balance the whole charge to be equal.

$$AS_2S_3 + 20H_2O \rightarrow 2H_3ASO_4 + 3SO_4^{-2} + 34H^+$$

$$AS_2S_3 + 20H_2O \rightarrow 2H_3ASO_4 + 3SO_4^{-2} + 28\bar{e} + 34H^+$$

$$ClO_3^{-1} + 6H^+ \rightarrow Cl^- + 3H_2O$$

$$\downarrow \qquad\qquad \downarrow$$

$$+5 \qquad\qquad -1$$

$$ClO_3^- + 6H^+ + 6\bar{e} \rightarrow Cl^- + 3H_2O$$

Now, $[ClO_3^{-1} + 6H^+ + 6\bar{e} \rightarrow Cl^- + 3H_2O] \times (14)$

$[AS_2S_3 + 20H_2O \rightarrow 2H_3ASO_4 + 3SO4^- + 34H^+ + 28\bar{e}] \times (3)$

$$14ClO_3^- + 84H^+ + 84\bar{e} \rightarrow 14Cl^- + 42H_2O$$

$$\left.\begin{array}{l} 3AS_2S_3 + 60H_2O \rightarrow 6H_3ASO_4 + 9 + 102H^+ + 84\bar{e} \\ \hline 3AS_2S_3 + 18H_2O + 14ClO_3 \rightarrow \\ 6H_3ASO_4 + 9SO_4^{-2} + 18H^+ + 14Cl^- \end{array}\right]\ \text{Balanced}$$

Detection of End Point

1. Internal Oxidation – Reduction Indicator
2. Self Indicator
3. External Indicator
4. Irreversible Redox Indicator
5. Dissaperance of Substance Titrated
6. Potentiometric Titration

1. Internal Oxidation – Reduction Indicators

- Oxi-Red. Indicator mark the sudden change in the oxidation potential in the neighborhood of the equivalence point in an oxidation reduction titration.
- The ideal oxidation-reduction indicator will have an oxidation potential intermediate between the values for the solution titrated and the titrant and it should exhibit a sharp, readily detectable colour change.

- An oxidation-reduction indicator (redox indicator) is a compound which exhibit different colors in the oxidized and reduced forms.

$$In_{ox} + ne \rightleftharpoons In_{red}$$

- The oxidation and reduction should be reversible. At a potential E, the ratio of concentration of two forms is given by Nernst equation,

$$E = E_{In}^{\theta} + \frac{RT}{nF} \ln \frac{[In_{ox}]}{[In_{red}]}$$

Where, E_{In}^{θ} = standard potential of indicator

- If the color intensities of two forms are comparable, a practical estimate of the color change interval corresponds of the change in the ration $(In_{ox})/(In_{red})$ from 10 to 1/10,

$$E = E_{In}^{\theta} \pm \frac{0.0591}{1} \text{ (at 25°C)}$$

- If the color intensities of two differ considerably the intermediate color is attained at a potential somewhat removed from E_{In}^{θ}. For a sharp color change at end point, E_{In}^{θ} should differ by at least 0.15V from the standard potentials of the other systems involved in the reaction.

Eg : 1, 10 – phenanthroline – iron (II)

With strong oxidising agents the complex ion is formed, which has a pale blue colour.

- The color change is very striking,

$$[Fe(C_{12}H_8N_2)_3]^{+3} + \bar{e} \rightleftharpoons [Fe (C_{12}H_8N_2)_3]^{2+}$$

    Pale blue   deep red

    (ferrin)   (Ferroin)

- The standard potential is 1.14 V. Color change – plae blue to deep red in HCl (1M) solution.

Eg. Diphenyl amine

- *Its disadvantage* it is slightly soluble in water. This can be overcome by use of soluble barium or sodium diphenyl aminesulphonate. The redox potential E_{In}^{θ} is 0.85V in 0.5 M H_2SO_4.

- Color changes to redish-violet color

- Used for detection of Fe^{+2} and $K_2Cr_2O_7$ as titrant.

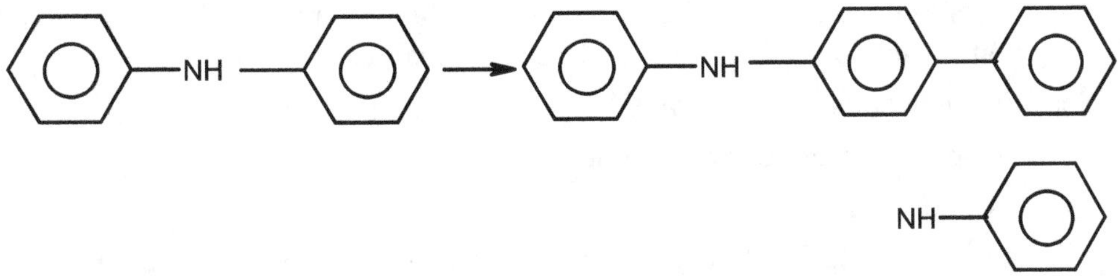

Diphenyl amine $+12H^+ + 12\,\bar{e}$

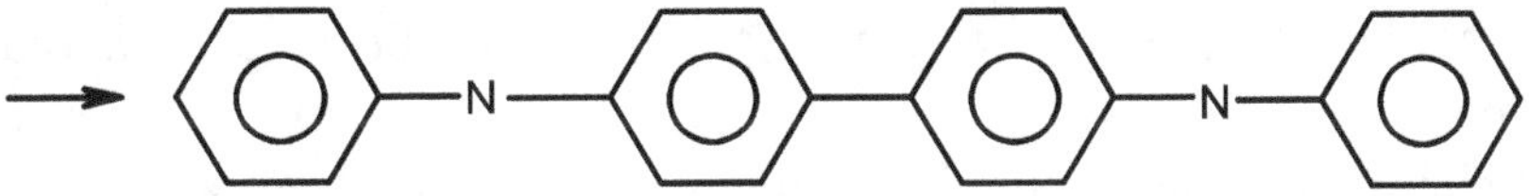

Diphenyl benzidine colourless solution

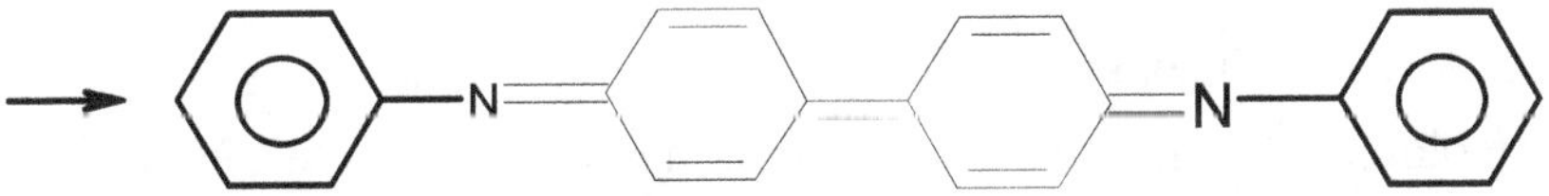

Violet Colour

- Oxidation of dichromate solution in excess therefore colour change from colourless to violet they give red-yellow precipitate.

    Eg. Ferrous dipyridine

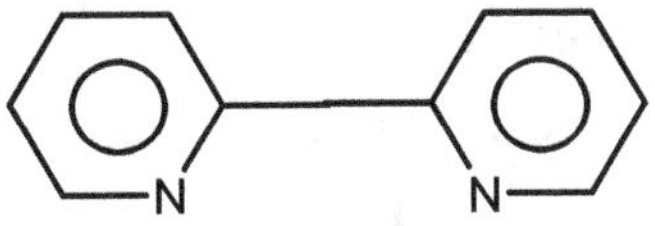

- With Fe^{+2} gives red color
- With Fe^{+3} gives blue color

Indicator	**Color change**	**Potential**
1. Diphenylamine	Violet $\rightarrow$ colorless	0.76
2. Methylene blue	Blue $\rightarrow$ colorless	0.52
3. N-phenylanthranilic acid	purple, red $\rightarrow$ colorless	0.89

2. Self – Indicator

- Potassium permanganate is a good example
- One drop imparts a visible pink coloration to solution, even in presence of colored ions like Fe III

- The colors of cerium (IV) sulfate and iodine solution have also been employed for detection of end points, but color change is not marked.
- Sensitive indicators are available

  Eg.   10-phenanthroline iron (II) ion

  N-phenylanthranillic acid

- Self indicating reagents have the draw back that an excess of oxidising agent is always present at the end paint.

3. External Indicators

- The best known example is, the spot test for the titration of ferrous ion with $K_2Cr_2O_7$.
- Near equivalence point, drops of solution are removed and brought into contact with dilute freshly prepared potassium ferricyanide solution on a spot plate.
- The end point is reached when first drop fails to give (blue) color.

4. Irreversible Redox Indicator

- Some colored organic compounds can undergo irreversible oxidation or reduction and can't be used as internal indicator.
- If colorchange is very sensitive to slight amount of titrant.

  Eg. (i)   Methyl red/orange

  Color – red, decolorized by strong oxidizing agent

  (ii)   Napthol blue/black

  Green $\rightarrow$ pink $\rightarrow$ colorless

  used for Arsenate dichromate titration.

5. Disappearance of Substance Titrated

Eg. Reduction of Fe^{+3} by Ti^{+3}

$$Fe^{+3} \rightarrow Ti^{+3}$$

$$Fe^{+3} + Ti^{+3} \rightarrow Fe^{+2} + Ti^{+4}$$

$$Fe^{+3} + \bar{e} \xrightarrow{\ Ti_{+3}\ } Fe^{+3}$$

Blue to Red, at end point color disappears.

6. Potentiometric Titration

- The potential of an indicator electrode is measured as a function of volume titrant added.

- The equivalence point of the reaction will be revealed by a sudden change in potential in the plot of e.m.f readings against the volume of the titrating solution; any method which will detect this abrupt change of potential may be used.
- 2 electrodes, one a reference electrode.

  Eg. SCE and indicator electrode and Magnetic stirrer and automatic burette.

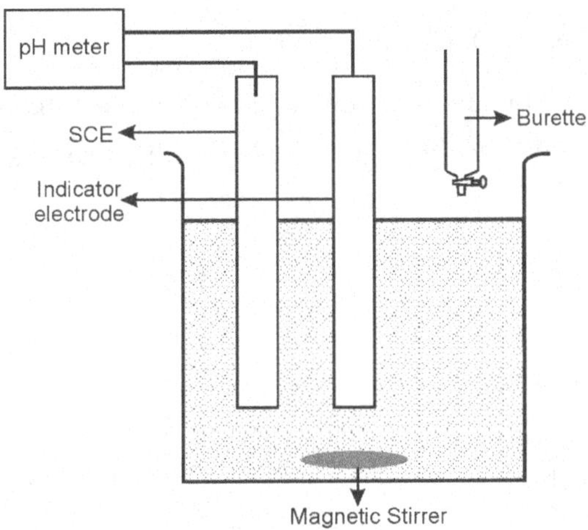

Fig. 8.3

e.g. Coloured solution for very dilute solution.

Eg. Iron (III) with potential permanganate or pot. Dichromate or cerium (iv) sulfate.

- The potential of increased electrode is thus controlled by the ratio of the Concentrations.

Redox Titrations

- Depending on the use of oxidizing agents, redox titration can be classified as :
    1. Permanganate titration

       (Titrations involving potassium permanganate).
    2. Iodine titration

       (Iodimetry and Iodimetry)
    3. Dichromate titrations
    4. Cerimetry

       (Titrations involving ceric ammonium sulfate)
    5. Titration involving potassium Iodate.
    6. Titrations involving potassium bromate.

1. Permanganate Titrations

- Manganese dioxide is present in solution of $KMnO_4$, catalyses the auto decomposition of the solution on standing,

$$4\ MnO_4^- + 2H_2O = 4MnO_2 + 3O_2 + 40H^-$$

- Permanganate is unstable in Mn^{+2} ion presence

$$2\ MnO_4^- + 3Mn^{+2} + 2H_2O = 5\ MnO_2 + 4H^+$$

- This reaction is slow in acid solutions and very rapid in neutral solution.
- Therefore it is usually freshly prepared, also sunlight causes its decomposition.

Preparation

- Weight   3.2-3.5 g $KMnO_4$

  Add 1– L water

  Close the breaker

  Boil gently for 15-30 min

  Allow to cool and filter through sintered glass crucible or funnel

Collect filtrate and store in a clean–glass stoppered bottle of dark brown glass.

Standardisation

PSC   (i) Sodium oxalate

(ii) Ansenic trioxide

- Sodium oxalate solution, acidified with dil H_2SO_4 and warmed to 80-90°C, it slowly titrated with permanganate solution with constant stirring until faint color is observed and temperature near end point falls below 60 °C.

$$2\ Na^+ + C_2O_4^{2-} + 2H^+ \rightleftharpoons H_2C_2O_4 + 2Na^+$$

$$2\ MnO_4^- + 5H_2C_2O_4 + 6H^+ = 2Mn^{+2} + 10\ CO_2 + 8H_2O$$

$$2KMnO_4 + 5Na_2C_2O_4 + 3H_2SO_4 \rightarrow K_2SO_4 + 2MnSO_4 + 10\ CO_2 + 5Na_2SO_4 + 8H_2O$$

Procedure

Dry   sodium oxalate at 105-110°C for 2 hours and allow to cool.

↓

Weigh 0.3 g of dry sodium oxaltate

↓

Add 240 ml distilled water

↓

Add 12.5 mL concentrated H_2SO_4 or 250 mL diluted H_2SO_4 (1M)

↓

Cool to 25-30°C and stir

↓

Add 90-95% $KMnO_4$ solution from burette.

↓

Heat to 55-60 °C

↓

Color change → faint pink color perists for 30 sec.

(ii) with Arsenious Oxide

Weight 0.25 g of arsenious oxide (Dry)

↓

+ 10 ml NaOH and 10 ml H_2O

↓

Allow to stand and stir continuously

↓

Add 100 ml H_2O + 10 ml concentrated HCl

Add 1 drop of 0.0025 M potassium iodide / iodate

↓

Add $KMnO_4$ from beaker

↓

Faint blue color persists for 30 secs.

PSC for $KMnO_4$

Anhydrous potassium Ferro cyanide, Ferrous Ammonium Sulphate and Potassium tetraoxalate.

2. Iodine Titration

- The direct iodometric titration method, sometimes called *iodimetry,* refers to titrations with standard solution of iodine.

- The indirect iodometric titration method, sometimes called *iodometry* deals with the titration of iodine liberated in chemical reactions.

$$I_2(s) + 2\bar{e} \rightleftharpoons 2I^-$$

- This equation refers to a saturated aq. solution in the presence of solid iodine, this half-cell reaction will occur towards the end of a titration of iodide with an oxidising agent such as potassium permanganate when the iodide ion concentration becomes relatively low.

- When an excess of iodide ion is present the triodide ion is formed,

$$I_2(aq) + I^- \rightleftharpoons 3I^-$$

- Since iodine is readily soluble in a solution of iodide.

$$I_3^- + 2\bar{e} \rightleftharpoons 3I^-$$

- Iodine or the tri-iodide ion is therefore a much weaker oxidizing agent than potassium. Permanganate, potassium dichromate and cerium (IV) sulfate.

- In most of direct titrations with iodine (iodimetry) a solution of iodine in potassium iodide is employed and the reactive species is therefore the tri-iodide ion I_3^-.

- Strong reducing agents such as tin (II) chloride, sulphurous acid, hydrogen sulphide and sodium thiosulfate, react completely and rapidly with iodine even in acid solution.

- Weaker reducing agents eg. Arsenic (III) or antimony (III), complete reaction occurs only when the solution is kept neutral or very faintly acid, under these conditions the reduction potential of the reducing agent is minimum or its reducing power is maximum.

- Strong oxidizing agent is treated in neutral or acid solution with a large excess of iodide ion, the iodide ion reacts as a reducing agent and the oxidant will be quantitatively reduced.

- In these cases an equivalent amount of iodine is liberated and is then titrated with a standard solution of a reducing agent usually sodium thiosulfate.

- The normal reduction potential of the iodine-iodide system is independent of the pH of the solution, so long as the pH is less than about 8, at higher pH iodine reacts with hydroxide ions to form iodide and the extremely unstable hypoiodite, which is rapidly transformed into iodate and iodite by self-oxidation and reduction.

$$I_2 + 20H^- = I^- + IO^- + H_2O$$

$$3IO^- = 2I^- + IO_3^-$$

- The reduction potential of certain substances increase considerably with increasing hydrogen ion concentration of the solution.

- Many weak oxidising anions are completely reduced by iodide ions if their reduction potentials are raised considerably by the presence in solution of a large amount of acid.

Conditions for Iodometric Determination

1. As the potential of the $I_2/2I^-$ system is not high many iodometric reactions are (revesible) and don't go to completion.

   Only if suitable conditions are provided, go to the end.

2. Since iodine is volatile, titration is conducted in the (cold, condition). Also, sensitivity of starch diminishes with rise in temperature.

3. Iodometric titration cannot be performed in strongly alkaline solution as it forms hypo iodide which is strong oxidizing agent.

   $$2NaOH + I_2 \rightarrow NaOI + NaI + H_2O$$

   If the reaction results in formation of H^+ ion, they must be removed to ensure that reaction proceeds practically to completion in required direction.

   $$HCO_3^- + H^+ \rightarrow H_2CO_3 \rightarrow H_2O + CO_2\uparrow$$

4. Since the solubility of iodine in water is low a considerable excess of KI must be used.

   $$KI + I_2 \rightarrow KI_3$$

   or $I + I_2 \rightarrow [I_3]^-$

5. Despite the use of large amounts of KI and acid the rate of reaction between oxidant and I^- ions is usually too slow and sufficient time should be given before titration.

6. The reaction mixture is kept in a dark place, because light accelerates the side reaction in which I^- ions are oxidized to I_2 by atmospheric oxygen.

   $$4I^- + 4H^+ + O_2 \rightarrow 2I_2 + 2H_2O$$

Preparing 0.05 M Iodine Solution

- Dissolve 20 g of iodate free KI

    ↓

    + 30-40 ml of water in a glass stoppered 1 L graduated flask.

    ↓

    12.7 g of iodine weigh

    ↓

    Transfer to flask

    ↓

    Close flask with glass stopper and shake in cold

    ↓

    Add water upto mark with distilled water.

Standardizing Iodine Solution

- Standard substance (i) sodium thiosulfate against iodate (ii) Arsenious oxide Transfer 25 ml of the iodine solution to 250 ml conical flask.

    ↓

    Dilute 100 ml

    ↓

    Add std. thiosulfate solution from a burette until the solution has a pale yellow color.

    ↓

    + 2 ml starch solution

    ↓

    Solution → colorless.

Preparation and use of Starch Solution

- Make a paste of 0.1 g of soluble starch with a little water and pour the paste with constant stirring into 100 ml of boiling water.

    ↓

    Boil for 1 min

    ↓

    Allow the solution to cool

    ↓

    2-3 g of potassium iodide

    ↓

    Keep the solution in a stoppered bottle.

- If the starch solution is added when the iodine concentration is high some iodine may remain absorbed even at the end point.

- Only freshly prepared starch should be used.

- Starch must not be added until just before the end point reached. Apart from the fact that the fading of the iodine color is a good indication of the approaching end point.

(ii) Standardization with Arsenious Oxide

Weigh accurately 2.5 g of powdered arsenious oxide, dissolve it in concentration sodium hydroxide solution.

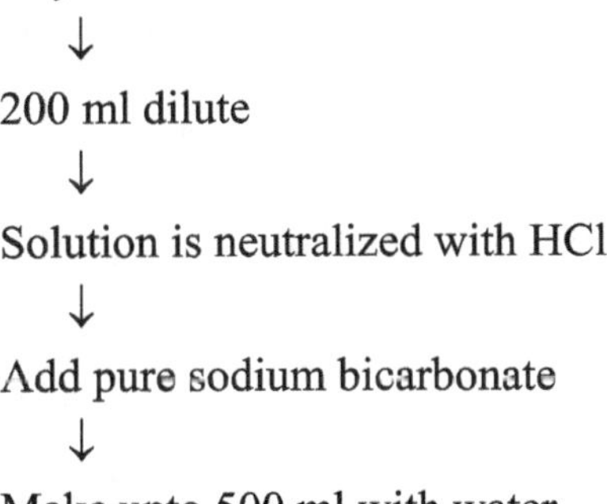

$\downarrow$

200 ml dilute

$\downarrow$

Solution is neutralized with HCl

$\downarrow$

Add pure sodium bicarbonate

$\downarrow$

Make upto 500 ml with water.

- Measure out the fixed volume of arsenious oxide solution in conical flask and titrate it against iodine solution to get the end point by use of starch as indicator.

Difference

Iodometry	Iodimetry
Indirect titration	Direct titration
Need of iodine flask for few minutes in dark	Sample is directly titrated with iodine and carried out in simple flask
Sample is reacted with KI and kept in dark for complete reaction	No need of KI
Iodine used in flask and back titrated with $Na_2S_2O_3$ and starch indicator	Iodine in burette
More accurate	Not so accurate

Praparing 0.1 M Sodium Thiosulfate

- Sodium thiosulfate ($Na_2S_2O_3.5H_2O$) is readily obtainable in a state of high purity, but there is always some uncertainly as to the exact water content because of the efflorescent nature of the salt and for other reasons. Therefore used as primary standard.

$$2S_2O_3^{2-} \rightleftharpoons S_4O_6^{2-} + 2\bar{e}$$

- 0.1M solution is prepared by dissolving about 25 g $Na_2S_2O_3$ in 1L of water in a graduated flask.

Procedure: 25 g of sodium thiosulfate crystals

$$\downarrow$$

Dissolve in boiled and cooled distilled water

$$\downarrow$$

1L $\rightarrow$ Dissolve with boiled H_2O

$$\downarrow$$

Solution kept for few days

$$\downarrow$$

$+ 0.1g$ of Na_2CO_3.

(Na_2CO_3 is added to keep pH 9 to 10 because as bacterial activity is least)

Standardising $Na_2S_2O_3$

1. with potassium iodate

- 99.9% pure and dried at $120^{\circ}C$

$$IO_3^- + 5I^- + 6H^+ \rightarrow 3I_2 + 3H_2O$$

- Relative molecular mass is 214.

$\therefore$ 0.02 M $\rightarrow$ 4.28 g of potassium iodate per litre.

Weight 0.14-0.15 g potassium Iodate

$$\downarrow$$

Dissolve in 25 ml water

$$\downarrow$$

Boiled and cooled water used

$$\downarrow$$

$+2$ g iodate – free potassium iodide

$$\downarrow$$

$+5$ ml of 1 M sulphuric acid

$$\downarrow$$

Liberated iodine titrated with thiosulfate solution $\rightarrow$ shake

$$\downarrow$$

Pale yellow color

$$\downarrow$$

Add 200 ml distilled water + 2 ml of starch

$\downarrow$

Blue $\rightarrow$ colorless.

2. with Potassium Dichromate

- PSC – potassium dichromate. (oxidizing agent)
- Known quantity of potassium dichromate

$\downarrow$

Dissolve in water

$\downarrow$

Acidified with HCL

$\downarrow$

Excess of potassium Iodide is added

$\downarrow$

Potassium dichromate is added in excess.

$\downarrow$

Potassium dichromate oxidizes KI to iodine and liberated iodine is then titrated with thiosulfate using starch indicator till pale green color.

$$K_2Cr_2O_7 + 6Kl + 7H_2SO_4 \rightarrow Cr_2\,(SO_4)_3 + 3I_2 + 4K_2SO_4 + 7H_2O$$

$$Cr_2O_7^{2-} + 14H^+ + 6\bar{e} \rightarrow 2Cr^{+3} + 7H_2O$$

$$6I^- \rightarrow 3I_2 + \bar{e}$$

Equivalent wt. of $K_2Cr_2O_7 = \dfrac{\text{Mol. wt}}{7} = 49.03.$

3. Dichromate Titration

- (oxidising agent) Potassium dichromate is pure, it is stable up to its fusion point.
- Standard solution of exactly known concentration can be prepared by weighing out the pure dry salt and dissolving it proper volume of water.
- Potassium dichromate is used only in acid solution, and is reduced rapidly at the ordinary temperature to green chromium (III) solution.
- It is not reduced by cold hydrochloric acid, provided the acid concentration doesn't exceed 1 or 2M.
- They are less easily reduced by organic matter and they are also stable to light.

- Potassium dichromate is therefore of particular value in determination of iron in iron ores, the ore is usually dissolved in HCl, the iron (III) reduced to iron (II) and the solution then titrated with standard dichromate solution.

$$Cr2O_7^{2-} + 6Fe^{+2} + 14H^+ \rightarrow 2Cr^{+3} + 6Fe^{+3} + 7H_2O$$

- It is available in pure form as its excellent PSC.

- In acid solution, the reduction of $K_2Cr_2O_7$:

$$Cr_2O_7^{2-} + 14H^+ + 6\bar{e} \rightleftharpoons 2Cr^{+3} + 7H_2O$$

- Green color due to Cr^{+3} ions formed by the reduction of $K_2Cr_2O_7$ makes it impossible to ascertain the end point.

Suitable external indicators include :

- N-phenylanthranilic acid 0.17% solution in 0.005 M NaOH

- Sodium diphenylamine sulfonate 0.2% aq. solution.

- Sodium diphenylamine sulfonate must be used in presence of phosphoric (V) acid.

Preparation 0.02M potassium dichromate

Powder 6 g of $K_2Cr_2O_7$ in mortar

↓

Heat for 30-60 min in over at 140-150°C

↓

Allow to cool in a closed vessel in a desiccator

↓

Weigh out accurately about 5.88 g of dry potassium dichromate

↓

Dissolve it upto 1 litre mark with water

4. Ceriometry

- It is powerful oxidising agent. It can be used only in acid solution, as solution is neutralised, cerium (IV) hydroxide or basic salts precipitated.

- The solution has an intense yellow color and in hot solution the end point is detected by suitable indicators.

Advatanges

1. Stable over prolonged periods, not to be protected from light. An acidic solution of cerium (IV) sulphate exceeds stability of permanganate solution.

2. Cerium (IV) sulphate used to determine reducing agents in presence of concentrated HCl

$$Ce^{+4} + \bar{e} \rightleftharpoons Ce^{+3}$$

3. In 0.1M solution are not too highly colored to abstract vision.

   - Solution of cerium (IV) sulfate in dil H_2SO_4 are also stable, even at boiling temperature.

Preparation 0.1M Cerium (IV) Sulfate

- 35-36 g of pure cerium (IV) sulphate

  56 ml 1:1 solution mix of H_2SO_4 and water

  Stir and gentle warm

  Dilute upto 1L with distilled water
- Weigh about 64-66 g of amm. cerium (IV) sulphate

  Add 28 mL of concentrated H_2SO_4 + 500 ml water

  $\downarrow$

  Dilute upto 1L
- Mol. Wt of $Ce(SO_4)_2 - 333.25$

  Mol. Wt of $(NH_4)_4 [Ce(SO_4)_4].2H_2O - 632.56$

Standardisation

1. with Arsenious oxide

   0.2 g of Arsenious oxide and transfer to a 400 ml beaker

   + 20 ml of 2N NaOH solution

   Warm to dissolve arsenious oxide

   Add 100 ml water

   + 25 ml 5 N sulfuric acid

Add 3 drops of 0.01 M osmium tetraoxide solution

$\downarrow$

+ 0.5 ml N-phenylanthranilic acid

$\downarrow$

Titrate with ceric sulfate

$\downarrow$

Sharp color change occur

2. with Anhy. potassium Ferro cyanide

$\downarrow$

Add 50 ml $4NH_2SO_4$

$\downarrow$

0.5 ml N-phenylanthranilic acid solution

$\downarrow$

Titrate against ceric sulfate

5. Titrations with potassium iodate

- Potassium iodate is powerful oxidizing agent.
- The reaction between Potassium iodate and reducing agents such as iodide ion or arsenic (III) oxide in solution of moderate acidity (0.1–0.2 M HCl) stops at the stage when the iodate is reduced to iodine.

$$6\,IO_3 + 5I^- + 6H^+ = 3I_2 + 3H_2O$$

$$2IO_3^- + 5H_3ASO_3 + 2H^+ = I_2 + 5H_3ASO_4 + H_2O$$

- With a more powerful reductant

  Eg. Titanium (III) chloride, the iodate is reduced to iodide.

$$IO_3^- + 6Ti^{3+} + 6H^+ = I^- + 6Ti^{+4} + 3H_2O$$

Preparation

Dry potassium iodate at 120 °C for 1h

$\downarrow$

Weigh 5.350 g powdered potassium iodate

$\downarrow$

Add about 400-500 ml of water

$\downarrow$

Make upto 1L $\rightarrow$ shake well.

Titration with Potassium Bromate

- Potassium bromate is a powerful oxidizing agent, which is reduced smoothly to bromide.

$$BrO_3^- + 6H+ + 6\bar{e} \rightleftharpoons Br^- + 3H_2O$$

- At end of titration free bromine appears,

$$BrO_3^- + 5Br^- + 6H^+ \rightleftharpoons 3Br_2 + 3H_2O$$

Examples,

$$BrO_3^- + 3H_3ASO_3 \xrightarrow{(HCl)} Br^- + 3H_3ASO_4$$

$$2BrO_3^- + 3N_2H_4 \xrightarrow{(HCl)} 2Br^- + 3N_2 + 6H_2O$$

$$BrO_3^- + NH_2OH \xrightarrow{(HCl)} Br^- + NO_3^- + H^+ + H_2O$$

Preparation

Dry some finely powdered potassium bromate for 1-2 h at $120^{\circ}C$.

$\downarrow$

Cool

$\downarrow$

Weigh out 3.34 g potassium bromate

$\downarrow$

Dissolve in 1 L flask

Examples

1. The given cell,

$$Cu+2 + 2\bar{e} \rightarrow Cu$$

$$\frac{Zn \rightarrow Z^{n+2} + 2\bar{e}}{Cu^{+2} + Zn \rightarrow Zn^{+2} + Cu}$$

$E_R (cu/cu^{+2}) = 0.337$

$E_o (Zn/Zn^{+2}) = + 0.763$

Method

- Draw cell diagram
- Calculate cell potential

- State whether cell is spontaneous or not

$$E_{cell} = E^o_{(auode)} - E^o_{(cathode)}$$

$$= +0.763 - 0.337$$

$$= 0.426$$

$$E_{cell} = +ve, \therefore \text{ Spontaneous}$$

Cell Diagram

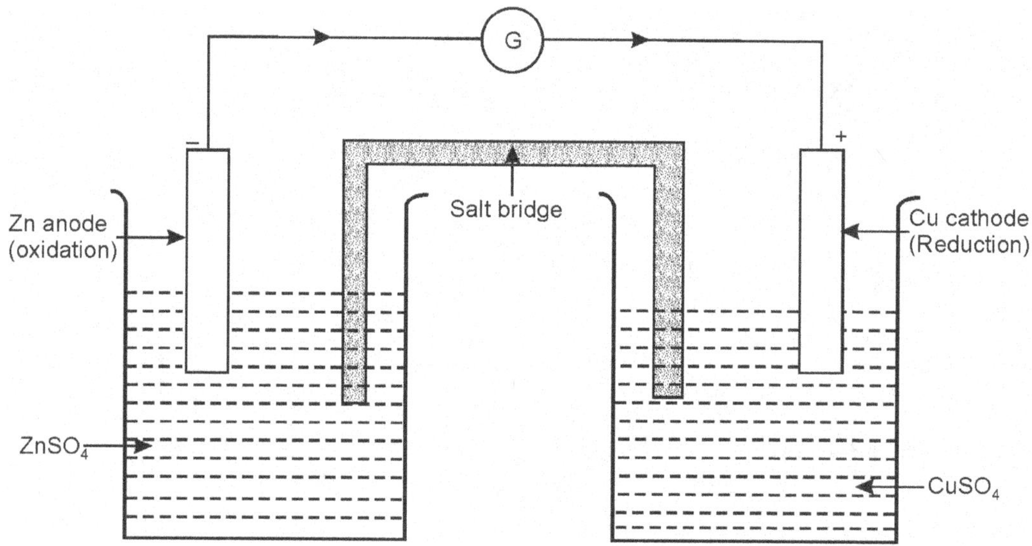

Fig. 8.4

2. Given that,

$$E^oCu, Cu^{+2} = -0.39 \text{ V (Oxi potential)}$$

$$E^oZn, Zn^{+2} = 0.76 \text{ V (oxi potential)}$$

$$E^o \text{ Cell} = E^o_{(anode)} - E^o \text{ (cathode)}$$

$$= 0.76 + 0.39$$

$$= 1.1$$

$$E^o \text{ Cell} = +ve$$

$$\therefore \text{ Spontaneous}$$

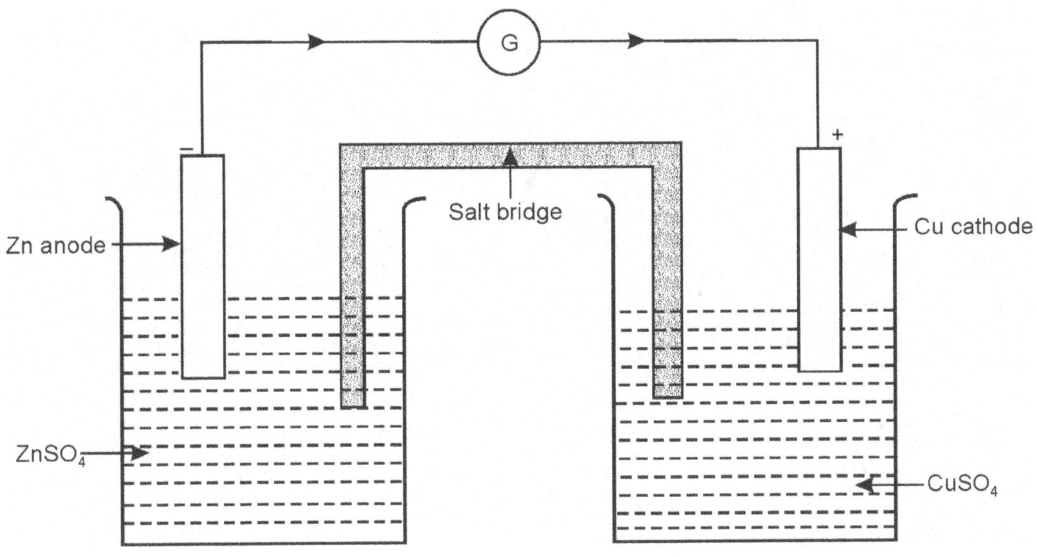

Fig. 8.5

3. The Given Cell,

$$Cr^{+2}(1m)/\ Cr^{+3}\ (0.001m)/\ V^{+3}_{(0.01M)}\ /\ V^{+2}_{(1M)}$$

$$\left.\begin{array}{l} E^{o}\ Cr^{+3}/Cr^{+2} = -0.41\ V \\[6pt] E^{o} = V^{+3}/V^{+2} = -0.26\ V \end{array}\right\} \text{Red Pot}$$

$$Cr^{+2} \rightarrow Cr^{+3} + \bar{e}\quad \text{(oxidation)}$$

$$V^{+3} + \bar{e} \rightarrow V^{+2}\quad \text{(Reduction)}$$

$$Cr^{+2} + V^{+3}\quad \rightarrow \quad Cr^{+3} + V^{+2}$$

$$E = Eo + \frac{0.0591}{n} \times \log \frac{[oxi]}{[Red]} \text{ - Nernst equation}$$

$$E^{o}Cr^{+3}/Cr^{+2} + \frac{0.0591}{1} \log \frac{[0.001]}{[1]}$$

$$E_{anode} = 0.41 + 0.0591\ (-3)$$

$$\qquad\quad = -0.41 - 0.1773$$

$$E_{anode} = 0.5873V$$

$$E_{cathode} = E^{o}_{V^{+3}/V^{+2}} + \frac{0.2592}{n} \log \frac{[Oxi]}{[Red]}$$

$$E_{cathode} = -0.26 + 0.0592 \log \frac{[0.01]}{[1]}$$

$$= -0.26 + (0.0592)(-2)$$

$$E_{cathode} = -0.3784 \text{ V}$$

As, both red. potential are given, convert them to Oxi. Potential

$\therefore E_{cathode} = 0.3784\text{V}$

$\therefore E_{anode} = 0.5873 \text{ V}$ } Oxi potential

$$E^o_{cell} = E_{anode} - E_{cathode}$$

$$= 0.5873 - 0.3784$$

$$= 0.2089 \text{ V}$$

$E^o_{cell} = +\text{Ve}, \quad \therefore \text{ Spontaneous}$

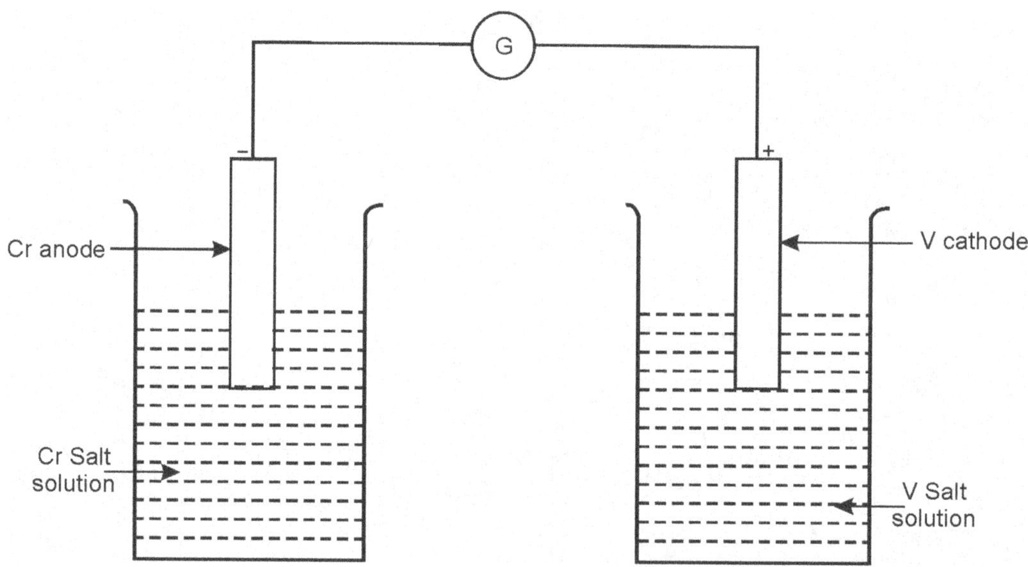

Fig. 8.6

4. Calculate the cell potential for the following cell and write cell eqn.

$$\text{Ni/Ni}^{+2} \text{ (0.44M)} \parallel \text{C}^{+2}_0 \text{ (0.6M)/Co}$$

$E^O_{Ni}, \text{Ni}^{+2} = 0.23 \text{ V}$

$E^O_{Co}, \text{C}^{+2}_0 = 0.28 \text{ V}$ } Oxi. Potential

$$Ni \rightarrow Ni^{+2} + 2\bar{e} \qquad \text{(Oxidation)}$$

$$\frac{Co + 2 + 2\bar{e} \rightarrow Co}{Ni + Co^{+2} \rightarrow Ni^{+2} + Co} \qquad \text{(Reduction)}$$

$$E_{anode} = E_O^o + \frac{0.0592}{n} \log \frac{[oxi]}{[red]}$$

$$E_{anode} = 0.23 + \frac{0.0592}{2} \log \frac{[0.44]}{[1]}$$

$$= 0.23 + \frac{0.0592}{2} \times (-0.3565)$$

$$= 0.23 - 0.0105$$

$$E_{anode} = 0.2195 \text{ V}$$

$$E_{cathod} = E_R^o + \frac{0.0592}{n} \log \frac{[oxi]}{[red]}$$

$$E_{cathod} = 0.28 + \frac{0.0592}{2} \log \frac{[0.60]}{[1]}$$

$$= 0.28 + \frac{0.0592}{2} \times (-0.2218)$$

$$= 0.28 - 0.0066$$

$$E_{cathod} = 0.2734 \text{ V}$$

$$E_{cell}^o = E_{anode} - E_{cathode}$$

$$= 0.2195 - 0.2734$$

$$E_{cell}^o = -0.0539 \text{ V}$$

$$E_{cell}^o = -Ve$$

$\therefore$ Non-spontaneous

5. Calculate equilibrium constant for reaction between 0.1 N Fe^{+3} and 0.1N ce^{+4}. Calculate the unionzed Fe^{+2} at stoichiometical point.

$$\left.\begin{array}{l} E^o \; Fe^{+3}, Fe^{+2} = 0.77 \\ E^o \; Ce^{+4}, Ce^{+3} = 1.61 \end{array}\right\} \text{Reduction potential}$$

$$\left.\begin{array}{l} E^o \; Fe^{+2}, Fe^{+3} = -0.77 \\ E^o \; Ce^{+3}, Ce^{+4} = -1.61 \end{array}\right\} \text{Oxidation Potential}$$

$$Fe^{+2} \rightarrow Fe^{+3} + \bar{e} \ (Oxidation) \ A$$

$$\underline{Ce^{+4} + \bar{e} \rightarrow Ce^{+3} \ (Reduction) \ C}$$

$$Fe^{+2} + Ce^{+4} \rightarrow Fe^{+3} + Ce^{+3}$$

At equivalence point, $E_R = E_O = E_{cell}$

$\therefore E_{cell} \ E_R - E_O = 0$

$$E_R^o - E_O^o = \frac{0.0591}{n} \left(\log \left(\frac{Oxi}{Red} \right)_o \left(\frac{Red}{Oxi} \right) \right)_R$$

$$1.61 - 0.77 = 0.0591 \ (\log(K))$$

$$\therefore \log K = \frac{0.84}{0.0591} = 14.21$$

$$K = 1.633 \times 10^{14}$$

$$K = \left[\frac{Oxi}{Red} \right]_O \left[\frac{Red}{Oxi} \right]_R$$

$$K = \left[\frac{Fe^{+3}}{Fe^{+2}} \right] \left[\frac{Ce^{+4}}{Ce^{+3}} \right]$$

At equivalence point,

$$Red_1 = Oxi_2$$

$\therefore Fe^{+3} = Ce^{+3}$ and

Similarly, $Fe^{+2} = Ce^{+4}$

$$K = \frac{[Fe^{+3}]^2}{[Fe^{+2}]^2}$$

$$\frac{Fe^{+3}}{Fe^{+2}} = \sqrt{K} = 1.277 \times 10^7$$

At equivalence point

Fe^{+3} reduces to Half. $Fe^{+3} = 0.05M$

$$Fe^{+2} = \frac{0.05}{1.277} \times 10^{-7}$$

$$= 0.03915 \times 10^{-7}$$

$$Fe^{+2} = 3.915 \times 10^{-9} \, M$$

6. 50 ml of 0.1N Sn^{+2} is titrated with 0.1N of Ce^{+4}. Calculate Equation.

$$E^o\ Sn^{+4}/Sn^{+2} = 0.15\ V$$
$$E^o\ Ce^{+4}/Ce^{+3} = 1.61\ V$$
$\left.\right\}$ Std. Red. Potential

$$E^o\ Sn^{+2}/Sn^{+4} = -0.15\ V$$
$$E^o\ Ce^{+3}/Ce^{+4} = -1.61\ V$$
$\left.\right\}$ Std. Oxi. Potential

$$Sn^{+2} \rightarrow Sn^{+2} + 2\bar{e} \qquad\qquad \text{(Oxidation)}$$

$$\underline{2Ce^{+4} + 2\bar{e} \rightarrow 2Ce^{+3}} \qquad \text{(Reduction)}$$
$$2Ce^{+4} + Sn^{+2} \rightarrow Sn^{+4} + 2Ce^{+3}$$

At equivalence, $E_O = E_R = E_{cell}$

$$E_{cell} = E_R - E_O = 0$$

$$E_R^o - E_O^o = \frac{0.0592}{n}\ \log \left[\frac{Oxi}{Red}\right]_O \left[\frac{Red}{Oxi}\right]_R$$

$$E_R^o - E_O^o = \frac{0.0592}{2}\ \log K$$

$$+ 1.61 - 0.15 = \frac{0.0592}{2} \times \log K$$

$$\log K = \frac{1.46}{0.0592} \times 2 = 49.32$$

$$K = 2.08 \times 10^{49}$$

$$\text{Now, E equation} = \frac{n_1, E_R^o + n_2\ E_O^o}{n_1 + n_2}$$

$$= \frac{2(0.15) + 1(1.61)}{2 + 1}$$

$$= \frac{0.30 + 1.61}{3}$$

$$= \frac{1.91}{3}$$

$$\text{E equation} = 0.635\ V$$

CHAPTER 9

PRECIPITATION TITRATIONS

- Based on reactions that yield ionic compound of limited solubility.
- There are only few agents for precipitation titrations because of slow rate of formation of most precipitates.

  Eg: Silver nitrate for determination of halides, CN^-, SCN^-, CNO^-, mercaptans, fatty acids and inorganic anions.

- Titimetric methods based on silver nitrate are sometimes called argentometric methods.

Indicators for Argentometric Titrations

- Three types of end points are encountered in titrations with silver nitrate.
    1. Chemical
    2. Potentiometric
    3. Amperometric

1. Chemical

   Three chemical indicators are used, they are chromate ion, adsoption indicators and iron (III), ions

2. Potentiometric

   - End points are obtained by measuring the potential between silver electrode and reference electrode whose potential is constant and independent of added reagent.

3. Amperometric

   - The current generated between a pair of silver microelectrodes in the solution of analyte is measured and plotted as a function of reagent volume.

- The end point produced by chemical indicator usually consists of a colour change and appearance or disappearance of turbidity in the solution being titrated.

Requirements of an Indicator of Precipitation Titrations

- Colour change should occur over a limited range in P-function of reagent or analyte. (–log)
- The colour change should take place within the steep portion of titration curve.

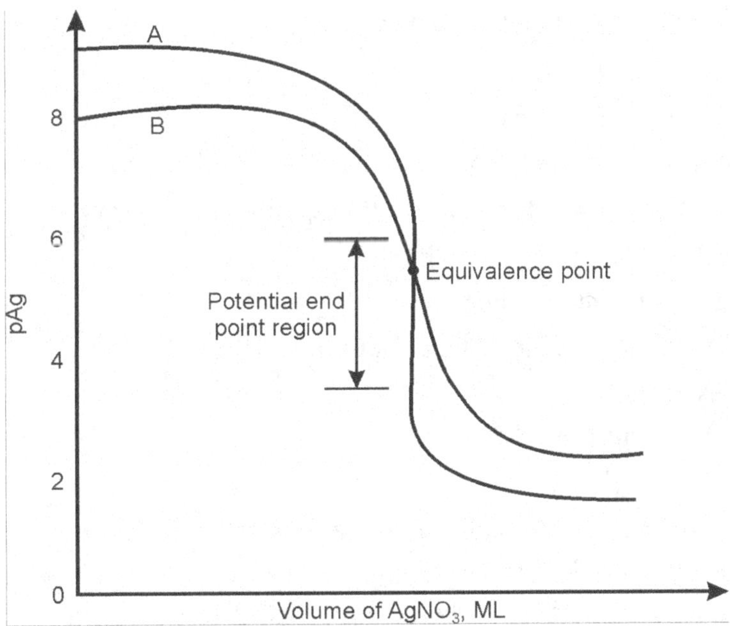

Fig. 9.1 Titration curve.

(A) 0.05 M Nacl with 0.1 M AgNO₃

(B) 0.005 M Nacl with 0.01 M AgNo₃

- Thus end point region for Cl^- ion is limited to PAg of about 4.0 to 6.0.

Applications of Ag NO₃ solution (Standard)

- Some typical precipitation reactions, $AgNO_3$ is standard solution. Mostly for these Volhard's method is used.
- $AgNO_3$ is hygroscopic and standardised against potassium thiocynate.

Precipitation Titration

- Solubility is the concentration of dissolved solution in moles/litre, when the solution is in equilibrium with a solid solute.
- In the solid state the solute molecules occupy space in a fixed repeating pattern to form a crystal of solid.

Solubility Product

- Consider an aq. solution of slightly soluble salt BA in equilibrium with excess of the solid at constant temperature.
- The equilibrium can be represented by

$$BA\,(s) \rightleftharpoons B^+ + A^-$$

Where,   BA(s) – Solid phase

- In dilute aq. sol. essentially no undissociated BA will be present in the solution.
- Since the activity of solid is constant, the equilibrium constant.

$$K_{sp} = [\,B^+\,]\,[\,A^-\,] \quad \text{unit : gm. mole/litre}$$

where, K_{sp} = solubility product

Constant for a given solute, solvent and temperature.

- In complex cases,

$$Bm\,An\,(s) \rightleftharpoons mB^{n+} + nA^{m-}$$

$$K_{sp} = [B^{n+}]^m\,[A^{m-}]^n$$

- Solubility product is important as it permits the calculation of one of the ion concentration if the other is known.
- A substance precipitates out when the product of ionic concentration exceeds K_{sp} value.

Molar Solubility

- Concentration of dissolved solute in mole per litre when the solution is in equilibrium with the solid state.
- Depends on solvent temperature

$$K_{sp} = [\,Ag^+\,]\,[\,Cl^-\,]$$

$$K_{sp} = [s]\,[s]$$

$$= S^2$$

$$Eg : Cacl_2 \rightleftharpoons Ca^{+2} + 2\,Cl^-$$

$$K_{sp} = [ca^+] [Cl^-]^2$$
$$= [s] [2s]^2 = s.4s^2$$
$$= 4s^3$$

Molar Conc = ICP

$\therefore$ $I_{cp} < K_{sp} \rightarrow$ unsaturated solvent

$I_{cp} = K_{sp} \rightarrow$ Saturated solvent

$I_{cp} > K_{sp} \rightarrow$ Super Saturated solvent

Common Ion Effect

- The solubility of any slightly soluble salt can be decreased by adding an excess of either of its ions.

    Eg : Dissociation of slightly soluble salt BA,

    $$BA_{(s)} \rightleftharpoons B^+ + A^-$$
    $$K_{sp} = [B^+][A^-]$$

- This is equilibrium condition
- An excess of B^+ or A^+ are added in the form of another salt whose solubility is greater than that of BA, then the ionic concentration of $[B^-/A^-]$ will exceed the solubility product and hence BA will precipitate.
- The common ion effect provides a valuable method for controlling the concentration of the ions furnished by a weak electrolyte.

Effect of pH on solubility

- The solubility of salt will increases by decrease in pH, the anion of the salt is a conjugated base of weak acid.

    Eg : consider the slightly soluble salt BA the anion of which (A^-) is conjugated base of W.A. HA

    $$BA(s) \rightleftharpoons B^+ + A^- \qquad \qquad .....(1)$$
    $$HA \rightleftharpoons H^+ + A^- \qquad \qquad .....(2)$$

- The equilibrium shifts towards left in (2) right in (1).
- Solubility of BA increases with increase of H^+ or decrease in pH.

- The equilibrium expressions are

$$Ksp = [B^+][A^-]$$

$$Ka = \frac{[H^+][A^-]}{[HA]}$$

- Molar solubility of BA is equal to [BT] = total concentration of $[A^-]$,

$$\therefore S = [B^+] = [A^-] + [HA]$$

$$Ka \; \frac{[H^+]Ksp}{[B^+][HA]}$$

$$[HA] = \frac{H^+Ksp}{B^+Ka} \quad A^- = \frac{Ksp}{B^+} \quad \therefore S = [A^-][H_A]$$

Thus,

$$S = [B^+] = \frac{Ksp}{[B^+]}\left(1 + \frac{[H^+]}{Ka}\right)$$

$$S = \sqrt{KSP\left(1 + \frac{[H^+]}{ka}\right)}$$

- If salt whose cation is conjugated acid of weak base, solubility increases with increase in pH.

Effect of Temperature on Solubility

- The solubility increases with increase in temperature

Solubility of	AgCl	at	10°C	1.72	mg/L
			100°C	21.1	mg/L
	BaSO$_4$	at	10°C	2.2	mg/L
			100°C	3.9	mg/L

Effect of Solvent upon Solubility

- Solubility decreases on addition of organic solvents such as

$$\left.\begin{array}{l} \text{methyl} \\ \text{ethyl} \\ \text{n-propyl} \end{array}\right\} \text{alcohols}$$

Eg: Lead Sulfate

on addition of 20% ethanol, solubility negligible.

Fractional Precipitation

- When a precipitation reagent is added to solution containing two anions, both of which form slightly soluble salts with the same cation.

  Eg : when silver nitrate solution is added to a solution containing both chloride and iodide.

- The question which arises here is which salt will precipitate first and how completely will first salt be precipitate before the 2nd ion begins to react with the reagent.

- The solubility products of silver chloride and silver iodide is 1.2×10^{-10} and 1.7×10^{-16} respectively.

$$[Ag^+][Cl^-] = 1.2 \times 10^{-10}$$

$$[Ag^+][I^-] = 1.7 \times 10^{-16}$$

- It is evident that the solubility product of silver iodide being less will be exceeded first and hence, AgI will be precipitate first. i.e. $[Ag^+]$ exceeds the value $\dfrac{1.7 \times 10^{-16}}{[\bar{I}]}$ before it exceeds $\dfrac{1.2 \times 10^{-10}}{[\bar{Cl}]}$

- AgCl will precipitate when the latter value exceeds.

- After both ions will be precipitated simultaneously

- The Ag^+ ions will then be in equilibrium with both the salts.

$$[Ag^+] = \frac{Ksp\,(AgI)}{[\bar{I}]} = \frac{Ksp\,(AgCl)}{[\bar{Cl}]}$$

$$\frac{[I^-]}{[Cl^-]} = \frac{Ksp\,(AgI)}{Ksp\,(AgCl)} = \frac{1.7 \times 10^{-16}}{1.2 \times 10^{-10}} = 1.41 \times 10^{-6}$$

So, when the concentration of iodide ions is about one millionth part of the chloride ion concentration, silver chloride will precipitate.

Drugs		**Assay methods**
→ Aminophylline	-	Volhard's method
→ Chlorbutol	-	Volhard's method
→ Ethionamide	-	Volhard's method
→ Silver nitrate	-	Volhard's method

$\rightarrow$ Sodium chloride   -   Volhard's method

$\rightarrow$ Dialysis fluid   -   Mohrs method

$\rightarrow$ KCl   -   Mohrs method

Determining End Points in Precipitation Reaction

1. Formation of coloured precipitates (Mohr's)
2. Formation of soluble coloured (Volhard's) compound.
3. Use of Adsorption indicator (Fajan's)
4. Turbidity method (Gay Lussac)

Formation of Coloured Precipitates

- This may be illustrated by the Mohr procedure for the determination of chloride and bromide.
- In the titration of a neutral solution of chloride ions with silver nitrate solution a small quantity of potassium chromate solution is added to serve as an indicator.
- At end point, the chromate ions combine with silver ions to form silver chromate, red in colour and sparingly soluble.

Theory

- This is a case of fractional precipitation.
- Two sparingly soluble salt,

  0.1M silver chloride

  0.1 M Silver chromate and dilute solution of potassium chromate.
- AgCl is less soluble salt, therefore initially Cl^- concentration is high. Therefore AgCl will precipitate.

$$K_{AgCl} = [\,Ag^+\,]\,[\,Cl^-\,] = 1.2 \times 10^{-10}$$

$$K_{Ag_2}\,CrO_4 = [\,Ag^+\,]^2\,\big[Cr\,O_4^{2-}\big] = 1.7 \times 10^{-12}$$

- at first point, red silver chromate is just precipitated therefore both salts are in equilibrium.

$$[\,Ag^+\,] = \frac{K_{AgCl}}{[Cl^-]} = \sqrt{\frac{K_{Ag2}O_4}{[CrO_4^{-2}]}}$$

$$\therefore\ \frac{[Cl^-]}{[CrO_4^-]^{1/2}} = \frac{K_{AgCl}}{\sqrt{K_{Ag_2}\,CrO_4}} = 9.2 \times 10^{-5}$$

- At equivalence point,

$$[Cl^-] = \sqrt{K_{AgCl}} = 1.1 \times 10^{-5} \qquad \because [Ag^+] = [Cl^-] \therefore K_{AgCl} = [Cl^-]^2$$

- If silver chromate is to precipitates at this chloride ion concentration, then,

$$[CrO_4^{2-}] = \left(\frac{Cl^-}{9.2 \times 10^{-5}}\right)^2$$

$$= 1.4 \times 10^{-2}$$

- So, a slight excess of silver nitrate solution must be added before the red colour of silver chromate is visible.

$$[Ag^+] = \left(\frac{K_{Ag2}CrO_4}{CrO_4^{2-}}\right)^{1/2} = \left(\frac{1.7 \times 10^{-12}}{1.4 \times 10^{-3}}\right)^{1/2}$$

$$= 1.1 \times 10^{-5}$$

- The titration is carried out in neutral solution or in very faintly alkaline solution within pH range 6.5 to 9.

- In acid solution, the following reaction occurs,

$$2CrO_4^{2-} + 2H^+ \rightleftharpoons 2HCrO_4^- \rightleftharpoons Cr_2O_7^- + H_2O$$

- $HCrO_4^-$ is a weak acid, so the chromate ion concentration is reduced and the solubility product of silver chromate may not be exceeded.

- The solubility product of silver chromate increases with rising temperature, the titration should be therefore performed at room temperature.

- By using a mixture of potassium chromate and dichromate in preparations to give a neutral solution, the danger of accidentally raising the pH of an unbuffered solution beyond the acceptable limits is minimised, the mixed indicator has a buffering effect, and adjusts pH of solution to 7 ± 0.1.

- In the presence of ammonium salts, the pH must not exceed 7.2 because of the effect of appreciable concentration of ammonia upon the solubility of silver salts.

Mohr's Method

Prepare indicator solution by dissolving 5 g of potassium chromate in 100 ml of water.

- 1 ml of indicator is used and concentration in actual titration is 0.005 – 0.0025.

- Dissolve 4.2 g potassium chromate and 0.7 g potassium dichromate in 100 ml and use 1 ml of this mixed indicator for titration.

- Pipette 2.5 ml of standard 0.1 mL solution of NaCl prepared by dissolving 2.922 g of salt in 500 mL water, into conical flask,

↓

Add 1 ml indicator

↓

Titrate against silver nitrate

↓

Faint reddish brown colour obtained

- $NaCl + AgNO_3 \rightarrow AgCl + Na\,NO_3$
- $Ag\,NO_3 + K_2\,CrO_4 \rightarrow Ag_2CrO_4 + 2KNO_3$
- $Ag_2CrO_4 \rightarrow$ reddish brown precipitation
- As, solubility of AgCl is less therefore AgCl precipitates first but on adding excess of $AgNO_3$ reddish brown precipitate formed.

Limitations of Mohr's Method

- Applicable to Cl^- and Br^- only and not applicable to I^- and SCN^-.
- Titration with I^- and SCN^- is not carried out because AgI and AgSCN absorb chromate ion and hence false result is obtained.
- Applied at room temperature only because change in temperature changes solubility of AgCl and Ag_2CrO_4.
- They are applied at neutral pH only, at an acidic pH the chromate ion or Ag_2CrO_4 is converted to dichromate and at alkaline pH $AgNO_3$ will precipitate out as $Ag(OH)_2$.

$$2CrO4^- + 2H^+ \rightleftharpoons 2HCrO_4 \rightleftharpoons Cr_2\,O_7^{-2} + H_2O$$

- Iodides can't be titrated by Mohr's method because of absorption phenomena and the difficulty of distinguishing the colour change of the potassium chromate.
- Eosin is a suitable absorption indicator.

Volhards Method

- This method is applied to anions which are completely precipitated by silver and are sparingly soluble in dilute nitric acid.

      Eg : Cl^-, Br^-, I^-

- Excess of $AgNO_3$ is added to solution containing free Nitric acid and residual $AgNO_3$ solution is titrated with standard thiocynate solution. This is residual titration.

- Anions whose silver salts are slightly soluble in water but which are soluble in nitric acid may be precipitated in neutral solution with an excess of $AgNO_3$ solution.

     Eg : Phosphate, arsenate, chromate, sulphide and oxalate.

- The precipitate is filtered off, washed, dissolved in dilute HNO_3 and the silver titrated with thiocyanate.

Indicator used

Ferric Alum or

Ferric Ammonium sulphate

Reaction

$$NH_4Cl + AgNO_3 \rightarrow AgCl + NH_4NO_3$$

$$AgNO_3 + NH_4SCN \rightarrow AgSCN + NH_4NO_3$$

$$NH_4SCN + Fe(NH_4)(SO_4)^2 \rightarrow Fe\ SCN + 2NH_4SO_4$$

Procedure

10 ml of NH_4Cl + 10 ml HNO_3 + 25 ml $AgNO_3$ + 5 ml Nitrobenzene $\rightarrow$ Titrate with Ammonium thiocyanate.

Use of Nitrobenzene

- According to solubility product, AgSCN will precipitate first. So, to prevent precipitation of AgSCN, the precipitate of AgCl are coagulated with nitrobenzene. Hence, $AgNO_3$ and not AgCl will be reacted with Ammonium thiocyanate and formation of AgSCN.

Use of HNO_3

- This method is applicable at acidic pH. $AgNO_3$ is insoluble with HNO_3 therefore we get full precipitation of AgCl.

- HNO_3 prevents precipitation of carbonate and the phosphate as they act as impurity.

- It also prevents hydrolysis of ferric alum, changes in temperature changes solubility, therefore colour disappears and as ferric alum at alkaline pH gives $Fe(OH)_2$.

     Applications: applied at acidic pH, Cl^-, Br^-, I^- ion at acidic conditions.

- Cl^- ion can be determined without filtering as KspAgcl < KspAgSCN

Advantages

- Applicable at acidic pH.
- Indicator gives sharp end point
- Higher concentration of indicator used to ensure formation of detectable amount of red coloured complex by excess of SCN.

Standardisation of Thiocyanate

Preparation

- 8.5 g of Ammonium thiocyanate or 10.5 g of potassium thiocyanate and dissolve in 1 litre of water.

Standardization

- 0.1 M silver nitrate + 25 ml in 250 ml conical flask + 5 ml of 6 M nitric acid + 1 ml of iron indicator.

Titrate against thiocyanate

White precipitation produced, milky appearance of liquid and after adding few drops of thiocyanate, reddish brown precipitate forms.

At end point precipitation is flocculent.

Formation of a Soluble Coloured Compound

- This procedure is exemplified by Volhard's method for the titration of silver in the presence of free nitric acid with standard potassium thiocyanate or ammonium thiocyanate solution.
- The indicator is a solution of iron (III) nitrate or iron (III) ammonium sulphate.
- The addition of thiocyanate solution produces first a precipitation of silver thiocyanate.

$$Ag^+ + SCN^- \rightleftharpoons AgSCN$$

- When reaction is complete, the slightest excess of thiocyanate produces a reddish brown coloration, due to the formation of a complex ion.

$$Fe^{+3} + SCN^- \rightleftharpoons [FeSCN]^{2+}$$

- This method may be applied to the determination of chlorides, bromides and iodides in acid solution.

- Excess of standard silver nitrate solution is added, and the excess is back-titrated with standard thiocyanate solution.

- For the chloride estimation, we have the following two equilibria during the titration of excess of silver ions.

$$Ag^+ + Cl^- \rightleftharpoons AgCl$$

$$Ag^+ + SCN^- \rightleftharpoons AgSCN$$

- The two sparingly soluble salts will be in equilibrium with the solution, hence

$$\frac{[Cl^-]}{[SCN^-]} = \frac{K_{AgCl}}{K_{AgSCN}} = \frac{1.2 \times 10^{-10}}{7.1 \times 10^{-13}} = 169$$

- When the excess of silver has reacted, the thiocyanate may react with the AgCl since silver thiocyanate is the less soluble salt, until ratio $\dfrac{[Cl^-]}{[SCN^-]}$ in the solution.

$$AgCl^+ \ SCN^- \rightleftharpoons AgSCN \ \vert \ Cl^-$$

- The NaCl is filtered off before back titrating. Since at this stage the precipitation will be contaminated with absorbed silver ions, the suspension should be boiled for a few minutes to coagulate the silver chloride and thus remove most of the absorbed silver ions from its surface before titration. The cold filtrate is titrated.

- After the addition of silver nitrate, potassium nitrate is added as coagulant, the suspension is boiled for about 3 minutes, cooled and then titrated immediately.

- Desorption of Ag^+ occurs and on cooling readsorption is largely prevented by the presence of potassium nitrate.

- An immiscible liquid is added to 'coat' AgCl particles and thereby protect them for interaction with the thiocyanate.

- The most successful liquid is nitrobenzene. The suspension is well shaken to coagulate the precipitate before back titration.

$$\frac{[Br^-]}{[SCN^-]} = \frac{KAgBr}{KAgSCN} = \frac{3.5 \times 10^{-13}}{7.1 \times 10^{-13}} = 0.5$$

Use of Adsorption indicators.

Turbidity Method.

Gay-Lussac's Method

- The fact that occurrence of turbidity accompanies precipitation reaction is made use of in this method.

- After the equivalence, the precipitation reaction ceases and addition of an extra drop will not result in turbidity.

- The procedure may be exemplified by the titration of $AgNO_3$ with standard NaCl in the presence of free nitric acid and a small quantity of pure barium nitrate (to assist the process of coagulation).

- Weigh out accurately 0.4 g of silver nitrate in well stoppered bottle.

- Add about 100 ml of water, a few drops of concentration nitric acid and a small crystal of barium nitrate.

- Titrate with standard 0.1 M sodium chloride by adding 20 ml at once, stoppering the bottle and shaking vigorously until the precipitation of silver chloride has coagulated and settled leaving a clear solution.

- Still the silver ions are in excess.

- Continue to add NaCl solution, 1 ml at each time, stoppering and shaking after each addition till not turbidity is produced.

- Note the volume of NaCl consumed; consider it as pilot reading.

- Repeat the titration, add 1 ml less than the pilot reading initially and continue adding 0.02 ml after that.

- The end point is determined with the help of a Nephelo-turbidimetric method.

Mercurometric Methods

Titration using Mercuric nitrate

- Mercury ions are used as precipitates. Such titrations are not strictly of precipitation type.

- Although, these offer no advantages over the more common argentometric titration, mercurometric titrations can be regarded as an alternative method for the determination of chlorides, bromides, thiocyanates and cyanides.

- In these titrations diphenyl carbazone or a mixture of diphenyl carbazone and bromophenol blue can be used as indicator.

- At equivalence point the yellow colour of the solution becomes blue violet due to reaction of the excess of mercury ions with diphenyl carbazone.

- owing to their stability to react with diphenyl carbazone, complete absence of chromate and iron ions is a necessity, whereas other ions like Mg, Al, Mn, Zn, fluoride, sulphate, nitrate, acetate don't interfere at low concentration.

- The fact that in mercurometric titrations can be applied to diluted solution is the only possible upper edge they have over argentometric titrations.

- The end point obtained by mercurometry is not very sharp in aq. solution and hence it is advantageous to use 80% ethanolic medium.

(i) Preparation and standardization of Mercury nitrate solution (0.1 M)

- Dissolve 17 g of mercuric nitrate in 800 ml distilled water + 20 ml of 2M Nitric acid.

- Dilute to 1 litre which gives 0.1N solution.

- This is standardized in a process similar to that of $AgNO_3$ using diphenyl carbazone or mixture of diphenyl carbazone and bromophenol blue as indicator.

(ii) Diphenyl Carbazone mixture indicator

- Dissolve 0.1 g of Diphenyl carbazone in 100 ml water, to get indicator D.C.

- Mix 0.5 g diphenyl carbozone + 0.5 g bromophenol blue in 100 ml of 95% ethanol. We get mixed indicator.

Adsorption Indicator : Fajan's Method

- An Adsorption indicator is an organic compound that tends to be adsorbed onto the surface of the solid in the precipitation titration.

- Ideally, the adsorption occurs at equivalence point and results not only in a colour change but also in a transfer of colour from solid to solution or reverse.

  Eg: Fluorescein

- It is a typical adsorption indicator, used for titration of chloride ion with silver nitrate.

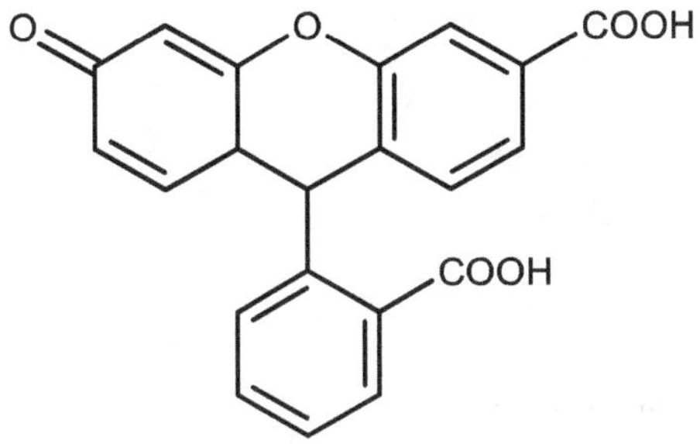

Fluorescein

(Used in various disease of retina, study of circulation in retina)

- In aqueous solution fluorescein partially dissociates into hydronium ions and negatively charged flouresceinate ions that are yellow-green.

- The fluoresceinate ion forms an intensely red salt of silver.

- Whenever this dye is used as indicator, its concentration is not large enough to precipitate as silver fluoresceinate.

- Titration of Cl^- with $AgNO_3$, the colloidal silver chloride particles are negatively charged because of adsorption of excess of chloride ion.

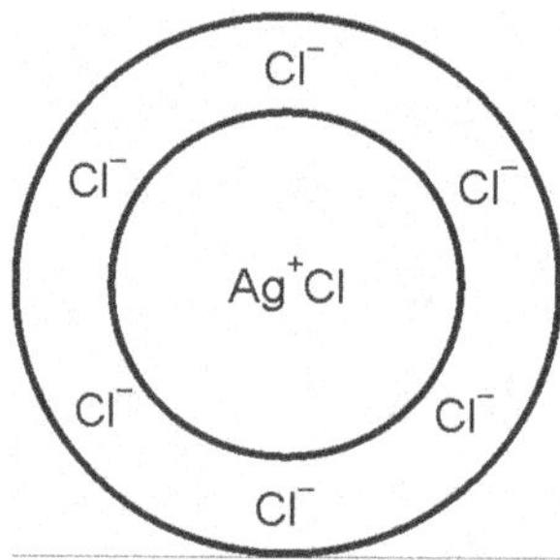

Fig. 9.2

- The dye anions repelled from this surface by electrostatic force and impart yellow-green colour to the solution.

- Beyond the end point, the silver chloride ions adsorb the silver ions thereby aquire a positive charge.

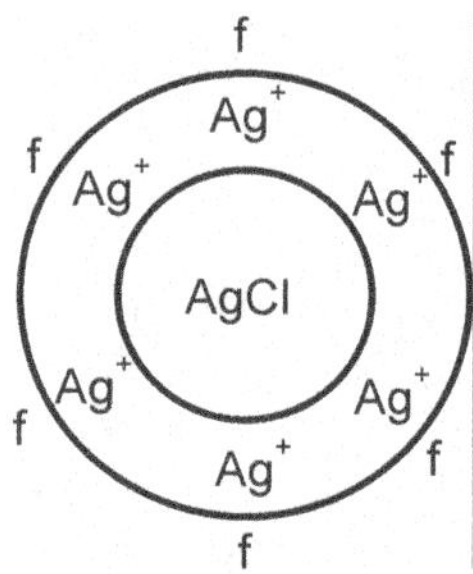

Fig. 9.3

- Fluoresceinate ions are now attracted into the counter-ion layer that surrounds the colloidal AgCl particle.

- The net result is the appearance of red colour of silver fluoresceinate in the surface layer of the solution.

- The adsorption is reversible, the dye being desorbed on back-titration with chloride ion.
- Titration involving adsorption indicators are
  - rapid
  - accurate
  - reliable

but applicable to limited reactions where colloidal precipitations are formed rapidly.

Indicator Solutions

Fluorescein – Dissolve 0.2 g of fluorescein in 100 ml of 70% ethanol or dissolve 0.2 g sodium fluoresceinate in 100 ml of water.

Procedure: Take 25 ml of standard 0.1 M NaCl in 250 ml conical flask

$\downarrow$

Add 10 drops of fluorescein indicator

$\downarrow$

Titrate against $AgNO_3$

$\downarrow$

Pink Colour

$\downarrow$

Add excess $AgNO_3$

$\downarrow$

Red Colour

Adsorption Indicators

Working

At the equivalence point, they are adsorbed by the precipitate and become changed, producing a new colour.

Conditions

- The precipitate should separate ideally in the colloidal condition.
- Coagulation should be avoided.
- The titration solution must be at a suitable pH for the indicator to be predominantly in the ionic form.
- Titration should be carried out in subdued light.

Indicator	Use	Colour Change	Expected conditions
1. Fluorescein	Cl^-, Br^-, I^- with Ag^+	Yellow green $\to$ pink	Neutal or weekly basic
2. Dichloro fluorescein	Cl^-, Br^- with Ag^+	Yellow green $\to$ red	pH range 4.4 to 7
3. Eosin (Tetrabromo fluorescein	Br^-, I^- with Ag^+	Pink $\to$ red violet	Best in ethanoic acid solution
4. Tartrazine	Ag^+ with I^- or SCN^-, $I^- + Cl^-$, excess Ag^+, back titration with I^-	Colourless $\to$ Green sol.	Sharp colour change in $I^- + Cl^-$, back titration

Examples

1. Solution product of $Mg(OH)_2$ is 3.4×10^{-11} mole^3/l. Calculate solution product in g/litre

   M.W of $Mg(OH)_2 = 58.3$

Sol:

$$Mg(OH)_2 \to Mg^{+2} + 2OH^-$$

$$Ksp = [Mg^{+2}][OH^-]^2$$

$$= [S][2s]^2$$

$$= 4s^3$$

$$4s^3 = 3.4 \times 10^{-11}$$

$$S^3 = \frac{3.4 \times 10^{-11}}{4}$$

$$S^3 = 0.85 \times 10^{-11}$$

$$= 8.5 \times 10^{-12}$$

$$S = 2.04 \times 10^{-4} \text{ mole/l}$$

Now to find in g/litre

$\therefore$ multiply by M.W

$$S = 2.04 \times 10^{-4} \times 58.3 = 118.932 \times 10^{-4}$$

$$= 1.18 \times 10^{-2} = 1.2 \times 10^{-2} \text{ gm/litre}$$

2. Will Ca^{+2} give precipitation on mixing the equal volume of 0.02 molar $CaCl_2$ and 0.04 molar Na_2SO_4 per litre of solution.

$$Ksp\, CaSO_4 \rightarrow 2.4 \times 10^{-5}$$

Sol: $CaCl_2 + Na_2SO_4 \rightarrow CaSO_4 + 2NaCl$

(0.01M)   (0.02 M)

$$CaSO_4 \rightarrow Ca^{+2} + SO_4^{-2}$$

(0.01)   (0.02)

$$I_{cp} = 2 \times 10^{-4}$$

$$Ksp = 2.4 \times 10^{-5}$$

$\therefore$ super sat. sol. as $I_{cp} > Ksp$.

$\therefore$ precipitation of $CaSO_4$ is formed

3. Calculate the concentration of $SO4^{-2}$ in 500 ml of saturated solution of Ag_2SO_4
M.wt = 311.76

$$Ksp = 1.74 \times 10^{-5}$$

Sol:

$$Ag_2SO_4 \rightarrow 2Ag^+ + SO_4^{-2}$$

$$Ksp = [Ag^+]^2 \ [SO_4^{-2}]$$

$$= [2s]^2 \ [s] = 4s^3$$

$$4s^3 = 1.74 \times 10^{-5}$$

$$S^3 = \frac{17.4}{4} \times 10^{-6} = 4.35 \times 10^{-6}$$

$$S = 1.63 \times 10^{-2} \text{ mole/litre}$$

To find in gm/500 ml $\therefore$ multiply by $\dfrac{mw}{2}$

$$\therefore S = 1.63 \times 10^{-2} \times \frac{311.76}{2} = 254.08 \times 10^{-2}$$

$$= 2.54 \text{ gm/500ml}$$

4. Calculate the solution Ag_2CrO_4 in 0.001 M $AgNO_3$ and 0.01 M of K_2CrO_4 solution.

Ksp $Ag_2CrO_4 = 1.7 \times 10^{-12}$

Sol:

$$2AgNO_3 + K_2CrO_4 \rightarrow 2KNO_3 + Ag_2CrO_4$$

(0.01)   (0.02)

$$Ag_2CrO_4\ 2Ag^+ + CrO_4^{-2}$$

$$\therefore Ksp = 4s^3$$

$$4S^3 = 1.7 \times 10^{-12}$$

$$S^3 = \frac{1.7}{4} \times 10^{-12} = 0.425 \times 10^{-12}$$

$$S = 0.751 \times 10^{-4}$$

$$S = 7.51 \times 10^{-5} \text{ mole/litre}$$

If given concentration of $AgNO_3$ then

$$Ksp = [Ag^+]^2\,[CrO_4^{-2}]$$

$$[CrO_4^{-2}] = \frac{Ksp}{[Ag^+]^2} = \frac{1.7 \times 10^{-12}}{10^{-6}}$$

$$= 1.7 \times 10^{-6} \text{ mole/litre}$$

If given concentration of K_2CrO_4 then

$$[Ag^+]^2 = \frac{Ksp}{CrO_4^{-2}} = \frac{1.7 \times 10^{-12}}{0.01} = 1.7 \times 10^{-10}$$

$$= 1.30 \times 10^{-5} \text{ mole/litre}$$

CHAPTER 10

FUNCTIONAL GROUP ANALYSIS

Introduction

A number of organic compounds contain one or several functional groups such as amino, hydroxyl, aldehyde, keto, carboxylic acid, esters, phenolic and sulphonamide. The above mentioned groups may be present in aliphatic, aromatic, cyclic, polynuclear or heterocyclic systems. The analysis of functional groups for quantitative determinations is very vast. In some cases it is very simple and in other cases it is highly complicated. A good number of methods based on chemical reactions of functional groups can be used for their estimations.

To be useful in quantitative analysis, a reaction must meet the following requirements:

1. It must give a quantitative yield of product of known composition.
2. It must be specified for a given group, ion or radical.
3. The extent to which the reaction takes place must be determinable by measuring either the quantity of the reagent employed in its formation on the quantity of the product produced.
4. It must proceed with reasonable rapidity under easily achievable laboratory conditions.

In this chapter, some simple and routinely adapted methods which are commonly used for estimation are discussed.

Determination of Amino Group

There are four methods which can be employed for the estimation of amino group. They are as follows :

1. Acetylation method

2. Bromination method

3. Titration in aqueous or non-aqueous media

4. Determination of equivalent weight of amine by conversion to picrate and its titration in non-aqueous media.

1. Acetylation Method

Generally amines undergo acetylation reaction in presence of excess of acetic anhydride in pyridine at room temperature. The excess of acetic anhydride is decomposed with water and the acetic acid generated is determined by titration with a standard solution of alkali. Simultaneously a blank determination is also performed. The difference between the two readings gives the quantity of acetylating agent consumed by amine. The chemical reactions in this process can be written as follows

$$RNH_2 + (CH_3CO)_2O \rightarrow RNHCOCH_3 + CH_3COOH$$

$$R_2NH + (CH_3CO)_2O \rightarrow R_2NCOCH_3 + CH_3COOH$$

In the reaction the amine is kept in contact with acetylating agent for about 30 minutes at room temperature. In general double the quantity of acetylating agent is added than theoretically required. The experimental conditions may vary from one amine to another one. Some amines may require longer time for acetylation than others. If substituent groups like nitro-methyl or halogen are present then amino group may undergo diacetylation. At higher temperatures, there is a danger of deacetylation and that is why acetylation is performed at room temperature only. A large number of $1°$ and $2°$ aliphatic, aromatic and heterocyclic amines are determined by this method of acetylation.

2. Bromination Method

Bromination method is generally applicable to primary aromatic amines. In this particular method the amine under investigation is treated with excess of brominating reagent (standard $KBrO_3 - KBr$ solution) in presence of hydrochloric acid. The bromine liberated in this reaction causes bromination of the amine. The excess bromine is then allowed to react with excess of KI solution, where by an equivalent amount of iodine liberated. The liberated iodine is titrated with standard solution of sodium thiosulfate employing starch mucilage as indicator. A blank is also performed simultaneously. The difference between the two readings gives the amount of bromine consumed by the amine.

The reaction may be represented as follows by taking the example of aniline (primary aromatic amine).

$$KB_rO_3 + 5KBr + 6HCl \rightarrow 3Br_2 + 6KCl + 3H_2O$$

$$\text{C}_6\text{H}_5\text{-NH}_2 + 3\text{Br}_2 \longrightarrow \text{(2,4,6-tribromoaniline)}$$

$$\text{Excess of Br}_2 + 2\text{KI} \rightarrow \text{I}_2 + 2\text{KBr}$$

$$\text{I}_2 + 2\text{Na}_2\text{S}_2\text{O}_3 \rightarrow \text{Na}_2\text{S}_4\text{O}_6 + 2\text{NaI}$$

3. Titration in Aqueous and Non–aqueous Media

Amines can be titrated directly as bases in aqueous or non-aqueous media. The amines which are water-soluble, having the dissociation constant more than 10^{-6} can be titrated directly with standard acid using a suitable mixed indicator (methanolic solutions of 0.1% methyl red and 0.1% bromocresol green in the ratio of 1:5). Alternatively, the end-point can also be determined potentiometrically.

The amines which are weakly basic connot be estimated in aqueous medium. The basic nature of such weakly basic amines can be enhanced by using non-aqueous solvents like glacial acetic acid or dioxane. These substances are dissolved in glacial acetic acid and titrated with acetous perchloric acid using a suitable indicator like crystal violet or α-naphthol benzein. In Indian pharmacopoeia, a large number of drugs, which are weakly basic in nature, are analysed by this non-aqueous titration.

4. Determination of Equivalent Weight of Amine by Picrate Method

Picric acid reacts with several amines to form crystalline picrates. The picrates so obtained are separated, dried, dissolved in glacial acetic acid and titrated against acetous perchloric acid using visual indicator or potentiometric method to locate the end-point. The reaction involved can be represented as follows

The equivalent weight (EW) of the amine picrate and thus amine can be calculated by the formula

$$EW = \frac{\text{weight of picrate in grams} \times 1000}{\text{volume of acetous perchloric acid} \times \text{normality}}$$

Experimental Procedure

Determination of Amine by Acetylation

Introduce a weighted sample containing about 2 ml equivalent of amine into a glass stoppered iodine flask and dissolve in 10 ml of pyridine. Add 10 ml of acetate anhydride pyridine reagent and stopper the flask. Set the flask aside for 30 minutes with occasional agitate. Add about 10 ml of water and mix the contents. Rinse the sides of the flask and stopper with 10-15 ml in butanol. Titrate the contents of the flask with standard alcoholic sodium hydroxide solution (0.5 N) using mixed indicator and note the reading of titrant (A). Following the same procedure simultaneously within sample (blank) perform titration and note the reading (B).

$$\% \text{ of Amino group} = \frac{(B - A) \times 16.03 \times 500}{\omega \times 1000}$$

Where

    B = volume of alkali required for blank

    A = volume of alkali required for sample

    N = normality of alkali solution

    ω = weight of sample taken in grams

Primary aromatic amino group can be determined quantitatively by titrating with sodium nitrite solution.

Determination of Hydroxyl Group

The behaviour of the hydroxyl group varies depending on the molecule to which it is attached. On aliphatic chain (ROH), the hydroxyl group contributes to the molecule, the chemical characteristics attributed to alcohols. A compound with a hydroxyl group on a carbon containing a double-bond $RCH = CH$ classed as an enol. If there

$$\overset{\displaystyle \|}{\underset{\displaystyle OH}{}}$$

are hydroxyl groups on adjacent carbon atoms, $RCH - CR$, these are classified as glycols.

$$\underset{\displaystyle OH \quad OH}{|\quad\quad\|}$$

Hydroxyl groups on aromatic rings yield the properties/characteristics of phenols. Thus we have hydroxyl groups in different situations, each exhibiting a different set of characteristics.

The hydroxyl group present in a compound (alcohol) can be determined by the following methods :

1. Acetylation method

2. Phthalation method

3. Oxidation method

1. *Acetylation Method*

In this method, the sample (alcohol) is treated with excess anhydride pyridine reagent. The hydrogen of hydroxyl group is replaced by acetyl group. The excess of the reagent is then treated with water whereby acetic anhydride is converted to acetic acid. This acetic acid is then titrated with standard solution of an alkali. A blank determination is also performed simultaneously. The difference between the two readings gives the amount of acetylating agent consumed by alcohol. The reactions involved can be summarised as follows

$$R(OH)n + n(CH_3CO)_2O \rightarrow R(OCOCH_3)n + nCH_3COOH$$

$$(CH_3CO)_2O + H_2O \rightarrow 2CH_3COOH$$

$$CH_3COOH + NaOH \rightarrow CH_3COONa + H_2O$$

In the acetylation of alcoholic group pyridine acts as solvent and also as catalyst.

2. *Phthalation Method*

In this method, the reagent used is phthalic anhydride and the process is almost similar to acetylation. The reaction can be represented as follows :

R-OH+
C
C
O
COOH
COOR

The process of phthalation is slower when compared to acetylation and therefore a large excess of phthalic anhydride reagent is required for completion of reaction.

3. *Oxidation Method*

Oxidation with periodates is used in the case of polyhydric alcohol containing adjacent hydroxyl groups as in glycols, mannitol etc. The hydroxyl groups on adjacent carbon atoms are oxidised by excess of periodic acid or its salts. The general reaction can be represented as follows

$$-\overset{|}{C}-\overset{|}{C}- H_5IO_6 \rightarrow -\overset{\|}{\underset{O}{C}}-\overset{\|}{\underset{O}{C}}- + HIO_3 + 3H_2O$$

$$\underset{OH\ OH}{}$$

This reaction is known as "Malaprade" reaction. The various groups attached to the carbon bearing the hydroxyl group has a lot of influence on the reaction. The reaction with ethylene glycol and glycerol can be written as follows :

1.

$$CH_2 - CH_2 + H_5IO_6 \quad 2HCHO + HIO_3 + 3H_2O$$
$$\quad | \qquad |$$
$$\quad OH \quad\; OH$$

2.

$$CH_2 - CH - CH_2 + 2H_5IO_6 \quad 2HCHO + HCOOH + 2HIO_3 + 5H_2O$$
$$\quad | \qquad | \qquad |$$
$$\quad OH \quad\; OH \quad OH$$

Oxidation with periodic acid is employed in the N.F. for the assay of mannitol. In the analytical procedure 1 mole of manitol is oxidised to produce 2 moles of HCHO and 4 moles of HCOOH.

$$
\begin{array}{l}
CH_2OH \\
| \\
HOCH \\
| \\
HO\!-\!CH \\
| \\
HCOH \\
| \\
HCOH \\
| \\
CH_2OH \\
\text{Mannitol}
\end{array}
\quad + 5KIO_4 \quad \longrightarrow \quad 2HCHO + 4HCOOH + 5HIO_3 + H_2O
$$

The following procedure is employed for this purpose.

Transfer about 200 mg of mannitol to a 250 ml volumetric flask. Dissolve it in water and dilute to volume. Transfer 5 ml of the solution to a 250 ml iodine flask, add 50 ml of potassium periodate reagent (prepared by mixing 40 ml of sulphuric acid [1 in 20] with 60 ml of potassium periodate solution [1 in 1000] acidified with 3 to 5 drops of sulphuric acid). Heat the solution on a steam bath for 15 minutes. Cool to room temperature and add 1 gm of potassium iodide. Allow the flask to stand for 5 minutes, add starch indicator and titrate the solution with 0.02N sodium thiosulphate. Perform a blank determination, using water instead of mannitol solution. The difference in the titration values of the blank and the sample results from change in the periodate concentration due to oxidation of the mannitol. Each ml of 0.02 N sodium thiosulphate consumed in the titration is equivalent to 0.364 mg of mannitol ($C_6H_{14}O_6$).

Determination of Hydroxyl Groups in Phenols

The phenolic hydroxyl group can be determined by the following methods :

1. Non-aqueous titrimetric method

2. Acetylation method

3. Bromination method

1. *Non-aqueous Titrimetic Method*

Phenols are weakly acidic in nature. They can be titrated in non-aqueous media using basic solvent like ethylenediamine, dimethyl formamide or n-butylamine which enhances the acidity of phenols. Phenols in these solvents can be determined by titrating with standard sodium methoxide or potassium methoxide solution in benzene-methanol, using visual indicators or potentiometry for detection of end-point.

2. *Acetylation Method*

The basic concepts of acetylation method is similar to as described for acetylation of hydroxyl group in alcohols. The phenols when treated with acetylating agent undergo acetylation and excess of acetylating reagent is determined by titration with standard alkali solution. The reactions involved can be summarised as follows :

$$C_6H_5OH + (CH_3CO)_2O \longrightarrow C_6H_5OCOCH_3 + CH_3COOH$$

$$(CH_3CO)_2O + H_2O \rightarrow 2CH_3COOH$$

$$CH_3COOH + NaOH \rightarrow CH_3COONa + H_2O$$

3. *Bromination Method*

In bromination method, the sample is treated with $KBrO_3 - KBr$ solution under acidic conditions. The bromine liberated brominates the phenol and excess of bromine is determined by adding excess of potassium iodide solution. By this an equivalent amount of iodine is liberated which is determined by titrating with standard sodium thiosulphate solution. The reactions involved can be summarized as follows

$$KBrO_3 + 5KBr + 6HCl \rightarrow 3Br_2 + 6KCl + 3H_2O$$

$$\text{Excess of } Br_2 + 2KI \rightarrow I_2 + 2KBr$$

$$I_2 + 2Na_2S_2O_3 \rightarrow 2NaI + Na_2S_4O_6$$

Experimental Procedure

Acetylation Method

Accurately weigh about 1 to 2.5 milli quivalent of the phenolic sample and transfer to an iodine flask and add 3 ml of acetylating reagent. Insert the stopper. Heat the flask on steam bath for about 45 minutes. Add around 5-10 ml of water. Mix the contents and heat on a water bath for 2-3 minutes. Cool in ice water and rinse the stopper and walls of the flasks with about 10 ml of *n*-butanol and titrate with 0.5 N alcoholic sodium hydroxide solution using mixed indicator and note down the reading (A). Carry out a second titration using same quantities of reagents following same procedure simultaneously without sample and note the reading (B). The difference between two readings of standard alkali used corresponds to the phenol which has reacted.

The percentage of phenolic hydroxyl group can be calculated by the formula given below

$$\text{Percentage of phenolic OH group} = \frac{(B-A) \times 17.01 \times 100}{\omega \times 1000}$$

Where

B = volume of alkali used for blank

A = volume of alkali used for sample

N = normality of sodium hydroxide used

ω = weight of sample in grams.

Determination of Carboxyl Group

Carboxylic acids are generally moderately strong acids. The carboxylic group can be conveniently estimated by the following methods :

1. Direct aqueous titration method
2. Non-aqueous titrimetric method
3. Iodometric method

1. *Direction Aqueous Titration Method*

Water soluble carboxylic acids are determined by direct titration with standard solution of an alkali such as sodium hydroxide, potassium hydroxide, barium hydroxide using a suitable indicator like phenolphthalein. The titration of carboxylic acid with alkali is a neutralization reaction. During the titration process the salt produced undergoes hydrolysis and the resulting solution will be slightly alkaline in reaction with pH value above 7.0. Many of the carboxylic acids are neutralized at pH 8.4 and therefore the suitable indicator is phenolphthalein (pH range 8.0-10.0). In addition to phenolphthalein other indicators with alkaline pH ranges like thymol blue and thymolphthalein are used. The general reaction can be represented as follows

$$RCOOH + MOH \rightarrow RCOOM + H_2O$$

(where M = Na or K or Ba/2)

The carboxylic acid like benzoic acid or salicyclic acid are insoluble in water. So they can be titrated with standard alkali using a suitable indicator after dissolving the sample in neutral methanol or ethanol.

2. *Non-Aqueous Titrimetric Method*

Non-aqueous titrimetric method is used for the carboxylic acids which are either insoluble in water or which do not give sharp end point in water or hydro alcoholic solutions. In this method, the sample is dissolved in solvents like acetonitrile, dimethylformamide or phridine and titrated with a solution of sodium of potassium methoxide using a suitable indicator (Thymol blue, azo violet or *o*-nitroaniline).

3. *Iodometric Method*

When a solution of carboxylic acid is treated with a solution of mixture of KIO_3 and KI, an equivalent amount of iodine is liberated. The liberated iodine is estimated by titration with standard solution of sodium thiosulphate using starch indicator.

$$KIO_3 + 5KI + 6H^- \rightarrow 3I_2 + 3H_2O$$

Determination of Aldehydes and Ketones

Both aldehydes and ketones contain the carbonyl group (C = O) therefore, both undergo a number of similar reactions. Although aldehydes and ketones resemble closely each other in structure and in their chemical reactions, they may be distinguished by the relative ease with which aldehydes are oxidised to acids. The silver mirror formed when an aldehyde is treated with ammonical silver nitrate is not characteristic of ketones. This test has been widely used to distinguish between these two classes of compounds and to determine aldehydes in the presence of ketones.

Aldehydes and ketones can be determined by using the following reagents:

1. 2, 4-Dinitrophenyl hydrazine
2. Sodium bisulfite
3. Hydroxylamine hydrochloride-pyridine

1. 2, 4 Dintrophenyl Hydrazine

The reaction between carbonyl compounds and hydrazines has been employed for their analysis. It has been found that an excess of the hydrazine and higher than reflux temperatures may help in obtaining result, close to quantitative yields. The cause of the reaction can be measured by weighing the hydrazone produced. In general, the most widely used hydrazine is 2, 4-dinitophenyl hydrazine (2, 4-DNP).

2. Sodium Bisulfite

Aldehydes, methyl ketones can be analysed by their reaction with sodium bisulfite.

The above obtained bisulfite addition products are not determined gravimetrically. Instead, the quantity of bisulfite ion entering into the reaction is measured. In the reaction a measured excess of the bisulfite solution is employed, and the excess reagent is determined by its reaction with an excess of iodine (Iodometry).

$$NaHSO_3 + I_2 + H_2O \rightarrow NaHSO_4 + 2HI$$

$$I_2 + 2Na_2S_2O_3 \rightarrow 2NaI + Na_2S_4O_6$$

Another procedure utilizes sodium sulphate instead of sodium bisulfite. Here the same bisulfite addition product is obtained, but a slightly different chemical reaction occurs.

$$R - \overset{\overset{\displaystyle H}{|}}{C} = O + Na_2SO_3 \longrightarrow R - \underset{\underset{\displaystyle SO_3Na}{|}}{\overset{\overset{\displaystyle H}{|}}{C}} - OH + NaOH$$

Each milliequivalent of aldehyde reacting with sodium sulfite produces a milliequivalent of sodium hydroxide, which may be determined by direct titration with an acid. The end-point is determined potentiometrically.

3. *Hydroxylamine Hydrochloride-Pyridine*

Reaction of aldehydes or ketones with hydroxyl amine results in the formation of oximes. If proper conditions are present, the reaction will be quantitative. Although oximes are insoluble in dilute acids or in aqueous solutions, they are not usually quantitatively precipitated and therefore cannot be determined gravimetrically. The reaction is determined by titration of the liberated hydrochloric acid or by measuring the excess of hydroxylamine employed. The former is simpler and more frequently used. This method is employed for the assay of benzaldehyde in U.S.P.

$$\text{C}_6\text{H}_5-CHO + NH_2OH.HCl \longrightarrow \text{C}_6\text{H}_5-CH = NOH + H_2O + HCl^-$$

$$HCl + NaOH \rightarrow NaCl + H_2O$$

In this titration to locate the end-point, the best indicator is bromophenol blue.

Determination of Esters of Carboxylic Acids

A large number of derivatives of carboxylic acid are used in modern therapy. While most of these are esters of carboxylic acid. All these compounds undergo hydrolysis, forming the parent acid or its salt. In most cases, this reaction can be employed in their analytical determination.

Most esters are hydrolysed by water to form acids and alcohols. The rate of the reaction is increased at elevated temperatures and by the use of an acid or base catalyst.

When a base is employed it not only catalyses the reaction but also reacts quantitatively with the acid produced to give the corresponding salt.

$$R-\overset{\overset{\displaystyle O}{\|}}{C}-OC_2H_5 + NaOH \longrightarrow R-\overset{\overset{\displaystyle O}{\|}}{C}-+O^-Na^+ + C_2H_5OH$$

This reaction of the formed acid with the basic catalyst may be used to measure the extent of the hydrolysis and thereby determine the quantity of ester being hydrolysed. If a known volume of standardised base is employed as the catalyst for the hydrolysis of a weighed sample of ester, the quantity of base remaining after hydrolysis may be determined by titration with standard acid. Simultaneously a blank is also performed. The difference between the two readings represents the base consumed by ester.

If methyl paraben is hydrolysed in basic medium, each mole of ester in the reaction will utilise 1 equivalent of sodium hydroxide. Thus each ml of 1 N alkali employed in the reaction is equivalent to 1 millimole of methyl paraben.

$$HO-\langle\bigcirc\rangle-\overset{\overset{\displaystyle O}{\|}}{C}-OCH_3 + NaOH \longrightarrow HO$$

$$-\langle\bigcirc\rangle-\overset{\overset{\displaystyle O}{\|}}{C}-O-Na^+ + CH_3OH$$

The above reaction is employed for the assay of methyl paraben in U.S.P.

Determination of Salts of Amines and Salts of Carboxylic Acids

1. Determination of Salts of Amines

For the determination of slats of amines two methods are generally followed. One method is aqueous titration and the second one is non-aqueous titration.

If the salt of the amine is strongly acidic in nature, then it is dissolved in water and titrated with standard solution of alkali using phenolphthalein as indicator.

$$RNH_2\,HCl = RNH_2 + HCl$$

$$HCl + NaOH \rightarrow NaCl + H_2O$$

Several drugs are used in the form of halide salts which cannot be titrated satisfactorily in water. They can be successfully titrated in non-aqueous media.

The halide ions like chloride, bromide and iodide are too weakly basic to react quantitatively with acetous perchloric acid. Addition of mercuric acetate to halide salt replaces the halide by an equivalent quantum of acetate ion which is a strong base in acetic acid.

$$2RNH_2\,HCl = 2RNH_3^+ + 2Cl^-$$

$$(CH_3COO)_2\,Hg + 2Cl^- \rightarrow HgCl_2 + 2CH_3COO^-$$

$$2CH_3COOH_2^+ + 2CH_3COO^- \rightarrow 4CH_3COOH$$

(onium ion)

The drugs estimated using the above method includes chloroproguanil hydrochloride, lignocan, hydrochloride, ephedrine hydrochloride etc.

2. *Determination of Salts of Carboxylic Acid*

Non-aqueous titrimetric method is widely employed for the determination of slats of carboxylic acids. The salt of a carboxylic acid when dissolved in acetic acid behaves as a strong base and this can be titrated with acetous perchloric acid.

$$HClO_4 + CH_3COOH \rightarrow CH_3COOH_2^+ + ClO_4^-$$

$$RCOOM \rightarrow RCOO^- + M^+$$

$$CH_3COOH_2^+ + RCOO^- \rightarrow CH_3COOH + R-COOH$$

In Indian Pharmacopoeia for some of the compounds like sodium acetate, sodium benzoate and sodium citrate, this method is recommended.

Determination of Nitro and Azo Groups

The nitro of azo group can be determined by using titanous chloride or titanous sulphate solutions. These reagents quantitatively reduce the above groups. For quantitative analysis, depending on solubility, the sample is dissolved in water or alcohol or glacial acetic acid. In general excess of titanous chloride or titanous sulphate is added and refluxed for a specified period of time. The unreacted titanous salt solution is back titrated with standard solution of ferric ammonium sulphate using ammonium thiocyanate as indicator. A blank determination is also performed. The difference between the two readings is used to calculate the content of nitro or azo group.

Determination of Unsaturation

The chemical reactions of olefinic and acetylenic groups may be utilised for the analysis of unsaturated compounds. The methods used for the determination of unsaturation includes :

1. The addition of halogen

2. Hydrogenation

1. The Addition of Halogen

Both bromine and chlorine readily add to the non-aromatic multiple bonds of unsaturated compounds. Since chlorine is a gas and is often too reactive, it is not usually employed in an analytical determination. Although iodine does not add directly to multiple bonds, it will add rapidly in a solution of iodine monochloride or iodine monobromide.

The analytical procedure is best carried out by treating a weighed sample of the unsaturated compound with a measured excess of iodine monobromide solution and allowing the reaction to proceed for the prescribed period of time. The reaction mixture is then treated with potassium iodide. The excess iodine monobromide reacts with the iodide to liberate iodine, which may be determined by titration with sodium thiosulphate (A).

$$IBr + KI \rightarrow I_2 + KBr$$

At the same time perform a blank also (B). The difference between the millilitres of thiosulfate reacting with the blank and those reacting with the sample is equivalent to the millitres of iodine monobromide solution reacted with the sample. If 1 N iodine monobromide solution is used and the molecular weight of the compound and the number of double bonds are known, the percentage of the compound present can be determined, using the formula.

$$\frac{(B-A) \times \text{mol. wt. of sample} \times 100}{\text{weight of sample} \times 2000 \times \text{no. of double bonds}}$$

Since most fried oils and fats contain unsaturated glyceryl esters, this procedure provides a satisfactory method for assuming their purity and in detecting their adulteration.

2. *Hydrogenation*

Hydrogen in the presence of the proper metal catalysts will add to multiple bonds quantitatively to form the corresponding saturated compound. This reaction will take place at room temperature and at approximate atmospheric pressure.

$$\overset{\overset{\displaystyle H}{|}}{R-C}=\overset{\overset{\displaystyle H}{|}}{C}-R' + H_2 \overset{Ni}{\longrightarrow} R-CH_2-CH_2+R$$

A measurement of the hydrogen employed in the reaction may be used to determine the quantity of unsaturated compounds. Hydrogenation offers an excellent method for determining unsaturated compounds. In many cases, it may be the preferred method, since under the conditions of this method, hydrogen will not add to double bonds of aromatic rings.

Determination of Methoxy Group

The properties of methoxy group in the sample is determined by the 'Zeisel method'. The reactions involved in this method are as follows :

$$R.OCH_3 + HI \rightarrow ROH + CH_3I$$

$$CH_3I + CH_3COOH \rightarrow CH_3COO.CH_3 + HI$$

$$HI + 3Br_2 + 3H_2O \rightarrow HIO_3 + 6HBr$$

$$(Br_2 + H.COOH \rightarrow 2HBr + CO_2) \text{ Removal of excess bromine.}$$

Add KI,

$$HIO_3 + 5HI \rightarrow 3I_2 + 3H_2O$$

The liberated iodine is titrated with standard solution of sodium thiosulfate.

Method

The following is the apparatus (Fig. 10.1) employed for the determination of methoxyl group in drugs or pharmaceuticals.

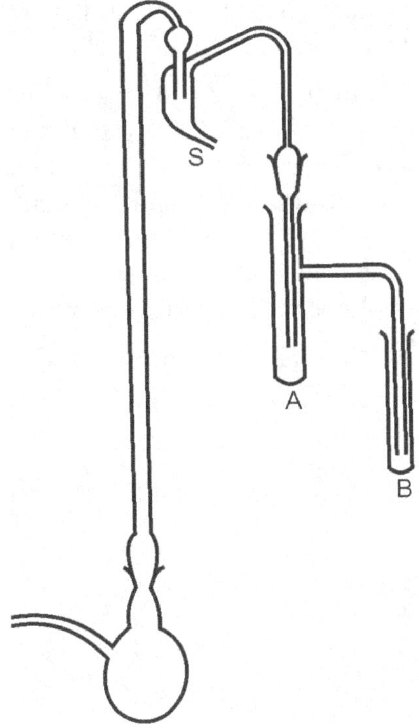

Fig. 10.1 Methoxyl determination apparatus.

The apparatus consists of 50 ml round–bottomed boiling flask into which is sealed a capillary side-arm, of 1-mm diameter, to provide an inlet for a stream of carbon dioxide. The flask is also fitted with an air condenser, approximately 25 cm in height and about 9 mm in diameter, bent through $180°$ at the top and terminating in a glass capillary, of 2 mm diameter, dipping into a small scrubber (s) containing about 2 ml of water. The outlet from the scrubber is a tube of about 7 mm in diameter, terminating in a removable tube of 4 mm diameter which dips below the surface of the liquid in the first of two receivers connected in series (A and B).

A quantity of the substance being tested, approximately equivalent to 50 mg of methyl iodide, is accurately weighed and placed in the boiling flask. A boiling rod, 2.5 ml of melted phenol, and 5 ml of hydroiodic acid are added, and the flask is connected with the remainder of the apparatus. The first receiver contains about 6 ml, and the second receiver about 4 ml, of a 10% w/v potassium acetate in glacial acetic acid to which 6 drops of bromine have been added. A slow uniform stream of carbon dioxide is passed through the capillary side-arm of the boiling flask, and the liquid is gently heated by means of a mantled microburner, at such a rate that the vapour of the boiling liquid rise half-way up the condenser. For most substances 30 minutes are sufficient to complete the reaction and sweep out the apparatus. The contents of the both receivers are then washed into a 250 ml conical flask which contains 5 ml of a 25% w/v solution of sodium acetate.

The volume of the liquid is then adjusted to approximately 125 ml and 6 drops of formic acid is added. The flask is rotated until the colour due to the bromine is discharged, 12 drops of formic acid are then added and the solution is allowed to stand for one to two minutes, 1g of potassium iodide and a few ml of dil. H_2SO_4 are added and the liberated iodine is titrated with 0.1 N sodium thiosulfate. The operation is repeated without the substance being tested (blank), and the volume of 0.1 N sodium thiosulfate required is deducted from the volume required in the determination of methoxyl.

Each ml 0.1 N $Na_2S_2O_3 \equiv$ 0.0005172 gm of methoxyl (CH_3O).

CHAPTER 11

POLAROGRAPHY

Introduction

- Polarography is a method of analysis in which the solution to be analysed is electrolysed in such a way that the graph of current against voltage shows what is in the solution and how much is present.

- If steady increasing voltage is applied to such a cell with two electrodes. It is possible to construct a reproducible current voltage curve.

- The electrolyte is an electro active dilute solution of material to be analysed in a suitable medium containing excess of differential electrolyte called base or supporting electrolyte. It is used to carry the bulk of the current and to raise the conductivity of the solution.

- The current-voltage curve, gives information about the nature and concentration of the material may be obtained.

- Thus, polarography is that method of instrumental analysis, which consists of the measurement of potential difference as current flows in solution and the result obtained can be thus interpreted in terms of nature and concentration of many substances.

- The value of current flowing through the cell at any applied voltage is measured with the help of an instrument known as polarography, (because, the curves obtained are graphical representation of the polarisation of dropping electrode) and the curves obtained with it are known as polarograms.

Apparatus

- Dropping mercury electrode consists of mercury reservoir from which mercury drops down as small drops through a capillary. This acts as cathode. It is known as indicator electrode or micro electrode.

- The anode consists of mercury pool at the bottom of the reservoir, which acts as a reference electrode and its area is larger, so that it is not polarised.

- Both cathode and anode are connected across the appropriate ends of a battery.

- The applied voltage can be changed by adjusting the sliding contact along the potentiometer wire EF.

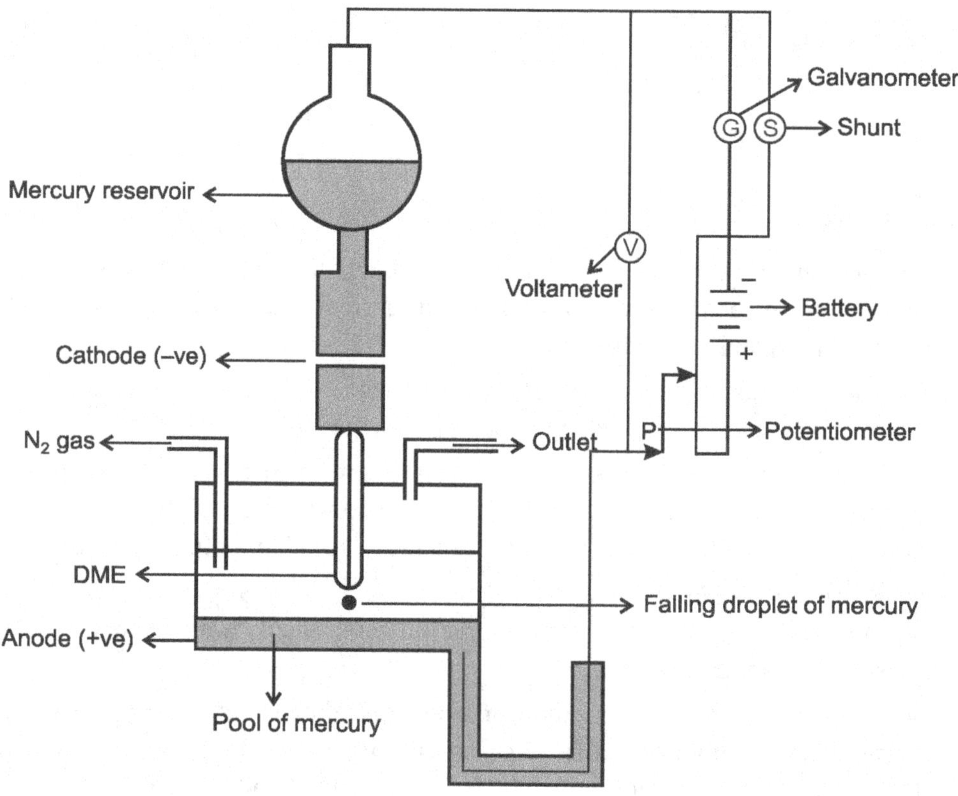

Fig. 11.1

Working

- Consider a polarographic cell, containing a solution of cadmium chloride, to which external EMF is applied.

- The positively charged ions present in the solution will be attracted to the dropping mercury electrode by an electrical force, and by a diffusive force resulting from the concentration gradient formed at the surface of the electrode.

- Thus, the total current flowing through the cell may be regarded as the sum of electrical and diffusive forces.

- When the applied voltage is increased and the current is recorded, a graph will be obtained.

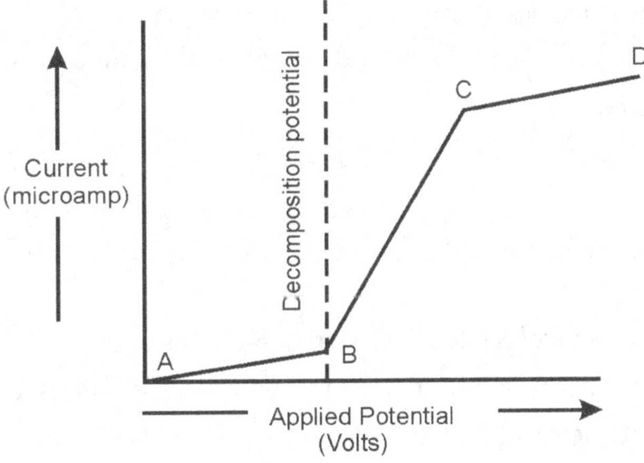

Fig. 11.2

- A to B, a small current flows. This is known as residual current and is carried by the supporting electrolyte and impurities present in the sample.

- At point B, the potential of the electrode becomes equal to the decomposition potential of Cd^{+2} ion.

- The current then increases along the curve BC.

- At point C current no longer increases linearly with applied voltage but reaches a steady limiting value at point D.

- After this, no increase in current is observed at higher cathode potentials.

- Thus, the current corresponding to the curve CD is known as limiting current.

- The difference between the residual current and the limiting current is called diffusion current and is generally denoted by i_d.

- The polarograph apparatus is manual polarograph.

Factors Affecting the Limiting Current

- Residual current
- Migration current
- Diffusion current
- kinetic current

1. Residual Current

- The current is not zero when no reducible ions are present. As the mercury drop grows, ions from supporting electrolyte gather around it.
- If the drop is negatively charged, these ions are positively charged.

2. Migration Current

- The electro active material reaches the surface of electrode by two processes.
- The first involves the migration of charged particles in the electrical field caused by the potential difference existing between the electrode surface and the solution.

  (b) The second involves the diffusion of particles.

  The current required for the above two processes is called migration current.

3. Diffusion Current

- The maximum current as shown as I_1 and I_2 is known as diffusion current.

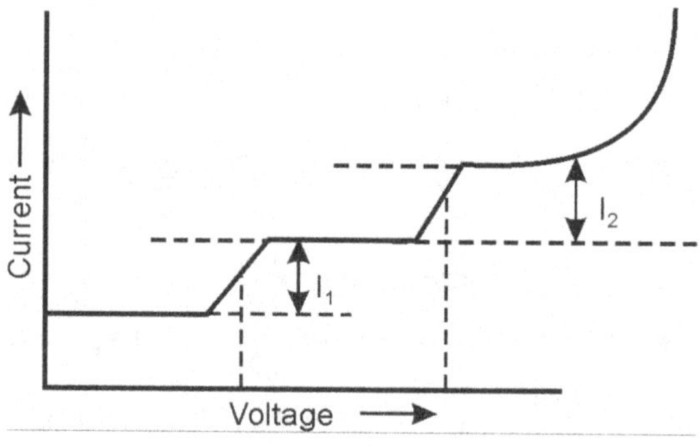

Fig. 11.3

- This current is directly proportional to the concentration of the substance being reduced or oxidised at the dropping mercury electrode.
- The observed diffusion current is directly proportional to the concentration of the electro active. This is the basis of quantitative polarographic analysis.

4. Kinetic Current

- The limited current may be affected by the rate of non-electrode reaction called the kinetic current.
- The kinetic current will be proportional to the rate constant and to the volume of the interface and therefore, is a direct function of size of the mercury drop but is independent of the velocity of the flow of mercury from the capillary.
- This current results if the oxidised or reduced form, of electro active species, is involved in a chemical equilibrium with other substances.

Form of Waves and Half Wave Potentials

- The half wave potential is polarography is a characteristic property of the electro active material.
- This potential is found on the steeply rising portion of the current – voltage curve and is one half of the distance between the residual and limiting currents. It is denoted by E_{12}.

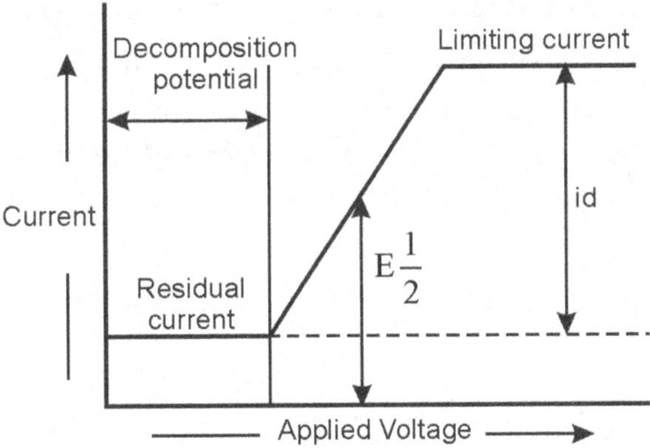

Fig. 11.4

- The importance of the half wave potential can be followed by considering the reduction taking place at the dropping mercury electrode which may be represented as follows

$$\text{Oxidant} + ne \rightleftharpoons \text{Reductant}$$
$$\text{(ox)} \qquad\qquad \text{(red)}$$

- The reversible potential of the system as it exists at the electrode-solution interface of the drop will be recorded on the polarogram.

- This electrochemical equilibrium may be represents by

$$E = E^\circ + \frac{0.0591}{n} \log \frac{[ox]}{[Red]} \qquad \ldots(i)$$

- Let us suppose that before the start of the current voltage curve, the solution at the electrode solution interface consists of oxidant only.

- As soon as the EMF becomes larger enough to reduce it, the concentration of the oxidant at the electrode surface begins to decrease.

- Some ions will move in form the bulk of the solution by means of diffusion, as the concentration of gradient builds up in the bulk of the volume around the electrode.

- The average current i, flowing through the cell, at any point of the wave is given by

$$I = K\,[(ox) - (ox)_o]\,D_{ox}^{1/2} \qquad \ldots(ii)$$

- where, K = capillary characteristics.

    ox   = conc. of reducible ions in bulk of the solution.

    $(ox)_o$ = conc. of oxidant at the electrode solution interface.

- When the current attains the limiting value represented by the diffusion current plateau i.e. the concentration of the oxidant at the electrodes, solution interface is reduced to zero.

$$\therefore\ i_d = K\,(ox)\,D_{ox}^{1/2} \qquad \ldots(iii)$$

From (ii) and (iii)

$$(ox)_o = \frac{i_d - i}{KD_{ox}^{1/2}} \qquad \ldots(iv)$$

- For metals which form amalgams with the dropping electrode, the concentration of metal amalgam is directly proportional to the current on the current voltage curve. So,

$$i = K\,[red]_o\,D_{red}^{1/2} \qquad \ldots(v)$$

- Substituting eq. (iv) and (v) in (i)

$$E = E^\circ + \frac{0.0591}{n} \log \frac{id - i}{i} + \frac{0.059}{n} \log \left[\frac{D_{red}}{D_{ox}}\right]^{1/2}$$

But by definition $i = id - i$ or

$$i = \tfrac{1}{2}\,id.$$

$$\therefore E_{1/2} = E^\circ + \frac{0.0591}{n} \log \left[\frac{D_{red}}{D_{ox}}\right]^{1/2} \qquad \qquad .....(vi)$$

where $E_{1/2}$ = half wave potential

- Thus from (vi) it is proved that the polarographic half wave potential is related to the standard reduction potential of oxidation-reduction system.

Application of Polarography

1. Applications to Inorganic Compounds

- Polarography can be used for the estimations of cations and anions in the presence of interfering ions.
- It is observed that the successful polarographic analysis of cations generally depends upon the employment of suitable supporting electrolyte.
- Polarography of aq. solutions of cations may be determined in the 10^{-2} to 10^{-6} M concentration range successfully.
- Ionic solutions of various elements can be determined directly. The mixtures of ions can be determined if half wave potentials of the ions are separated by 0.2V.
- This is essential in order to distinguish the height of two waves, otherwise the overlapping of the waves takes place.
- The polarographic analysis is also used in the determination of anions such as bromate, iodate, vanadate, selenite, nitrite and dichromate provided the central atom has two are more oxidation states.
- It is found that the polarograms for these substances are affected by the pH of the solution because the H ion is a participant in the reduction process.
- The technique has also been used successfully in the determinations of large no. of alloys.

2. Applications to Organic Compounds

- The reactions of organic compounds at a micro electrode are slow and more complex.
- Reversible organic reductions are generally confined to quinones and some other functional systems such as phenylene diamines.
- In organic polarography, solvents as glycols, dioxane alcohols, cellulose or glacial acetic acid have been employed. Supported electrolytes are often lithium salts or tetra alkyl ammonium salts.

- The estimation of sugars have been carried out in the range of 10^{-3} to 10^{-2} M using pH of 2.3 and supporting electrolyte hydrazine sulfate polarographically.
- The half wave potentials for organic compounds are markedly by pH dependent.

3. Determination of Dissolved Oxygen

- The determination of dissolved oxygen in aq. solution or in organic solvents can be carried out successfully with the help of polarography.
- Here, oxygen waves are measured and the dissolved oxygen determined.

4. Studies of the Complexes

- Polarography is a powerful tool in the study of the composition of complexes if the simple metal ion and complex of that metal ion in the same oxidation state give reversible electrode processes and involve the same no. of electrons.

5. Determination of Plant Contents

- The determination of plant contents is in general preceded by an extraction.
- A Polarographic analysis of the contents of essential oils can be carried out in most cases by dissolving oil in ethanol and diluted with a suitable aqueous buffer solution.
- Total content of mixture is obtained.

6. Applications to Pharmaceuticals

- Indirect polarographic determinations have been studied for frequently used analgesics and antipyretics.

Voltammetry

- Both current and potential are measured in voltammetry.
- The voltammetric experiment involves an indicator and reference electrode.
- A potential difference is imposed between these electrodes and current that flows because of electrochemical reactions is measured.
- The output consists of a record of current as a function of indicator electrode potential.
- In all these experiments one deals with heterogeneous reactions that occur at the surface of the working or indicator electrode.
- Since material must get from the bulk of solution to the electrode in order to react, a primary consideration in voltammetry is mass transport in solution.
- The transport of charged particles in solution can be explained on the basis of migration, convection and diffusion.

- The fact that diffusion and concentration are ultimately connected is the basis of analytical utility of voltammetry.
- The experiments are carried out in such a way that only diffusion makes an important contribution to the movement of material to the electrode.
- It is necessary to mention here that the term polrography is applied to a voltammetric experiment carried out using a dropping mercury electrode as the working electrode.

Chronopotentiometry

- Chronopotentiometry is a technique that involves the observation of electrode potential as a function of time.
- Moreover the technique requires the passage of constant current.
- Although chronopotentiometry can be used to determine the concentration of electro-active material in solutions, it has found little utilization for that purpose and has been restricted primarily to the study of electrode processes.
- It is usually carried out with a three electrode system.

Tensammetry

- In this technique the capacity current is derived form the process of adsorption or desorption or oscillatory motions of the dipole and the ions at the electrode surface.
- It was developed for the determination of tung states (10^{-3} M) in presence of different buffer solutions and is regarded as unusual derivative of A.C. polarography.

CHAPTER 12

ELECTRO-ANALYTICAL METHODS
OR
ELECTRO-CHEMICAL METHODS OF ANALYSIS

- These methods are generally directly or indirectly related to electricity.
  Here,

$$Drug + electricity \rightarrow Drug^* + electricity$$

  * indicates some modification

These methods are usually applied for analysis of drug. So, we pass the current through the solution of drug and then we measure the electricity before passing through the drug and after having passed through the drug.

The change in electricity tells us amount of drug to be analysed and type of that drug.

- In electro analytical method, different methods of drug analysis are included which are mentioned below:

  (i)   Conductometry

  (ii) Potentiometry

  (iii) pH metry

  (iv) Polarography

  (v)   Amperometry

  (vi) Biamperometry

Drugs are either organic or inorganic molecules.

Organic molecules like a simple molecule Amino acid and a complex molecule like Sulpha drug.

Inorganic molecules are generally in ionic form

E.g : $CaCl_2$, $ZnCl_2$, $FeSO_4$

In general, inorganic drug molecules are susceptible to electricity means they undergo oxidation and reduction or they undergo ion exchange.

E.g. $\qquad Fe^{+2} \rightarrow Fe^{+3}$

Organic molecules also primarily undergo oxidation–reduction

E.g., Phenol, ascorbic acid are easily oxidised and that can be measured by this method.

- **Electricity:** It is defined as the flow of electron ($\bar{e}$) from one place to another through the conductivity material.

  - Flow property of electron can be expressed as current.

  - Current: flow of electron is said to be current

    It is expressed as I or i

    It is measured in Ampere

- **One Ampre:** One ampere is the current which, when flows for one second, will cause deposition of 1.11800 mg Ag metal from $AgNO_3$ solution

$$[Ag^+ + \bar{e} \rightarrow Ag]$$

In other words,

One Ampere: It is about 6.26×10^{18} Number of electrons passing through any point in one second.

Quantity of Electricity: Coulomb discovered the quantity of electricity equal to one Ampere current flowing for one second.

$$6.26 \times 10^{18} \text{ electrons} = 1 \text{ coulomb}$$

$$1 \text{ Faraday} = 96,500 \text{ coulomb}$$

$$\therefore 1 \text{ Faraday} = 1 \text{ mole electrons}$$

$$\therefore 1 \text{ Faraday} = 6.023 \times 10^{23} \text{ electrons}$$

So, Coulomb and Faraday are used for expressing amount of electricity.

Faraday is easy and popular in SI system.

$$Na^+ + \bar{e} \rightarrow Na$$

$\therefore \qquad 1 \text{ mole of } \bar{e} = 1 \text{ Faraday} = 96,500 \text{ Coulombs}$

Electromotive Force (EMF) or Electrical Pressure or Potential Difference (P.D)

- *EMF* is the force which makes electrons to move. Generally it is referred to as potential

- *Potential difference:* It is not absolute value, it is relative difference between electrical pressure at two points.

- *$\bar{e}$ Pressure (electrical pressure):* It is defined as no. of $\bar{e}$ (electrons) or $\bar{e}$ density.

- *Driving force:* It is the force which makes electrons $\bar{e}$ to move or flow.

  It is expressed in terms of "volts."

  1 volt: It is electrical pressure required to flow 1 Ampere current through resistance of 1 Ω (ohms).

$$V = IR$$

- *Resistance:* Resistance is an inherent property of the substance to retard or oppose the flow of electricity. Certain materials have the high resistance toward electricity like chalk, wood, whereas metals have very low resistance. Resistance is expressed in unit of Ω (ohm).

- *1 Ohm ($1\,\Omega$):* $1\,\Omega$ is the resistance of Hg column (or mercury column) at $0°$ C at a uniform cross section and 106.3 cm long and containing 14.4251 gm pure Hg.

- *Ohm's law:* The current, flowing through any material, is directly proportional to potential and inversely proportional to resistance

$$\therefore I \propto E \quad \text{and} \quad I \propto \frac{1}{R}$$

$$\therefore I = \frac{E}{R}$$

Types of Current

(i)   A.C: Alternative current

(ii) D.C: Direct current

(i) AC

$\longrightarrow$ 50 cycles/sec

$-$ $\longleftarrow$ $+$

The direction of flow of $\bar{e}$ changes in no. of times in one second.

- How many times direction changes in one second is the frequency of $\bar{e}$.

  Normally the frequency seen in AC current is 50 Hzs.

(ii) DC

Here the flow of $\bar{e}$ is constant in one direction.

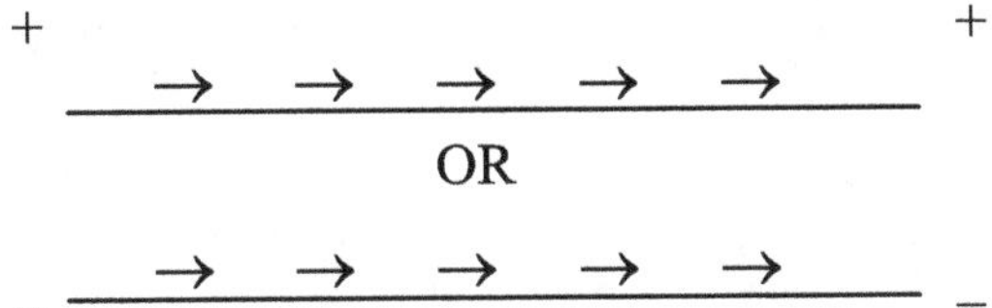

Here the $\bar{e}$ permanent remain in either positive or negative charged at the both sides.

- Here we do not need to know the frequency.
- Here is constant charge at any electrode.

- **Conductance (L) ($\mho$):** It is the inherent property of matter/material to allow electricity to pass through.

    So, it is opposite to resistance

    $$\therefore \qquad L = \frac{1}{R}$$

    The unit is Ohm^{-1} or Mho or Siemens

    $1\ Mho = 1\ Ohm^{-1} = 1\ Siemens$

    There are term μ siemens and milli siemens also exist.

Electrodes: (Terminology)

- Electrodes: electrodes are wire terminals made up of a metallic plate or a rod or a complicated device, capable of transferring electricity from circuit to the solution or from solution to the circuits.

- They can be classified in two ways:

    (i) Based on function

    (ii) Based on constituents

(i) **Based on Function**

(a) Working/Indicator/ Polarisable electrode

Reference electrode or Unpolarised electrode

- It does not posses any charge.
- It assumes positive or negative charge.
- It indicates the potential applied to the cell
- Working electrode is also called indicator electrode because it indicates potential produced by chemical reaction in solution.

    Thus, applied potential is expressed by this electrode.

There are Different Types of Reference Electrodes

(i) *Metallic electrode*

E.g: Platinum electrode

silver electrode

(ii) *Metal-Metal ion electrode*

E.g: $Cu/cuSO_4$ electrode.

(iii) *Amalgam electrode*

Mixture of mercury with any other metal

E.g: Na-amalgam

Na/Hg electrode

Cd/Hg electrode

Generally metals such as Na, Cd etc., are affected when exposed directly into the atmosphere. So, such metals cannot be used directly. Here we use mercury (Hg) to prevent the interaction of such metals with atmosphere.

(iv) *Gas electrode:* Here one component of electrode is a gaseous material

E.g: Hydrogen electrode

It is a standard electrode for all calculations

(v) *Micro-electrode:* It is of very small size

E.g.   (i) Dropping mercury electrode.

Here a very small drop of mercury is working as an electrode

(ii) Fibre electrode: It is a very small diameter tube.

- **What is reference electrode? How does it work?**

In reference electrode, the potential which we apply from the outside, the same potential is there in the solution

Or

If the solution has +ve charge then outside the electrode, there will be +ve charge.

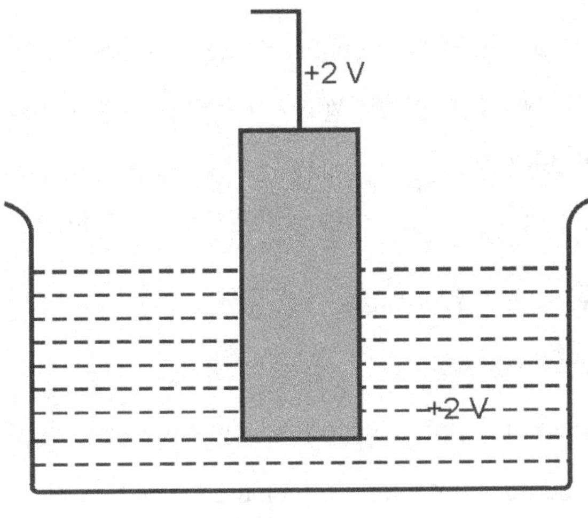

Fig.12.1

- Means there should be no change in potential when it passes through the electrode

- This electrode is not going to be polarised in any way whether the potential is given from outside or from the solution

- Thus, reference electrode maintains its state of being neutral or they are unpolarisable electrodes

Why These Types of Electrodes (Reference Electrodes) are Required Though they do not undergo any change?

- For completion of circuit, any chemical process requires two wires.

- All electrochemical processes involve both oxidation and reduction operations. And oxidation-reduction always exist simultaneously, it is a coupled process. In one electrode if the oxidation takes place simultaneously on the other electrode reduction takes place. So completion of chemical reaction is only possible by the use of reference electrode.

- Reference electrode itself changes its charge in oxidation–reduction process but does not express any change in the potential outside i.e., if we want to study only the oxidation of ascorbic acid, as per the rule oxidation and reduction process also takes place. In such case we use reference electrode, so that reduction process will take place on the reference electrode. And as reference electrode does not express any change in potential outside in spite of undergoing oxidation–reduction process.

- So, the cell potential will not get changed due to the reference electrode and due to reduction process. So, here whatever cell potential we get will be the oxidation potential of ascorbic acid

  e.g., of reference electrode is SCE (saturated Calomel electrode.

Applications of Reference Electrode

- It is applied in unit processes.

- In all the electrochemical processes one electrode is reference electrode.

- Reference electrode does not cause any change in potential.

- Used to study only one process either oxidation or reduction.

- If the electrode is very big (though it is not practically possible) the total voltage applied will not get affected because potential distributes and becomes negligible.

- As there is large enough concentration of reacting species of electrode, so the concentration undergoing change during reaction becomes negligible.

Most Commonly used Reference Electrode is Calomel Electrode

- Calomel electrode

  Here huge quantity of Hg, Hg^+Cl^-, K^+Cl^- is filled

  i.e., Hg^+Cl^- mercurous chloride or calomel electrode

  Now if we apply here negative charge from outside, excess $\bar{e}$ will react with Hg^+.

  $\therefore \qquad Hg^+ + \bar{e} \rightarrow Hg$

  Here the quantity of both Hg and Hg^+ is enough

- If we apply positive charge from outside, Hg^+ will be formed.

  $\therefore \qquad Hg \rightarrow Hg^+ + \bar{e}$

- But Hg and Hg^+ both are in sufficient quantity so the change in potential is not there.

- So, here potential is balanced within the electrode.
- But if we apply very high potential like 1000 V then there will be change in potential but for electro analytical purpose, we require very small potential.

- **Reference Electrode** is used to study only one process because electro chemical systems are redox couple systems. But sometimes we are only interested either in oxidation or in reduction process.

  i.e., oxidation of ascorbic acid.

  - So here we want to measure only one part of the redox reaction that is oxidation process.
  - But we can't block the reduction process, they both will occur simultaneously.
  - By using reference electrode with very high concentration, the change in potential will be negligible hence we can get the oxidation potential.
  - So, this is used to study only one process either oxidation or reduction.
  - So we can say that reference electrode is a buffer of electrochemical process.

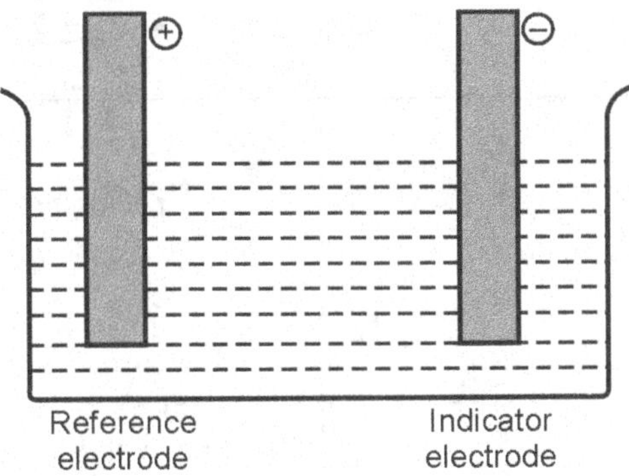

Fig 12.2

If we want to study only reduction, so we will consider gaining of $\bar{e}$ from the drug.

And if we want to study oxidation then we should consider $\bar{e}$ donated to the drug.

Electrochemical Cell: They are the devices or designs consisting of minimum two electrodes used to carry out electrolysis or to generate electricity by chemical reaction.

- So we can say that either of these two processes takes places here

  (i) Electrolysis [Hysis–break down; so break down of electricity]

  or (ii) Generation of electricity due to chemical reaction

Classification of Electrochemical Cell

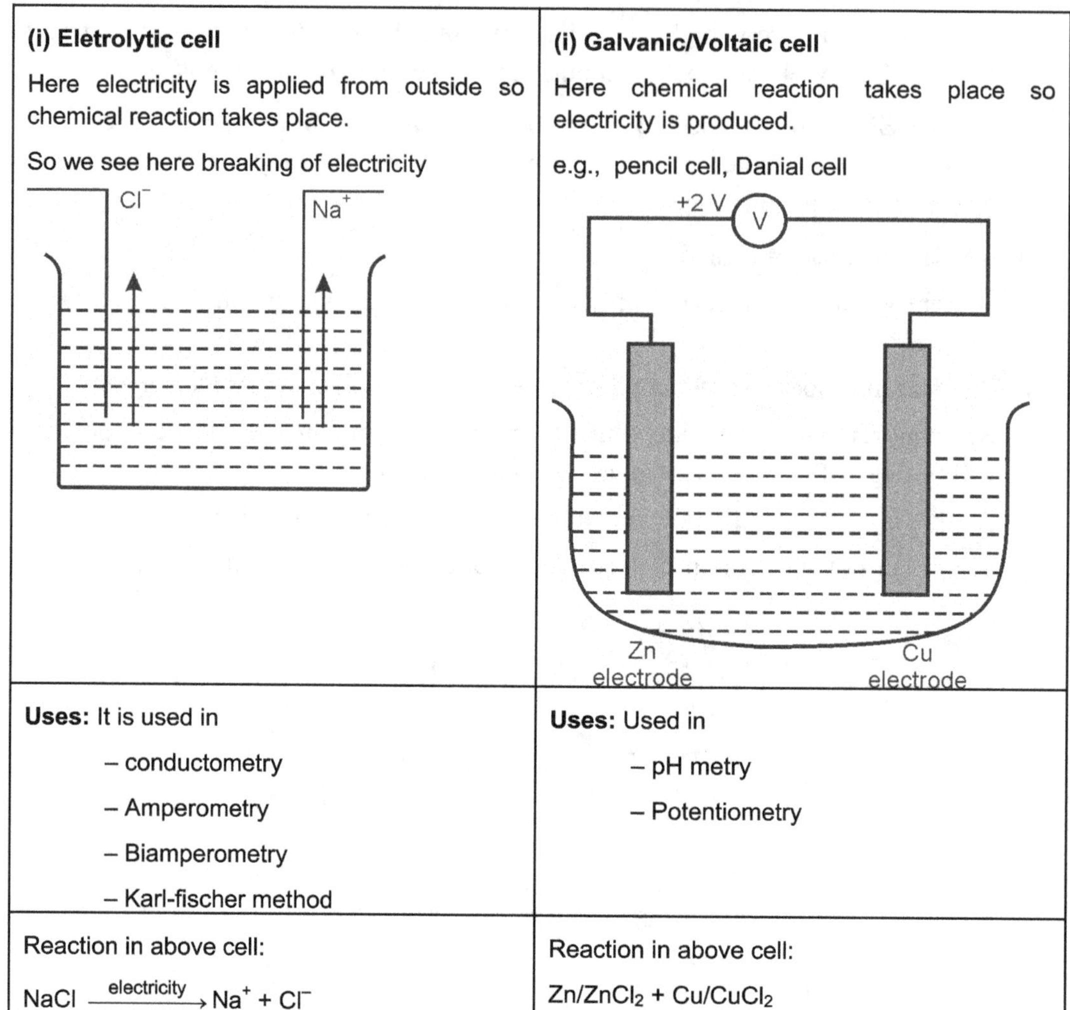

(i) Eletrolytic cell	(i) Galvanic/Voltaic cell

Uses: It is used in
   – conductometry
   – Amperometry
   – Biamperometry
   – Karl-fischer method
	Uses: Used in
	   – pH metry
	   – Potentiometry

Reaction in above cell: $NaCl \xrightarrow{\text{electricity}} Na^+ + Cl^-$	Reaction in above cell: $Zn/ZnCl_2 + Cu/CuCl_2$

Classification of Electrodes Based on Components

(i)   Metal electrode: Pt (Platinum) electrode

(ii)   Metal ion electrode

     e.g., $Zn/ZnSO_4$

     Danial cell Zn/Zn^{+2}, Cu/Cu^{+2}

(iii)   Amalgam electrode

     [Hg with any metal Hg-Cd Cell (Weston cell)]

     Na – amalgam cell

(iv) Gas electrode: One of the components in electrode is gas.

   i.e., Hydrogen electrode

   (standard electrode – reference electrode)

   • 0.00 volt cell potential

   • All the cells have potential in comparison to (or with reference to) H_2 electrode

(v) Micro or fibre electrode

   • here electrode is just like fibre

Here we can't write oxidation potential as standard potential because only reduction potential is universally accepted as the standard half cell or electrode potential.

E^0 = it indicates standard potential/ or standard reduction potential

- Each electrode has its own characteristic potential, it remains constant, mentioned as half cell potential.

- Standard potential of different electrodes is given in emf series in which standard potential values of electrodes or half cell potential is given with reference to standard electrode or H_2 electrode

- The potential of the whole cell is measured by taking the difference of standard cell potential

E^0/half Cell Potential: It is a potential of an electrode having unit activity of all the constituents in comparison with 0.00 volt potential of standard hydrogen electrode.

Or

It is defined as normal hydrogen potential when the system is under going reduction at STP (Standard Temperature and Pressure)

$$Fe^{+3} \rightarrow Fe^{+2}$$

$$Cu^{+2} \rightarrow Cu$$

CONDUCTOMETRY

- **Conductance:** It is the inherent property of material to pass the electricity through it.

- How the current passes through the metal depends upon the state of metal.

Solid	Solution
Conductance is very high and low resistance.	Conductance is very low and hence high resistance.
It is measured in mho and siemen.	It is measured in milimho, μ mho, or in mili or μ siemen.
When electricity passes through, there is no change in conductance or conductor.	When electricity passes through the solution, drastic change is seen (break down of mole).
The carrier of electricity is electrons ($\bar{e}$) means in solid themselves electrons $\bar{e}$ are moving and thus pass the electricity. $\bar{e}$ are very small and can move very fast and major portion is occupied by electrons as there are high number of $\bar{e}$ in solid.	Ions are carrier of electricity. **Ions are bulky and they are not alone but they are hydrated, so ions have to move with big crowd in the solution so they move slowly.**
Effect of temperature: As the temperature increases resistance in solid increases or conductance decreases due to, at higher temperature, atoms also start moving and cause hindrance (to retard) to movement of $\bar{e}$	**Effect of temperature:** As the temperature increases, conductance of the solution also increases due to decrease in viscosity of the solution
When electricity passes, solid does not undergo any change. Its proportion does not change	When electricity passes through the solution, we find considerable change in proportion of the solution because of oxidation and reduction of the metal.

Solution Conductance (L) : 1 Siemen is the conductance of a solution through which 1 ampere current flows when the potential difference is 1 volt.

- Siemen unit does not clarify or specify concentration of solution and diameter, area and thickness of the solution

    Units: ohm^{-1}, mho, siemen (SI unit)

- **Specific conductance: (L_s):** It is the conductance of a solution having 1 square cm area and 1 cm length. L_s can be co–related with only conductance.

$$\therefore \qquad L_s = L \times K$$

where L = measured conductance

K = cell constant of conduct measuring system

It can be indicated this way also

$$L_s = \frac{1}{\rho}$$

where ρ = specific resistance

$$\therefore \qquad L_s = \frac{l \times L}{A}$$

where L = conductance

A = cross sectional area of the solution

l = length of the solution

Now $$\frac{l}{A} = \text{constant} = K$$

$$\therefore \qquad L_s = K \times L$$

Here constant l and A are properties of electrode and in conductometry we have two electrodes with fixed l (length) and A (area).

$$\therefore \qquad K = \frac{l}{A} = \text{cell constant because cell has fixed dimensions}$$

- In all cells, distance between two electrodes is fixed.

- And specific conductance L_s is used to measure the conductance of solution.

Equivalent Conductance (λ)

It is the conductance of a volume of solution containing 1 gm equivalent (weight) of dissolved solute and this solution is placed between two parallel electrodes which are 1 cm apart from each other and are large enough to contain all the amount of solution between them.

Here
- amount of solute dissolved in the solution is fixed: 1 gm.

- Distance between two electrodes is specified: 1 cm.

- Volume of the solution is not specified or we can say it is not fixed.

(means 1 litre of solution containing 1 gm equivalence concentration also 1000 litre of solution containing 1 gm equivalence concentration).

So, amount of solute is here fixed every time that is 1 gm

- Concentration of the solution is not fixed

- Relation between specific and equivalent conductance

$$\Lambda = L_s \,.\, V$$

V = Volume of solution in ml containing 1 gm equivalant solute

$$\therefore \qquad \Lambda = \frac{L_s \times 1000}{C}$$

C = concentration of solute in 1 gm wt per litre or Normality

Units -   Siemen cm^{-2}

Mho cm^{-2}

Ohm–1 . cm^{-2}

Molar Conductance : (μ)

Molar conductance is the conductance of a solution containing 1 M solute dissolved in solution and placed between two parallel electrodes 1 cm apart from each other and are large enough to contain all solution between them.

$$\therefore \mu = L_s \times V'$$

V$'$ = Volume of solution in ml containing 1 gm mole (or 1M) solute

$$\mu = \frac{L_s \times 1000}{C'}$$

C$'$ = Concentration in gm mole

unit - Siemen Cm^2 ; $Ohm+.cm^{-2}$; $Mho.cm^2$

Equivalance Conductance at Infinite Dilution : (λ_o)

It is symbolised as Λ_o. Here zero (Λ_o) indicates concentration.

(means 1 gm in 1000 million litre concentration is extremely small, negligible)

Equivalance conductance at infinite dilution (λ_o)

Or

Limiting ionic conductance

Or

Sonic conductance at infinite dilution

- Suppose we have 1 gm equivalent solute present in 1000 million litre solution, then concentration of solute in the solution will be theoretically definite but practically the concentration is zero.

- At infinite dilution, the total concentration of solute remains same but the distance between solute particles increase tremendously than other particles.

  e.g.,: NaCl as solute, so in the solution there will be Na^+ and Cl^- ions.

$$
\therefore \quad
\begin{array}{c}
Cl^- \\
Cl^- \ Na^+ \ Cl^- \\
Cl^-
\end{array}
\quad \text{and} \quad
\begin{array}{c}
Na^+ \\
Na^+ \ Cl^- \ Na^+ \\
Na^+
\end{array}
$$

- Then if Na^+ wants to perform some activity, then it is affected by Cl^-, so it can't do desirable activity.

- While at infinite dilution individual ions are free from influence of other ions.

- And in solution phase ions are the carrier of electricity.

- So, conductance becomes higher here than the conductance at finite dilution.

- Ionic conductance at infinite dilution is also known as a limiting ionic conductance as some highest upper limit is achieved here.

$$
\therefore \ \Lambda_o = \lambda_o^+ \quad + \quad \lambda_o^-
$$

  Individual   individual onion

  cation

Equivalent conductance at infinite dilution for solutes (λ_o : siemen.cm^2)

Concentration (normality)	HAC (λ_o : seiemen cm^2)	HCL (λ_o : Siemen cm^2)
0.001	48.63	421.36
0.005	22.80	415.80
0.01	16.20	412.00
0.05	7.36 *Big change*	399.09 *Small change*
0.1	5.20	391.82

- As the concentration increases, equivalent conductance decreases, so inverse relationship exists here.

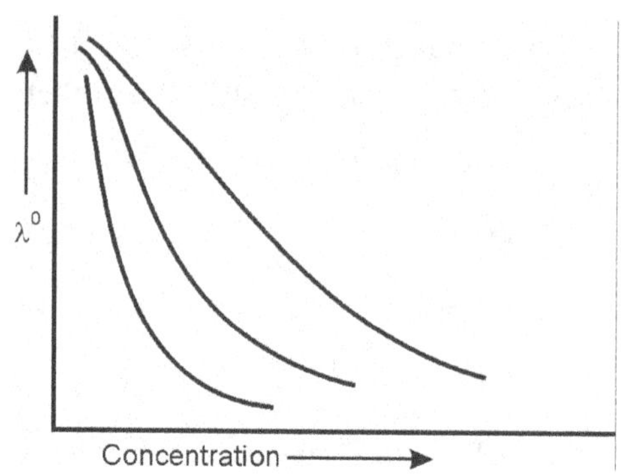

Fig 12.3

Conclusion

(i) As the concentration increases equivalence conductance decreases.

(ii) Equivalant conductance at any concentration of a strong electrolyte has more Λ_o as compare to weak electrolyte.

(Because of strong electrolyte no. of dissociated ions increases) means strong electrolyte completely dissociates while weak electrolyte dissociates partially).

F.W Kohlrausch's Law or Law of Independent Migration

- **Law :** At infinite dilution each ion contributes a definite amount of conductance to the total conductance of the electrolyte irrespective of the nature of the counter ion or other opposite ion.

  Eg : conductance of Na^+ ion is fixed in any form like $NaCl$, $NaBr$, Na_2SO_4 etc., here Cl^-, Br^-, SO_4^{-2} are counter ions.

How we derive this law ?

Λ_o at infinite dilution

Sub	Λ_o	Sub	Λ_o	Difference
KCl	130.0	NaCl	108.9	21.1
KNO_3	126.3	$NaNO_3$	105.2	21.1
$\frac{1}{2}k_2SO_4$	133.0	$\frac{1}{2}NaSO_4$	111.9	21.1

Conclusion : Law is derived from similar type

- Λ_o between Na^+ and k^+

- $-ve$ ion is same here

- Conductance due to Cl^-, NO_3^-, SO_4^- is same if we are adding infinite dilution, each ion is contributing fixed amount of conductance. Standard value of conductance remains constant for each ion.

$$\therefore \qquad \Lambda_o = \Lambda_o^+ + \Lambda_o^-$$

where Λ_o = equi. conductance at infinite dilution of any substance

and Λ_o is the sum of equi. conductance of infinite of any anion and cation

$\Lambda_o + \Lambda_0^-$ They are std value available in books

Ionic Conductance at Infinite Dilution $(\Lambda_o^+ \text{ or } \Lambda_o^-)$

Cation	Λ_o^+	anion	Λ_o^-
H^+	349.82	OH^-	198.5
K^+	73.52	Br^-	78.4
Na^+	50.11	I^-	76.8
NH_4^+	73.4	Cl^-	76.3

Factors affecting Conductance

(i) Types of electricity

D.C : Conductance measurement is not possible because constantly one electrode remains +ve at one end and –ve at the other.

- Constant deposition of ion
- constant change in property of electrode.
- it is time dependent measurement.

A.C : Here electrode remains constantly uniform in its property.

- Three types of frequency is seen in A.C current

    a > 50 Hz (cycles/sec)

    b > 1000 Hz

    c > high frequency current

- As the frequency of current increases, conductance also increases.

(ii)   Strength of current

- expressed in terms of volts
- At low volts (or at low voltage) or at low Ampere, conductance is low.
- As the volts increases, conductance also increases
- Maximum attainable conductance is the equivalence conductance.

(iii)   Solute

$$Ca > \text{Concentration} \left(\Lambda \propto \frac{1}{c} \right)$$

- L is ordinary conductance
- $L \propto C$ (generally). (This is not possible when solute concentration is very high).

When concentration is less, no. of ions available to pass the electricity is less so conductance is less.

- $L_s \propto c$ because between two electrodes, as the no. of ions are more conductance is more $-L_s \propto c$ (This is not possible when solute concentration is very high).

- Now based on detailed study done by these three scientists, Debye, Fruckel, Onsager

$$\Lambda \propto \frac{1}{c}$$

Why such relationship exists here ?

They gave explanation for this relationship based on two points.

Asymetric effect

   Or

Relaxation effect

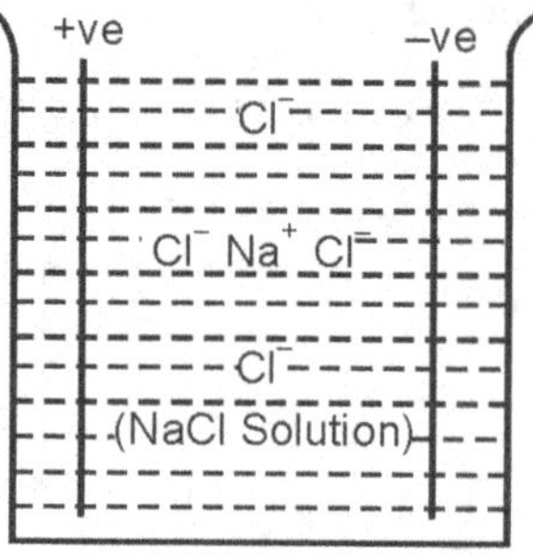

Fig 12.4

- If we have two electrodes, anode and cathode between which NaCl solution is filled up.
- Now each Na^+ ion is surrounded by no. of Cl^- ions and each Cl^- ion is surrounded by no. of Na^+ ions.
- So, if Na^+ wants move to the $-ve$ electrode, it has to break this surrounding complex.
- This effect decreases conductance at high concentration.
- Because at high concentration, the interaction between Na^+ and Cl^- ions will be more.

Electrophoretic Effect

(a) As Na^+ ion is surrounded by no. of Cl^- ions, there is equal possibility of Cl^- ion to move towards another Na^+ ion.

- So, there the movement of Na^+ is time consuming.
- So, here conductance decreases.
- These both asymmetric and electrophoretic effects do not take place in a very dilute solution.

(b) Type of solute : strong electrolyte has high conductance than weak electrolyte

(c) charge or ions or solute

$$Eg : \qquad KCl \rightarrow k^+ + Cl^-$$

$$K_2SO_4 \rightarrow 2\,k^+ + So_4^{-2}$$

$$\mu_o = \Lambda_o \times n$$

where μ_o = molar conductance at infinite dilution

n = no. of charge.

- two $-ve$ charge acts as double ions and carries two cations.

If ions are bivalent $\rightarrow \Lambda_o$ will be double.

- If Molar conductance μ_o is double than Λ_o (conductance at infinite dilution) will be double.

$$[k_2sO_4 \rightarrow \Lambda_o \qquad \text{if } \tfrac{1}{2}\ k_2SO_4 \rightarrow \frac{1}{2}\ \Lambda_o].$$

(d) **solute property** : Size of $+ve$ or $-ve$ ion also plays an important role in conductance.

- As the size or volume of ion increases ($\uparrow$), conductance decreases. ($\downarrow$)

- All the ion are not moving or existing independently.
- H_2O cannot exist as a single ion.

- It acts as a solvated ion.

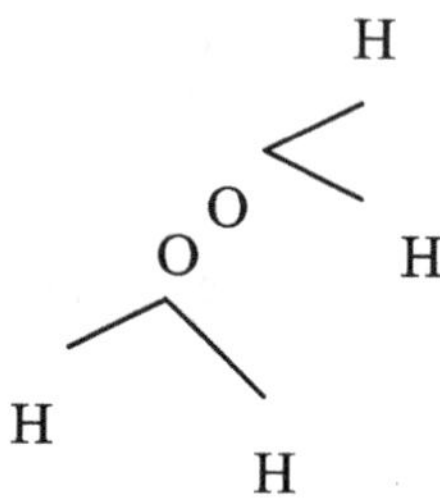

- so here ions move as solvated ions.

(e) Mobility of ion or ionic speed

The absolute velocity of any ion under a fall of potential of one volt per cm is called as ionic mobility.

Unit : cm/sec [It is the rate by which ion moves]

Ion	Ionic mobility
H^+	36.2×10^{-4}
K^+	7.61×10^{-4}
Ba^+	6.6×10^{-4}
OH^-	20.2×10^{-4}
SO_4^{-2}	8.27×10^{-4}
Cl^-	7.91×10^{-4}

- Ionic mobility decides overall conductance.
- H^+ has the highest value.
- So, equivalence conductance of H^+ is very high.

iv Solvent Types

- Normally water is used as solvent.
- But if we use solvent other than H_2O, following factors should be considered.

  (a) **Polarity of Solvent :** Solvents with low polarity are having very low conductance

- Solvents with low polarity don't allow solute ion to be soluble in them.
- So, in such solvents, solutes are insoluble or partially soluble.

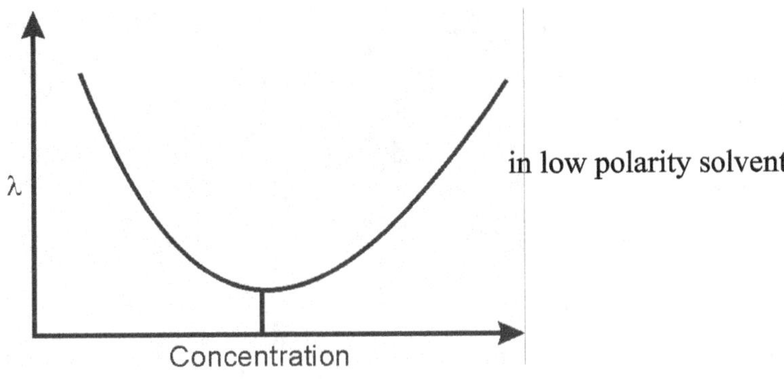

Fig.12.5

- The curve indicates that initially as the concentration increases, conductance decreases.
- But a point comes after which increase in concentration increases the conductance.
- Between the concentration range of increasing and decreasing conductance a point comes where there is the lowest conductance.
- Here at this particular concentration ions start joining with one another.

    E.g : $(+ - +)^{+} \rightarrow$ single +ve charge

    If 5 ions join then $(-+-+-)^{-} \rightarrow$ here −ve charge.

- So, due to joining of ions, conductance becomes very low.
- And after this particular point, dissociation of ions starts so conductance increases.

C_{min}: It is minimum concentration at which solute and solvent ions come together and act as single ion.

(b)Viscosity : It is the inherent property of liquid to resist or oppose flow current.

- As viscosity increases conductance decreases.

Walden's Rule

$$\Lambda_o \, \eta = \text{constant}$$

$$\therefore \; \Lambda_o \propto \frac{1}{\eta} \; ; \text{ as the viscosity of the solution is low, conductance is high.}$$

Limitation : This is applicable to non-solvated ions only.

$\eta \propto \dfrac{1}{\text{temp}}$. So, as the temperature increases, viscosity of the solution decreases and hence conductance increases.

Generalization : $1°$ rise in temp causes about 2.1 decrease in viscosity and hence 2.1 increase in conductance.

Instruments

By any instrument, using ohm's law, we can derive

$$E = ir$$

$$\therefore \qquad i = \frac{E}{R} = \frac{\text{Potential difference}}{\text{Re sis tan ce}}$$

But $\dfrac{1}{R} = L$ (conductance)

$$\therefore \qquad i = EL$$

So, we can measure the conductance covering entire system including wire, meter etc, and we can remove the error here using comparison method.

Wheatston Bridge

Measurement of conductance and measurement of resistance is same only units are different.

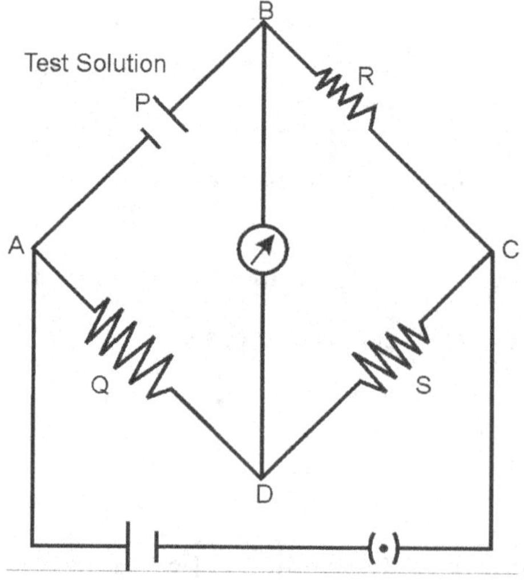

Fig.12.6

Here, P = unknown solution whose conductance is to be measured.

- here A.C current is passed through the circuit

$$\therefore p = \frac{R}{S} \times Q$$

Cell

Here cell is known as conductivity cell or conductometer cell.

- It is the device having minimum two electrodes and which allows to pass electricity through it.
- Here both electrodes are polarisable or working.
- They are generally made up of platinum which is a highly inert metal.
- Platinum metal is used in form of plate so dimension and area are also important.
- It is coated with PtO (platinum oxide)
- It is black in colour and known as platinum black coated plate.
- The distance between two point electrodes is fixed and remains same.

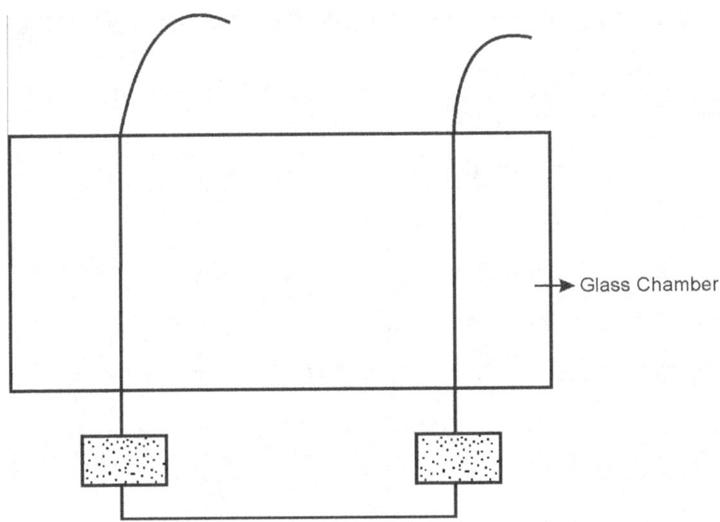

Fig.12.7

- Each cell is having characteristic constant that is cell constant = k

$$K = \frac{l}{A}$$

where   l = distance between two electrodes

A = area

- K is a fixed value for each cell and cell conductance or sp. conductance

$$L_s = L \times K$$

Scientific Measurement of Conductance

- Dip the conductance cell in 0.1 N KCl solution and measure the conductance.

- Then, use formula

$$K \text{ (Cell constant)} = \frac{0.01286}{\text{measured conductance in siemens}}$$

Use of cell constant: to find out specific conductance from the measured conductance.

Applications of Conductometry

- In industry to evaluate purity, strength etc., of states of matter

- In drug analysis conductometry is used to find out electrical potential of drugs.

Purity of Water

Pure water contains very low conductance because in purest H_2O, ions are absent.

Ionic impurity causes conductance.

Specific conductance of ultra high purified water is

$$L_s = 0.06 \ \mu scm^{-1}$$

Specific conductance of equilibrium water

$$L_s = 0.8 \ \mu scm^{+}$$

Purest water is obtained by distillation.

Specific conductance between the range of 30 to 40 μscm^{-1} is acceptable in industry.

Suppose we want to measure conductance of NaCl

Conductance of NaCl soln = X

Conductance of water = Y

$\therefore$ Actual Conductance of NaCl = X – Y

2. Finding conductance of unknown compound

Principle used in finding out conductance is addition or subtraction. Here we add or subtract the conductance.

e.g., $BaAc_2$

To find out conductance of $BaAc_2$

we add equivalent conductance of

$$\frac{1}{2} Ba^{+2} + 2Ac^-$$

$$= 63.64 + 2(40.g)$$

$$= 145.44$$

Find equi. conductance of HAC from NaAc, HCl, NaCl equi. conducatance

∴ $HCl + CH_3COONa$ NaCl + HAC

Or NaAc

∴ equi. conductance of HAC = $(\lambda_0)_{Hcl} + (\Lambda_0)_{NaAc} - (\Lambda_0)_{NaCl}$

$$= 419 + 91 - 120$$

$$= 390 \text{ siemen}$$

∴   HCl = 41g

NaAc = 91

NaCl = 120

3. Detection of solubility and K_{sp} of sparingly soluble compound

- This is applicable to only sparingly soluble compound. eg : $BaSO_4$, AgCl, $Al_3(PO_4)_2$
  (sparingly that is partially, so to dissolve the compound completely the amount of solute should be negligible or very less)
- Whatever small amount we dissolved gets completely ionized (10^{-5}, 10^{-8}gm equi (litre).
- The ionic concentration is so low that we can imagine it as infinite dilution.
- For any compound

$$\Lambda_0^+ + \Lambda_0^- = \Lambda_0$$

- Equivalent conductance is then equal to

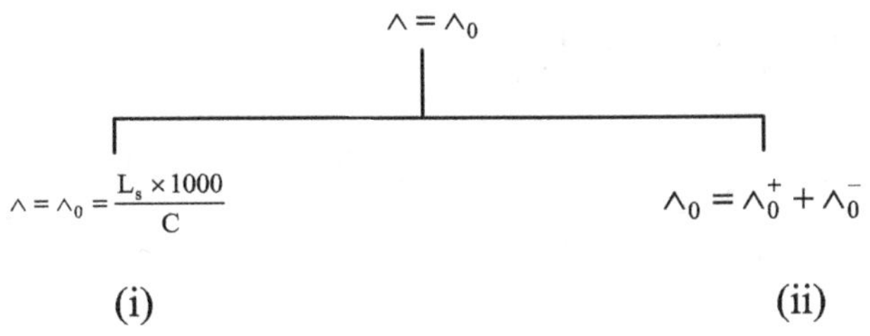

- Final formula for ionic conductance at infinite dilution can be given from (i) and (ii)

$$\therefore \; \Lambda_0 = \frac{L_s \times 1000}{C} \quad \text{and} \quad \Lambda_0 = \Lambda_0^+ + \Lambda_0^-$$

$$\therefore \; \Lambda_0^+ + \Lambda_0^- = \frac{L_s \times 1000}{C}$$

Where C = concentration in gm/litre

Now S = gm equi. solute in litre solution and C is replaced by S.

$$\therefore \; \Lambda_0^+ + \Lambda_0^- = \frac{L_s \times 1000}{S}$$

Examples on solubility and conductance

1. BaSO$_4$ has conductance of 2.7 µs, conductance of water is L = 0.5 µs, cell constant

   k = 1.1 cm^{-1}, equi. conductance of $\frac{1}{2}$ Ba^{+2} = 63.6 and $\frac{1}{2}$SO$_4^{-2}$ = 80

(a) Calculate solubility of BaSO$_4$ in terms of gm. equi/litre.

(b) Solubility pdt of BaSO$_4$

(c) Solubility pdt in terms of mole/litre

(i) conductance of BaSO$_4$ = 2.7 – 0.5

$$= 2.2 \; \mu s$$

Specific conductance $L_s = L \times k$

$$= 2.2 \times 1.1$$

$$= 2.42 \; \mu s \; cm^{-1}$$

Λ_0 Conductance of BaSO$_4$ = $(\Lambda_0)\frac{1}{2}$ Ba^{+2} + $(\Lambda_0)\frac{1}{2}$SO$_4^{-2}$

$$= 63.6 + 80$$

$$= 143.6$$

Now, $\qquad \Lambda_0 = \Lambda = \dfrac{2.42 \times 10^{-6} \times 1000}{S}$

$$\therefore \qquad 143.6 = \frac{2.42 \times 10^{-6} \times 1000}{S}$$

$$S = \frac{2.42 \times 10^{-6} \times 1000}{143.6}$$

$$\therefore S = 1.6 \times 10^{-5} \text{ gm equi/litre}$$

(ii) K_{sp} = pdt of solubilised part.

$$BaSO_4 \rightarrow Ba^{+2} + So_4^{-2}$$

$$\therefore \qquad K_{sp} = [Ba^{+2}] \left[So_4^{-2}\right]$$

$$= [1.6 \times 10^{-5}][1.6 \times 10^{-5}]$$

$$\therefore \qquad K_{sp} = 2.56 \times 10^{-10}$$

(iii)   Solubility in moles per litre

$$= \frac{\text{gm. equi / litre}}{2}$$

$$= \text{no. of moles of } BaSO_4$$

$$= \frac{1.6 \times 10^{-5}}{2} \text{ (Normality)}$$

$$= 0.8 \times 10^{-5} \text{ M}$$

(iv)   Determination of mode of ionization

- Complex compound ionizes in different manner
- Consider the e.g. of $K_4 [Fe (CN)_6]$

  This compound can ionize in three different manner

$$K_4 [Fe(CN)_6] \xrightarrow{\text{ionization}} k^+ \; K_3 [Fe(CN)_6]^- \qquad \ldots\ldots (a)$$

$$OR$$

$$2k^+ + K_2 [Fe(CN)_6]^{-2} \qquad \ldots.. (b)$$

$$OR$$

$$4k^+ + Fe(CN)_6^{-4} \qquad \ldots.. (c)$$

We find ionization of any type of these three types.

- ions are carrier of electricity.
- Double charged ions can carry double charge.
- Each and every single anion and cation has approximately conductance $\Lambda_0 = 60$ siemen cm^2

- This is an average value.
- Measured conductance is $\approx 120 = \Lambda$

$$\text{from} \quad \Lambda = \frac{L_s \times 1000}{c} \qquad \left[\because k^+ + k_3 \, [Fe(CN)_6]^{-2} = 60 + 60 = 120 \right]$$

- So, mode of ioniztion is of <a> type.
- If we get $\Lambda \approx 500$ then $<c>$ type of ionization is possible only.

Degree of ionization (α) = and ionization constant (K_a or K_b)

For weak electrolyte

Principle : The degree of ionization (α) can be measured by,

$$\alpha = \frac{\Lambda_c}{\Lambda_o} \quad \text{equivalent conductance at any definite concentration.}$$

To get the value of Λ_c put electrolyte with 'c' concentration.

5. Determination of Ka

$$K_a = \frac{\alpha^2 C}{1 - \alpha}$$

Example : HAC $= 0.015$ M has

conductance L $= 1.8$ ms, Conductance L for H_2O is 0.2 ms,

Cell constant (k) $= 0.6$ cm$^+$

Ionic conductance $H^+ = \Lambda^+$

$$Ac^- = \Lambda^-$$

$$H^+ + Ac^- = 391 = \Lambda_0 \rightarrow \text{at infinite dilution}$$

Find out

(i) Degree of ionization (α);   (ii) ionization constant (K_a)

$$L \text{ for HAC is} = 1.8 - 0.2$$

$$= 1.6 \text{ ms}$$

Specific Conductance $L_s = L \times K$

$$= 1.6 \times 0.6 \times 10^{-3}$$

$$= 0.96 \times 10^{-3}$$

$$\therefore \qquad L_s = 9.6 \times 10^{-4} \text{ S}$$

$$\Lambda_c = \frac{L_s \times 1000}{C(=S)}$$

$$\therefore \quad \Lambda_c = \frac{9.6 \times 10^{-4} \times 1000}{0.015}$$

$\therefore \quad \Lambda_c = 64 \rightarrow$ equi. conductance in terms of Normality

Now degree of ionization

$$\alpha = \frac{\Lambda_c}{\Lambda_0}$$

$$= \frac{64}{391}$$

$$\therefore \quad \alpha = 0.164$$

$$K_a = \frac{\alpha^2 c}{1 - \alpha}$$

$$= \frac{(0.164)^2 (0.015)}{1 - 0.164}$$

$$= \frac{0.0004030}{0.836}$$

$$= 4.82 \times 10^{-4}$$

To find out Degree of Dissociation : To find out degree of dissociation of a compound, only conductometry is used.

- degree of dissociation of weak electrolyte

$\Lambda_0 \rightarrow 100\%$ ionization $\because$ infinite dilution

$\Lambda_c \rightarrow$ ionization at any concentration.

here Λ_0 indicates very low concentration of solute as it gets 100% ionized inspite of being a weak electrolyte.

$\alpha =$ fraction of solute undergoing ionization

(6) Determination of Reaction kinetics

Principle : The reaction involving the change in concentration of highly conducting species can be studied by measurement of conductance.

e.g., hydrolysis of ester

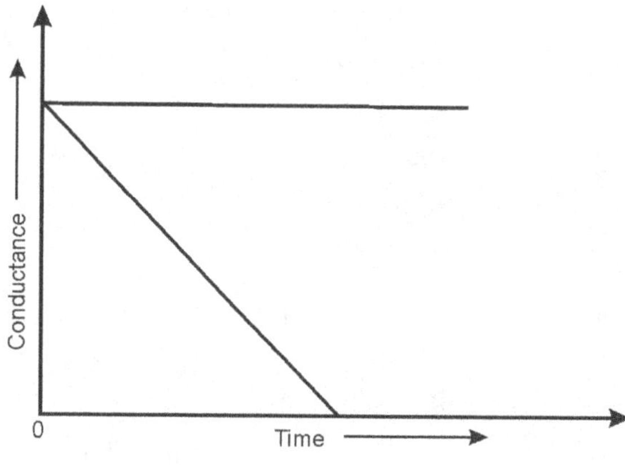

- Here solute is having very low conductance because it does not have any ion.
- OH^- has very high conductance.
- CH_3COOH has very low conductance because it is a weak electrolyte.
- CH_3OH has also very low conductance.

Fig.12.8

- It is a relative conductance as decreases with time.
- at o (zero) time $\rightarrow$ highest conductance of OH^-
- As the time passes, concentration of OH^- ions decreases hence conductance also decreases.

7. Conductometric Titration

Instead of using indicator (to determine endpoint of the titration) only conductometer is used to carry out titration.

Principle : Conductance before endpoint and after end point must be different.

Titrations which are based on this principle (means which show difference in conductance before and after endpoint) can only be carried out using conductometer.

Like pH metry, Acid–Base titration.

e.g., $HCl + NaOH \rightarrow H_2O + NaCl$ [acid–base titration]

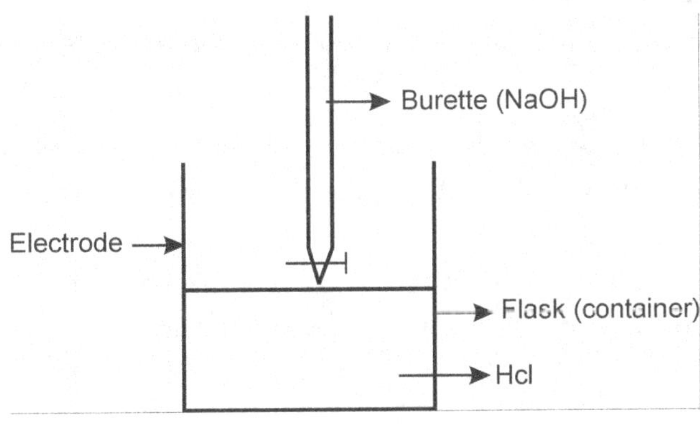

Fig.12.9

Here H_2O is formed so, H^+ ion concentration decreases so dilution of the solution takes place.

Now, NaCl will be formed which will get completely ionised in water. So, Cl^- concentration remains same and hence conductance due to Cl^- remains same.

- At zero time, when no NaOH is added in the flask, there is highest conductance due to unused H^+ ions.
- Initially we have Cl^- ions which have some conductance.
- As we add NaOH in the flask, H^+ ion concentration decreases.
- Here conductance due to Cl^- is constant and it remains constant even after addition of NaOH.
- Also, dilution takes place here [$\because$ H^+ decreasees and Cl^- remains same] because here NaCl will be formed which will get completely ionised in water.

There are Two Opinions

- Titrant should have minimum 10 times higher concentration than sample or titrant to compensate volume of sample or titrant.
- If volume of neither titrant nor titrant is prominent (more)
  Then

$$\Lambda_{actual} = \frac{\Lambda_{abs} + V(added\ volume)}{\Lambda_{obs}}$$

Λ_{obs} = Conductance observed

- Λ_{actual} can be calculated only when concentration of both the titrant and titrant is same.
- For compensating diluting effect, normally titrant is taken in higher concentration.
- At zero time $\rightarrow$ concentration of Cl^- decides total conductance.
  $HCl + NaOH \rightarrow NaCl + H_2O$
- Conductance due to H^+ ion concentration decreases with the passage of time because it forms H_2O which has minimum conductance

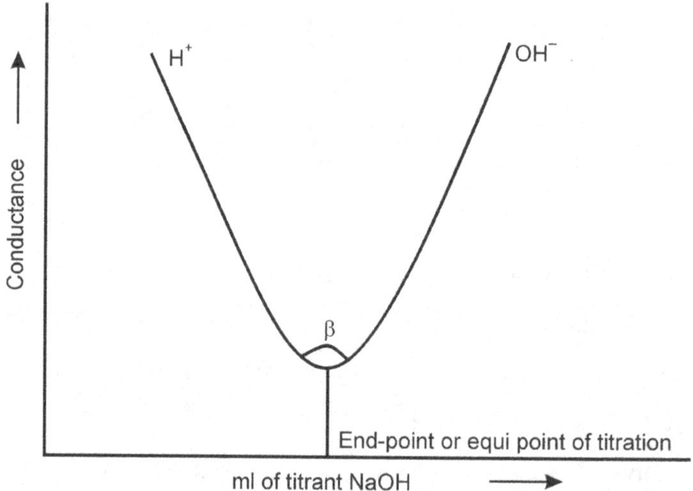

Fig.12.10 Titration Curve.

- Conductance due to Na^+ ion increases with passage of time and Na^+ is having normal conductance. So, because of $[Na^+] \rightarrow$ conductance increases initially at zero time.

$$[Na^+] = 0$$

- As we add NaOH to the flask,

$$\left[OH^-\right] \to \uparrow \text{ increases}$$

- So, conductance due to OH^- increases

- As the angle between 2 sides is narrow, accuracy is high and vice-versa.

  Question : What would be the shape of this titration curve ?

$$HAC + NaOH \to NaAC + H_2O$$

- Initially there will be low conductance because HAC is a very weak electrolyte.

  - Here $[H^+]$ is very low because being a weak electrolyte, HAC will not get ionized completely. It will partially get ionized. So $[H^+]$ concentration will be low.

  - When we add NaOH from the burette, Na^+ and part of HAC will react and will form NaAc buffer.

  - Which prevents change in pH or change in $[H^+]$.

  - As long as HAC is there, we will find some conductance in the solution.

  - When all HAC is used up, there won't be any conductance due to $[H^+]$. This is also called the end-point of the titration because at this time both the titrant and the titrand are in the same amount.

  - As no more HAC is there, the conductance will be the lowest at that time (at the end-point).

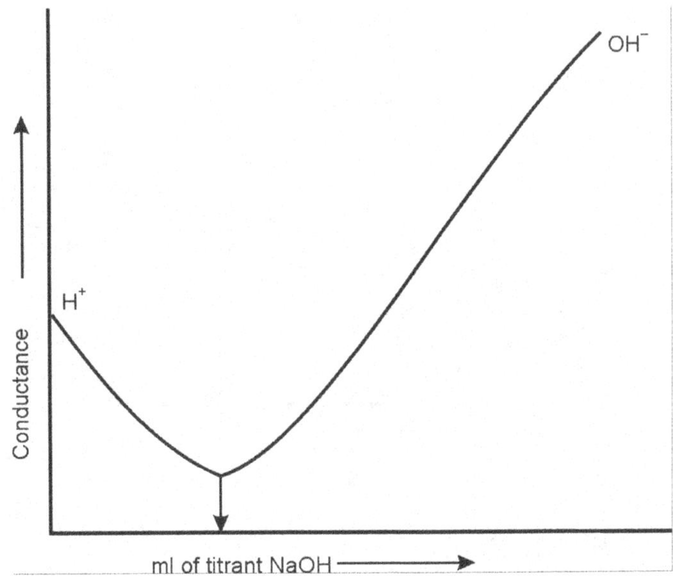

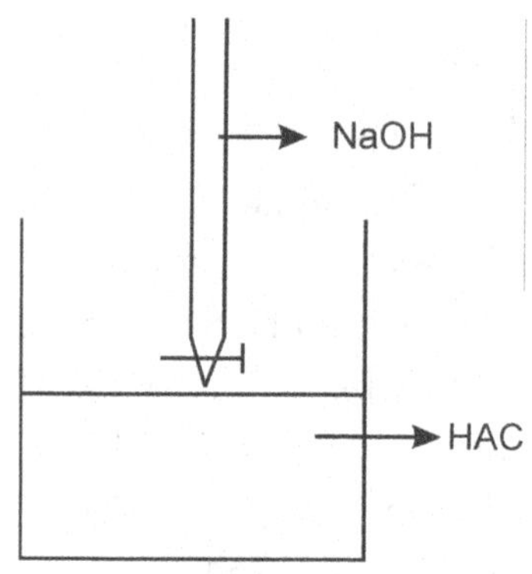

Fig.12.11

- Now on addition of more NaOH, there is no more HAC to react with it. So, NAOH will remain unreacted.
- Now, OH^- ion concentration will increase on addition of each drop of NaOH (titrant) .
- So, after endpoint, there will be increase in conductance on each addition of NaOH.
- So, the titration curve will be such that shown in Fig 12.7.

Question: How, the end-point of a mixture of weak acid and strong acid will be determined by using strong base NaOH ?

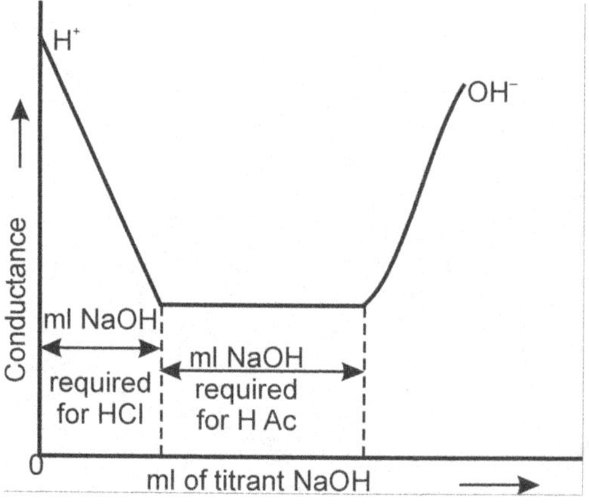

Fig.12.12

(i) $HCl + NaOH \rightarrow NaCl + H_2O$

(ii) $HAc + NaOH \rightarrow NaAc + H_2O$

- Titrand is a mixture of strong acid HCl and weak acid HAC and titrant is the strong base NaOH.
- So, when we add the NaOH, it will first react with HCl as the HCl is stronger acid than HAC.
- There won't be any reaction between NaOH and HAC as long as there is any HCl in the solution.
- When all the HCl is used up or consumed by NaOH, conductance will be lowest due to decrease in $[H^+]$.
- Now addition of NaOH will produce reaction between NaOH and HAC.
- So, there will be conductance due to $[Na^+]$ which will remain constant.
- When all HAC is consumed by NaOH, more drop of NaOH will increase the [OH].
- And as $[OH^-]$ increases, there will be increase in conductance.
- So, during this titration, initially conductance decreases, and a point comes hen it becomes lowest then it remains constant at its lowest limit and then it starts increasing.

8. Precipitation Titration

- Formation of insoluble compound
- Argentometry titration
- Titration involving $AgNO_3$ as one of the titrant.

Principle : Before and after end-point conductance difference is measured.

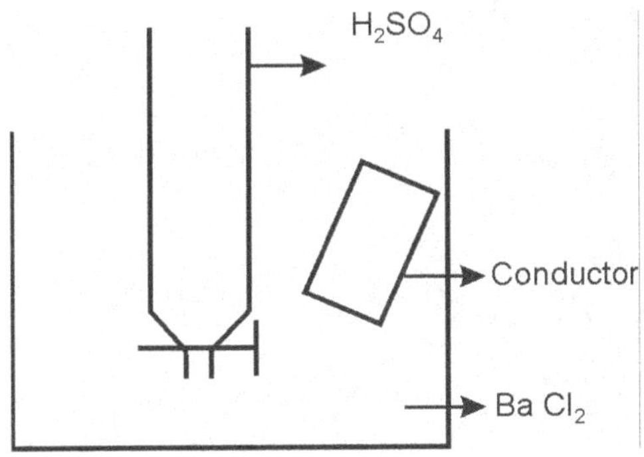

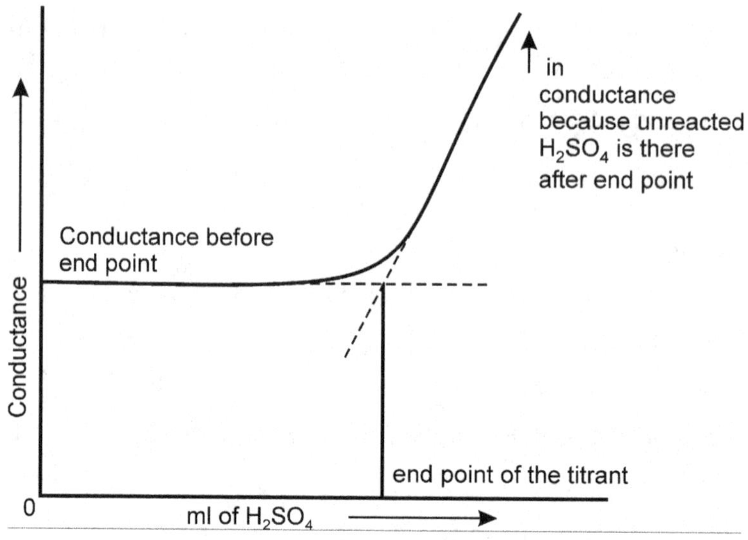

Fig.12.13

Here conductance due to $2Cl^-$ will remain same inspite of addition of H_2SO_4.

$$BaCl_2 \xrightarrow{\text{H}_2\text{SO}_4} BaSO_4 + 2HCl$$

Soluble compound   Highly insoluble Compound

Ionization100%   (will be precipitated out)

9. Salt Analysis

e.g., Here we can take any of these salts

   NH_4Cl

Or – chloroquine sulphate

Or – quinine sulphate

$$NH_4Cl \xrightarrow[\text{NaOH}]{\text{(titrant)}} NH_4OH + NaCl$$

(here all ions have nearly same conductance)

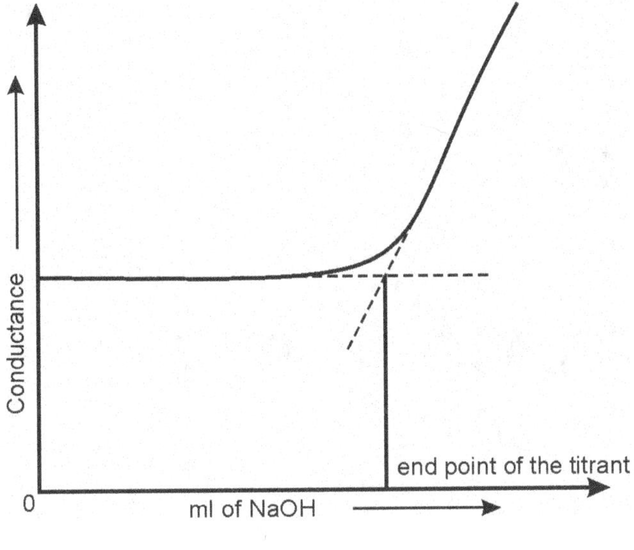

Fig.12.14

[mixture of NH_4OH and NH_4Cl will have a common ion effect, so buffer is formed. So ammonia does not get hydrolysed effectively].

CHAPTER 13

POTENTIOMETRY OR pH METRY

- Both potentiometry and pH metry are inter-related techniques.
- Most of the pH meters can function as potentiometers.

Principle of Voltaic or Galvanic Cells

- Different chemicals interact and produce electricity and the potential of generated electricity is measured.
- Potential measured here is actually potential difference or driving force, which makes electrons to move, it is also known as EMF [electro motive force].

  [Note : Degenerated potential depends upon the type of drug.
- Measurement of EMF during course of titration helps us in finding end point, which is used in potentiometric titration].

Standard Reduction Potential   OR
(E^0) Standard Potential

Definition

It is the potential of an electrode (half cell), when the concentration of involved species of electrode is unit (single) in comparison with potential of standard hydrogen electrode or normal hydrogen electrode as zero volt at NTP and when the system is undergoing reduction process.

- This is universal constant.
- Here reacting species of the electrodes have unit activity (unit concentration) at 25 °C.

- It is written as S.H.E (Standard hydrogen electrode).
- (N.H.E – Normal hydrogen electrode).
- Scientifically in all the calculations, activity should be considered but practically we can take concentration only because activity can't be measured practically.

$\downarrow$ Se in –Ve valancy $\rightarrow$ oxidation

$\uparrow$ Se in +Ve valancy $\rightarrow$ oxidation

$\downarrow$ Se in +Ve valancy $\rightarrow$ reduction

$\uparrow$ Se in –Ve valancy $\rightarrow$ reduction

Eg. $Fe^{+3} + \bar{e} \rightarrow Fe^{+2}$

Reduction Process

Standard reduction potential for this reduction process is + 0.77 volt.

$$E^o_{Fe^{+3}, Fe^{+2}} = + 0.77 \text{ volt}$$

Standard

Potential

Indicates
reduction
process

$$E^O_{Fe^{+2}, Fe^{+3}} = + 0.77 \text{ volt}$$

Indicates system is undergoing oxidation process i.e.,

$$Fe^{+2} \rightarrow Fe^{+3} + \bar{e}$$

- Before 10 years, there was a concept that physical chemistry scientists were using only oxidation potential, while analytical chemistry scientists were using only reduction potential.
- But now, only reduction potential is used universally.
- So, in all calculations, it is common to use reduction potential.
- So, if oxidation potential is given then convert it into reduction potential for calculation by changing its sign (+ to – or – to +)

Daniel / Denial Cell

- It is an electrochemical cell consisting of two electrodes and solution composed of the following components.
  - Zn-plate in $ZnSO_4$ solution (0.5 N)
  - Cu-plate in $CuSO_4$ solution (0.2 N)

- These two solutions are in electrical contact, but not mixed with each-other and the electrodes are connected externally by an electric conductor.

- The voltmeter "V" will indicate that a difference in electric potential exists between two species of metals (electrodes).

$$\therefore E^o_{Cu^{+2},\ Cu^o} = +0.34 \text{ volt}$$

$$E^o_{Zn^{+2},\ Zn} = -0.76 \text{ volt}$$

1. $Zn^{+2} + 2\bar{e} \rightarrow Zn^o$ -0.76

2. $Fe^{+2} + 2\bar{e} \rightarrow Fe^o$ -0.44

3. $Cd^{+2} + 2\bar{e} \rightarrow Cd^o$ -0.4

4. $2H^+ + 2\bar{e} \rightarrow H_2 \text{ (std)}$ 0.00

5. $S4O_6^{-2} + 2\bar{e} \rightarrow 2S_2O_3^{-2}$ $+0.88$

   (tetra thionate)

6. $Cu^{+2} + 2\bar{e} \rightarrow Cu^o$ $+0.34$

7. $Fe^{+3} + \bar{e} \rightarrow Fe^{+2}$ $+0.77$

8. $Cl_2 + 2\bar{e} \rightarrow 2Cl^-$ $+1.36$

9. $MnO_4^{-1} + 5\bar{e} \rightarrow Mn^{+2}$ $+1.51$

10. $HNO_2 + \bar{e} \rightarrow No$ $+1.00$

Significance of Standard Reduction Potential

- The one which is having higher reduction potential will be undergoing reduction process and oxidizing the counter part or working as oxidant or oxidizing agent.
  Eg. $Fe^{+2} + KMnO_4$

  Here $KMnO_4$ will undergo reduction and acts as oxidizing agent.

- The one which is having lower reduction potential will be undergoing oxidation process and reduces the counter part or works as reducing agent
  Eg. $Zn + Cu^{+2}$

  It will undergo oxidation and acts as reducing agent.

- This series is very important for selection of antioxidants.
  [We can decide stability of drug.]

- Major cause of decomposition of drug is oxidation and so to prevent oxidation of drug, we add antioxidant because if drug has been oxidized then it is ineffective].

- Antioxidants have very low E^o value, so antioxidants itself undergoes oxidation and prevents oxidation of drug.

  Eg. $NaHSO_3$: It is a very common antioxidant [sodium metasulphite]

  $$E^o = -\,0.93 \text{ V [which is very low]}$$

Design of Various Electrodes

1. **The Standard Hydrogen Electrode (S.H.E)**

   It is a type of reference electrode

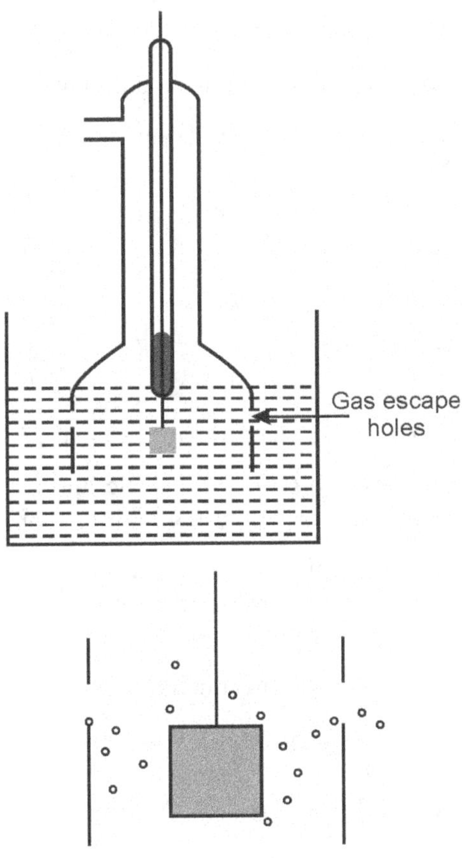

Fig. 13.1

- **Construction and Working**
  - It consists of a small piece of platinum foil, coated electrolytically with platinum black or platinum oxide, over which hydrogen gas is passed.

- The foil is covered with a close tube within which H_2 gas is continuously passed at 1 atmosphere pressure and concentration of gaseous substance is equal to pressure of gas.

  So activity of $H_2 = 1$ unit.

- Platinum black surface absorbs hydrogen more readily and the metallic surface constantly remains in contact with the gas.

- If it were an electrode of metallic hydrogen, only a half part of plantinum foil is immersed in the solution and the remaining half part is exposed to H_2 gas.

- Under this condition whatever potential we get is considered as 0.00 volt.

$$2H^+ + 2\bar{e} \rightleftharpoons H_2 \uparrow$$

$$E^\circ = 0.00 \text{ volt.}$$

- **Use :** It is used as a standard for all the calculations.

- All comparisons are made with reference to this electrode, considering it a standard electrode.

- It is universally accepted.

- **Advantages**

  - It exhibits no salt errors

  - It covers the entire pH range

- **Draw backs / Disadvantages**

  - It involves the used of gas and handling of gas is difficult.

  - Hydrogen is explosive i.e. highly exothermic and extremely faster so pressure should be maintained optimum and proper outlet should be provided.

  - The main disadvantage is that it easily gets poisoned by a large number of substances such as proteins, calomel, sulphides etc.

  - Serious errors are caused by oxidising and reducing agents as well as substances capable of being hydrogenated or reduced.

  - It is also unsatisfactory in the presence of salts of certain metals such as copper, silver and gold.

2. Saturated Calomel Electrode (SCE)

Type : Reference standard electrode.

- **Design**

  - It is most widely used reference electrode due to the constancy of its potential and ease of preparation.

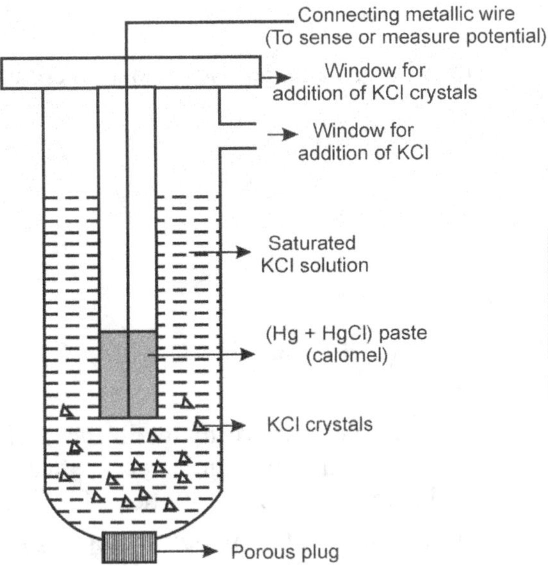

Fig. 13.2

- **Construction**
    - The electrode is made up to two glass tubes.
        (i) Inner glass tube
        (ii) Outer glass tube
    - In the inner narrow glass tube, paste of Hg + HgCl is filled in sufficiently high amount and on the top of this tube eg. on upper part, excess of Hg is filled.
    - In the outer tube saturated KCl solution is filled in which KCl crystals are added.

- **Working principle**
    - This electrode may undergo oxidation or reduction process but potential change will not occur.
    - If $\bar{e}$ density is more then

    $$Hg^+ + \bar{e} \rightarrow Hg \downarrow$$

    - and if there is deficiency of $\bar{e}$ then

    $$Hg \rightarrow Hg^+ + \bar{e}$$

    - But both Hg^+ and Hg are present in enough concentration so that above changes will not effect its concentration hence potential remains unchanged.

- **Standards**

  - The potential of calomel electrode depends upon the concentration of KCl in the cell.

		Potential
• Saturated KCl	$\rightarrow$	+ 0.250 V
• 1 N KCl (normal conc.)	$\rightarrow$	+ 0.286 V
• 0.1 N KCl (decinormal conc.)	$\rightarrow$	+ 0.388 V

  - In laboratory during experiment, if we maintain the KCl solution saturated all the time even then the potential will change because when this electrode is kept into sample solution, due to porous plug, dilution of kCl solution occurs.

  - So, to overcome this problem, take enough quantity of KCl solution and add KCl crystals.

  - If after a very long term use, if all KCl crystals gets exhausted then there is a facilitated window for addition of water and kCl crystals.

Advantage

- Constancy of potential
- Easy to prepare.

- **Uses**

  - Its use is unavoidable
  - It is necessary reference electrode for all the electrochemical processes, where we want to study only one part of redox reaction.

- **Relation between pH and Voltage**

  $$E = -\,0.0591\ pH$$

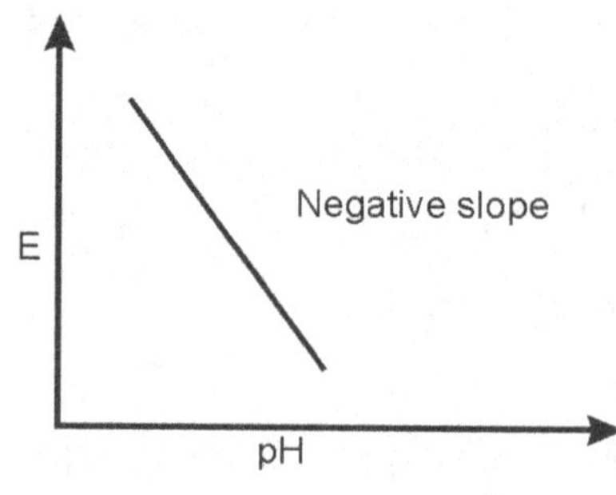

Fig. 13.3

3. Silver – Silver Chloride Electrode

OR

Ag/AgCl Electrode

- **Type :** Reference electrode
  - It is more difficult to prepare but is very convenient to use as calomel electrode.

- **Design**

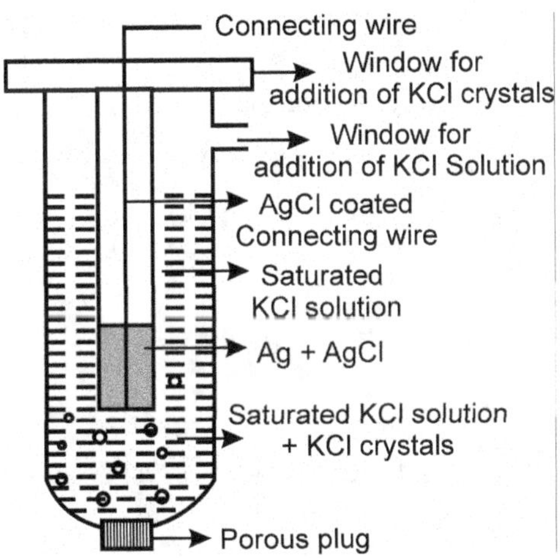

Fig. 13.4

Design is same as calomel electrode. Just take Ag + AgCl instead of Hg_2^+ + HgCl.

- It consists of a silver coated electrolytically with silver chloride, which is dipped into a solution of potassium chloride or KCl solution having definite strength.

- Thus it contains

  Ag – in excess amount

  AgCl – in excess amount

  Saturated KCl solution – too much excess.

- Working Principle - Same as calomel electrode.

- If there is more $\bar{e}$ density then,

  $$Ag^+ + \bar{e} \rightarrow Ag$$

- And if there is deficiency of $\bar{e}$, then

$$Ag \rightarrow Ag^+ + \bar{e}$$

- But both Ag and Ag^+ are present in enough concentration so there is no change occurs in the potential of the electrode thus it acts as a reference electrode.

- **Standards**

  - The potential of this electrode depends upon the concentration of KCl in the cell.

    Potential as compared to S.H.E

  - Saturated KCl solution $\rightarrow$ 0.200 V
  - 1 N KCl solution $\rightarrow$ 0.235 V

    (normal concentration)

  - 0.1 N KCl solution $\rightarrow$ 0.288 V

    (decinormal concentration)

  - for constant potential, add extra KCl crystals and keep the KCl solution saturated all the time.

  - If after the use of long time, KCl crystals get exhausted then there is a facilitated window for addition of KCl crystals.

- **Use** : It is used as a reference electrode in electrochemical processes.

4. Mercurous Sulphate Electorde

- **Type :** Reference electrode

  - This electrode is similar in construction to the calomel electrode but utilises dilute sulphuric acid saturated with mercurous sulphate.

  - **Use :** It is used in solution, where silver or lead ions are present.

5. Glass Electrode

- Type : Indicator electrode

  (polarisable or working)

- **Design**

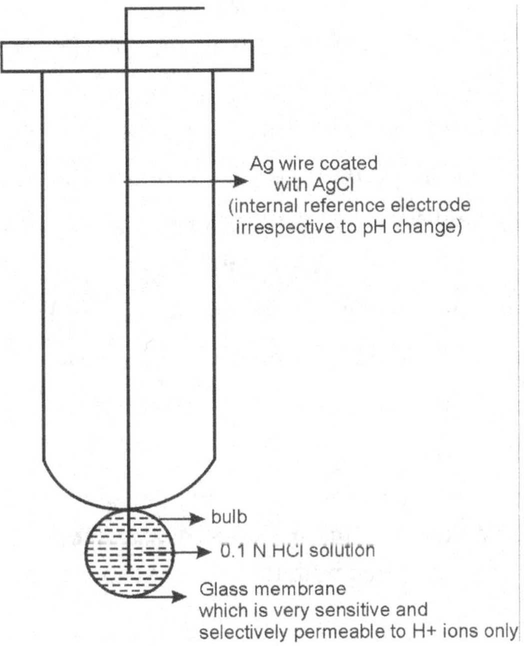

Fig. 13.5

- It is mode up of a glass tube and a bulb at the bottom and a conducting wire in the middle of this assembly.

- Glass membrane of the bulb is extremely thin and chemically it is made up of alumino silicate containing Ca^{+2} or Na^+ ions.

Working Principles

- This membrane is very unique and specific which allows only H^+ ions to go outside or to come inside.

- So, it is considered as "H^+ ions selective electrode".

- So, if we want to measure H^+ ions, then only it is useful.

- So, it selective electrode for measuring pH.

- Glass bulb contains 0.1 N (decinormal concentration), of HCl solution.

- Electrical contact with this solution is usually made with a silver wire coated with silver chloride, thus it acts as internal reference electrode (i.e. unresponsive to pH change).

- Here uniform coating i.e. 100% uniform coating is required, which can be achieved by electro coating method, which gives 100 % uniform coating.
- The potential of a glass electrode when immersed in a solution is given by following equation

$$E = K + 0.0592 \ (pH_1 - pH_2) \ (at \ 25°C)$$

pH_1 is the pH of sol^n in bulb pH_2 is the pH of test solution.

- Now, pH_1 is constant for given electrode so,

$$E = K - 0.0592 \ pH_2$$

where; K = constant = asymmetry potential value of k depends on.

(i) thickness of glass bulb (ii) composition of solution etc.

- **Advantages**
  - Response is very rapid
  - It is not affected by the presence of oxidising or reducing agents, dissolved gases, highly coloured liquid, colloids, suspended matter or moderate concentration of many salts, with the main exception of sodium salts.

- **Use**
  - It is a useful indicator available for pH measurements.

- **Difficulty or Disadvantages**
  - It is extremely fragile so careful handling is required because even a minute scratch on the bulb makes it useless.
  - It has very high internal resistance, normally in terms of $M\Omega$ (mega ohm) i.e. 1 to 10 $M\Omega$ so even very low current can pass through it. So proper modification e.g. proper amplification is required to compensate high resistance and getting proper readings.
  - So, glass electrode cannot be used for potentiometry; it is used in pH metry generally.

6. Combined Electrode

- Before measurement of pH, electrode should be dipped into distilled water for 24 hours to activate the membrane and then only it is ready for sensing H^+ ions

  [use of modern Lithia-silica glasses enables pH measurement to be valid over practically entire pH range. Some glass electrodes, however only respond linearly over the pH range 2 to 9].

Type : Both reference and indicator electrode.

- It is made up of two electrodes
  (i) glass electrode
  (ii) Calomel electrode
- So, it is rather easy in handling
- It is called combine electrode.

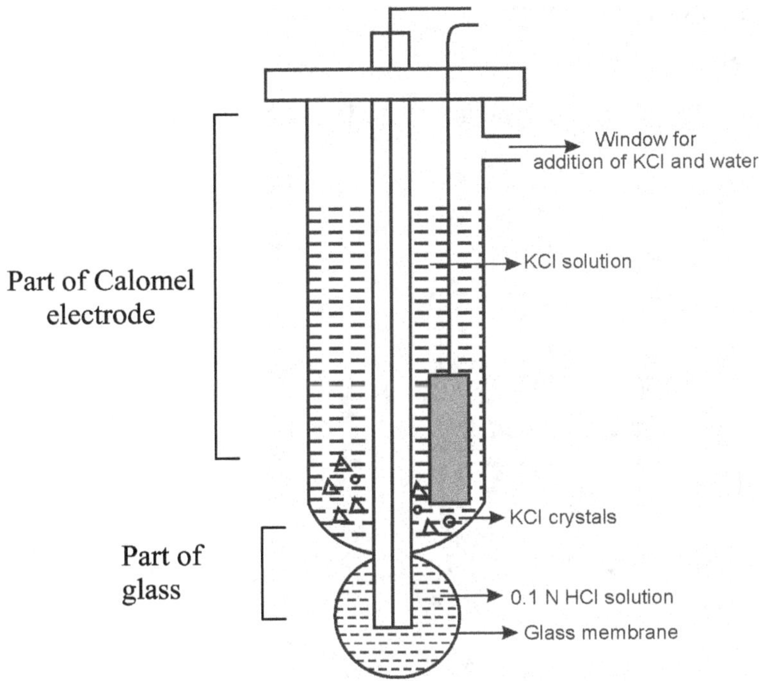

Fig. 13.6

7. Ion Selective Electrode (ISE)

Type : Indicator Electrode

- This is extension of concept of glass electrode.
- Glass electrode is H^+ ion selective electrode. So, from this concept we can think about electrode which can sense only Cl^- ions only Ca^{+2} ions or only Na^+ ions.
- Thus, we can make electrode which is specifically permeable to specific types of ions only and other ions are resisted.

Definition : An electrode which is capable of sensing only one cation or anion in a complex mixture.

- This electrode should not sense any ion other than that one particular ion.

Use : It is used to measure specific type of particular ionic concentration in the sample which is a mixture of 1000 of compounds.

- Now-a-days varieties of ion selective electrodes are available in the market.
- Thus, this is used for selective measurement of a particular ion.

Varieties or Types of ion Selective Electrode

(a) Solid Membrane ISE

- Here a solid substance of crystal structure is used to select any ion.

Design

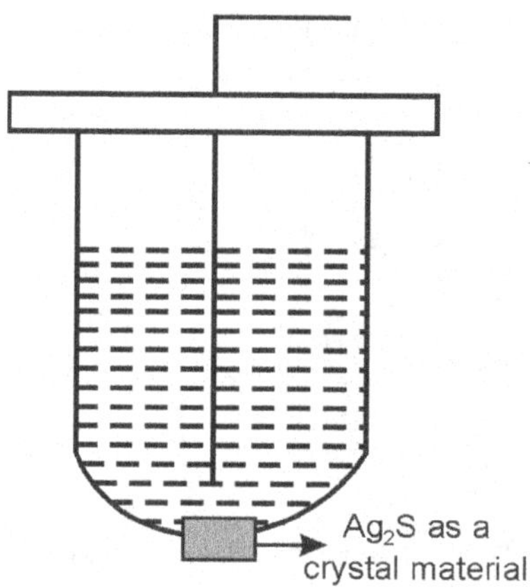

Fig. 13.7

- Here specifically designed liquid is filled in specific plastic material or resin material, which has semi permeable membrane, which is highly selective for particular ion so, we get selective measurement for particular ion.

- **Principle**
  - Crystal structure is highly pure and solid and it allows only ions similar to it to move and penetrate and thus it measures the concentration of that particular ion in the given solution.
    Eg. Ag^+ ISE
  - It consists of highly pure and solid Ag_2S at the bottom, which is crystalline material and it will be sensing only Ag^+ ions in the solution and so it can't give entry to ions other than Ag^+

(b) Liquid Membrane ISE

Design

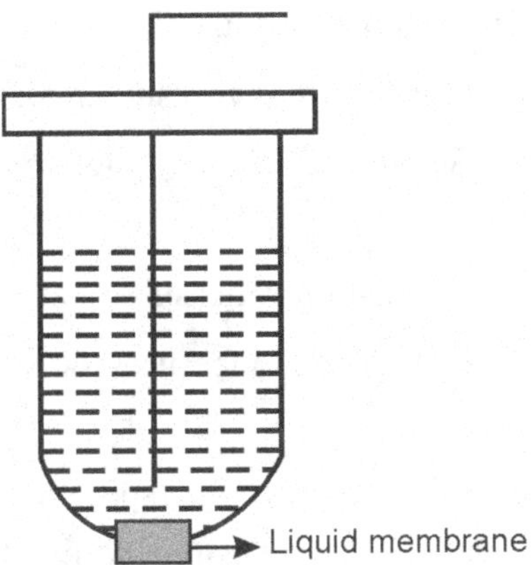

Fig. 13.8

- Here, specifically designed liquid is filled in specific plastic or resin material, which has semi permeable membrane which is highly selective for particular ion. So, we get selective measurement of particular ion.

(c) Enzyme Electrode

Design

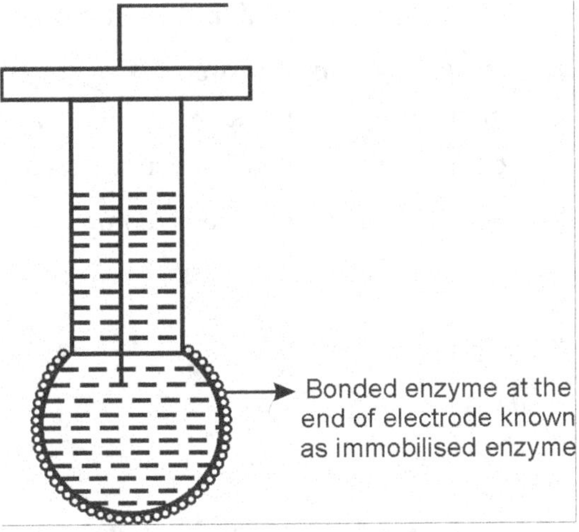

Fig. 13.9

- This electrode has other design same as other electrodes but here, enzyme is chemically bonded to some inner surface and once it is bonded permanently to surface, then we can have repeated ultisation.
- They are very selective for reaction with substrate.
  - So, this become a "Substance selective electrode" OR "Compound selective electrode".
  - Thus, this electrode is useful for measurement of insulin or adrenaline etc.

    Eg. Urea-enzyme Electrode: It measures only concentration of urea in the sample.
  - Thus, this is highly selective or highly specific electrode and so in a complex mixture also we can measure desired compound and there is no need of separation of that complex mixture for measurement of that particular compound.

7. Micro-Electrodes OR Fibre Electrodes

- If above any electrode is made very small (i.e, smaller than the needle of syringe) then that electrode is named as micro-electrode.
- If ion-selective electrode is used as micro-electrode then we can measure particular ion concentration in body without any withdrawal of blood fluid from body.
- The enzyme electrode is made up of micro-size type, so we can measure concentration of any body fluid from the body. (e.g. a scientist has found out concentration of diazepam in brain by some specific enzyme micro electrode).
- So, by uses of this, concentration of various compounds within body, without disturbance is possible.

8. Quinhydrone Electrode

Type : Indicator electrode

Design

- This electrode is used as a substitute of hydrogen electrode to overcome its disadvantages.

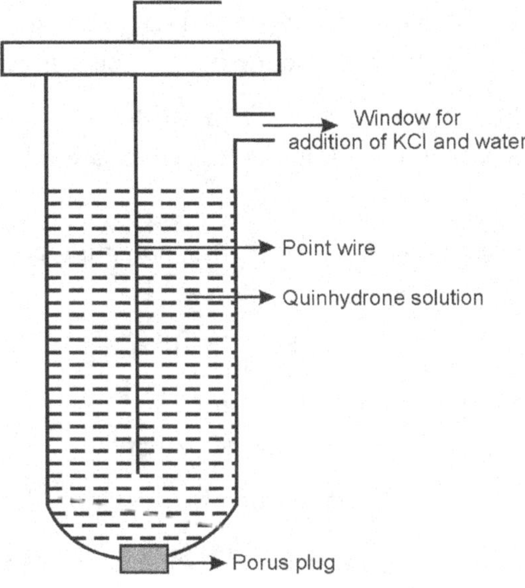

Fig. 13.10

- This electrode consists of a bright platinum wire dipped into the test solution which has been saturated with quinhydrone.

- In the solution, quinhydrone is almost completely dissociated into p-benzoquinone and hydroquinone in equimolecular proportion.

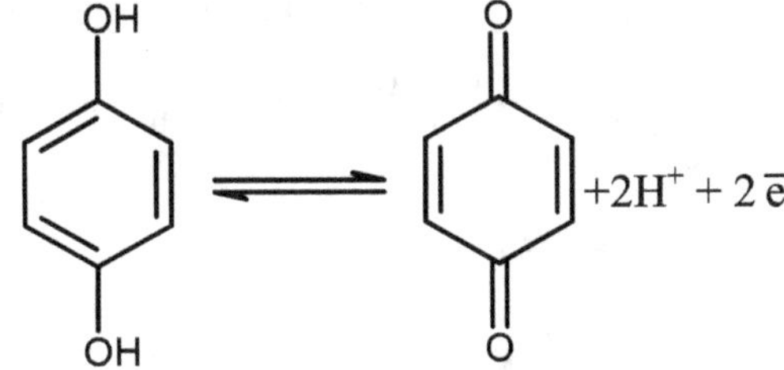

Hydroquinone   p-benzoquinone

& quinhydron <u>dissociation</u> → P- benzoquinone + hydroquinone

- Now consider that quinhydrone has unique activity or unique concentration so the concentration of benzoquinone and hydroquinone are equal.

So,

$$E_Q = 0.699 + \frac{0.0592}{2}$$

- Hydroquinone can undergo oxidation and P-Benzoquinone undergoes reversible oxidation–reduction process in acidic media and gets converted into hydroquinone.

- The pH of the solution can be determined by the use of this oxidation–reduction system because reduction to hydroquinone or oxidation to benzoquinone involves the hydrogen ion.

- For an oxidation-reduction electrode, the potential at 25°C is given by the expression :

$$E_Q = E_Q^O + \frac{0.0592}{n} \log \frac{[\text{oxi}]}{[\text{Red}]}$$

Where, $[\text{oxi}]$ = concentration of oxidant

$[\text{Red}]$ = concentration of reductant

N = No. of $\bar{e}$ gained by the oxidant is being converted into the reductant

$E_Q^O = 0.699$ volts at 25°c

$$\therefore E_Q = 0.699 + \frac{0.0592}{2} \log \frac{[\text{Benzoquinone}][\text{H}^+]_2}{[\text{Hydroquinone}]}$$

Now, consider that quinhydrone has uique activity or unique concentration and so the concentration of benzoquinone and hydroquinone are equal so,

$$E_Q = 0.699 + \frac{0.0592}{2} \times 2 \log [\text{H}^+]^2$$

$$\therefore E_Q = 0.699 + 0.0592 \log [\text{H}^+]$$

$$\therefore E_Q = 0.699 - 0.0592 \text{ pH}$$

This is the relationship between pH and potential of quinhydrone electrode.

- Suppose we use quinhydrone electrode with calomel electrode then relation between pH and potential can be given as follows.

$$\text{pH} = \frac{0.454 - E_{cell}}{0.0592}$$

This indicates co-relation between cell potential and pH.

- **Specificity of Quinhydrone Electrode**

It is very easy to prepare we just have to mix and dissolve in water and use it.

- **Advantages over Hydrogen Electrode**
  - Rapid in response.

    It can be used for many solutions which are not suitable for the hydrogen electrode.

    Eg : $KMnO_4$, Nitrite, Ferric system because they react with H_2.
  - It does not get readily in activated like hydrogen electrode.

Limitation

This electrode is unstable and so can't be prepared and stored for long time, because hydroquinone is readily oxidizable by O_2 of air. Quinhydrone electrode can't function in alkaline pH because above pH 8, apart from redox reaction, it also forms salt with hydroquinone. It can produce complex with boron compound, so with it, it can't be used because of alteration of properties.

G. Platinum Electrode

Type : working (indicator) electrode

It is the most simple electrode.

Design

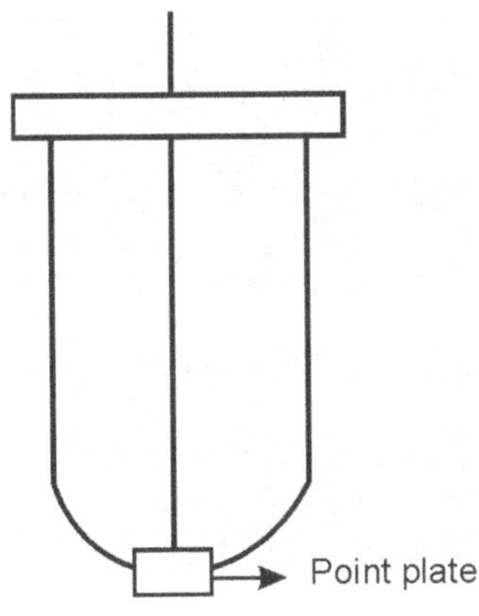

Fig. 13.11

- It has a platinum plate or platinum wire terminal or platinum ring.
- Platinum is the most inert and non reactive metal which is a good character for stable electrode.

Use : It is used in all redox titrations.

Potentiometers

Potentiometers are used to measure potential of given voltaic or galvanic cell. It is capable of measuring potential.

Potentiometer consists of two electrodes :

(i) saturated colomel electrode

(ii) Platinum electrode.

(here glass electrode can't be used because it is having very high resistance to potential, so it is replaced by platinum electrode or any other metal electrode.)

Basic Principle

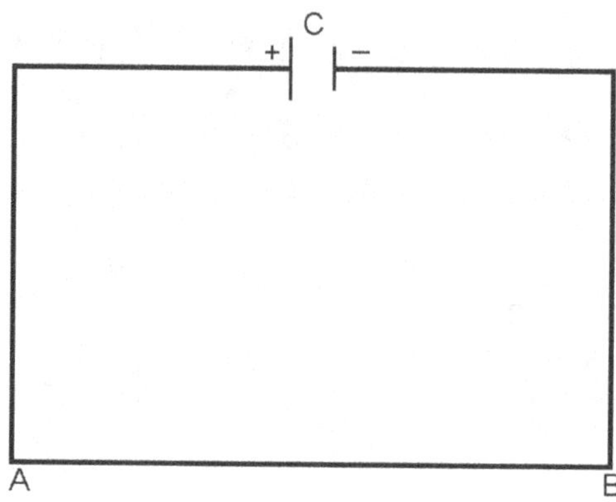

Fig. 13.12

C = D.C power supply (current supply) in which one electrode remains permanently +ve and other electrode remains permanently −ve and it requires 1.5 volt = 2 volt (cell generally).

AB = long wire with a perfect uniform cross section.

Each segment of the length of wire is expressing a definite potential.

(i)   Most commonly used principle in the measurement of potential is

   Length of wire α voltage

   Suppose we are supplying 2v power, then it is distributed to the entire length of AB wire

$$\therefore\ AB \rightarrow 2\ \text{meter} \rightarrow 2\ \text{volts} \rightarrow \left[\frac{2}{2}\right]$$

$$\downarrow$$

Each meter will express 1 volt

(ii)   If we want to measure smaller value of potential more accurately,

$$AB \rightarrow 20 \text{ meters} \rightarrow 2 \text{ volt} \rightarrow \left[\dfrac{2}{20}\right]$$

$$\downarrow$$

Each segment will be expressing still

Smaller value of potential : 0.01 volts.

Thus, as the length increases, sensitivity and accuracy of measurement of potential also increases.

(iii)   But practically it is not possible to increase the too much length of wire. So, coil is used.

(wire is rounded) on very small inert material)

Measurement of Potential of an unknown Cell

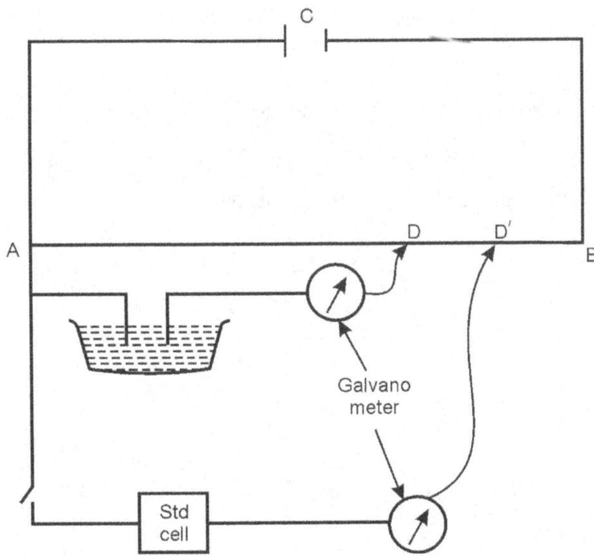

Fig. 13.13

- When potential on both sides become equal, potential of segment of wire and potential of solution becomes equal. This is called Null point.

- Generally Weston cell is used as a standard cell.

- Find out the proper distance by moving jockey key when zero in galvanometer is achieved that is the point when potential on both sides of wire becomes equal. This is called nul point.

- AD' has the length required for balancing the potential of standard cell.

- AD has the same potential as that of standard cell potential.

Thus,

Standard potential = E_s (comparable to AD 1th)

- D is the null point for unknown cell.

- Greater is the length, greater is the potential.

Now, potential $\propto$ length

$$E_u \propto AD$$

$$\text{And } E_s \alpha AD$$

$$\frac{E_u}{E_s} = \frac{AD}{AD^1}$$

$$\therefore E_4 = \frac{AD}{AD^1} \times E_s$$

Thus, potential of an unknown solution can be found out by comparison method.

E.g : A standard Weston cell having potential 1.012 volts gives null point at 42 cm length. If an unknown produce null point at 58 cm, calculate potential of unknown solution.

E_s = 1.012 volts

AD^1 = 42 cm

E_u = (?)

AD = 58 cm

$$\frac{Eu}{Es} = \frac{AD}{AD^1}$$

$$\therefore E_u = \frac{AD}{AD^1} \times E_s$$

$$\therefore E_u = \frac{58}{42} \times E_s$$

$$= \frac{58}{42} \times 1.012$$

$$= 1.397 \text{ volt}$$

Note : Number of complex instruments have this basic principle.

pH meters

pH meters are same as potentiometers

pH meters consists of two electrodes

    (i)   Saturated calomel electrode

    (ii) Glass electrode

Use : They are used to measure pH

  - Here we utilise same principle as potentiometer because

$E = -0.0591\ pH$

So,

We use the same instrument for both E and pH (E = potential that we measure here).

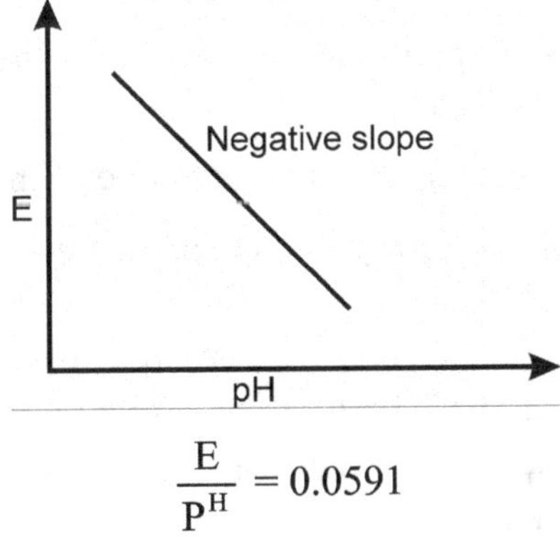

$$\frac{E}{P^H} = 0.0591$$

Fig. 13.14

- Here instead of platinum electrode, glass electrode is used.
- Because for measurement of pH, we want to measure selectively only H^+ ion concentration and glass electrode is "H ion electrode".
- It can't be used in potentiometry because it is selective only for H^+ ion and doesn't give reactions with any other substances and glass electrode has very high resistance in terms of $M\Omega$. So, some additional settings are made to compensate its high resistance.

Applications of pH Metry

For Accurate measurement of pH :

pH can be measured by several devices.

Litmus Paper

It is not an accurate method, it only indicates whether the pH is acidic or basic.

- ### pH – indicator

    E.g : Phenolphtheline : It has certain limitation i.e., they have specific pH range (generally 2 units) within which it shows colour change.

    pH range for phenolphtheline is 8.3 to 10 i.e below pH 8.3 it is colourless and above pH 10 it is pink coloured and between 8 to 10 pH, it shows colour change.

Simple Instruments

E.g : pH – comparator

It is a radio like instrument. Here, we have to use universal indicator or multiple range indicator.

- ### pH Strips

    Eg : pH papers : They have the pH range of 1 to 1.5 pH units.

- At different pH, different colours are produced on the strip and we can compare and judge the pH of the solution.

- All the above methods give range of pH, but none of them give accurate pH.

- So, pH meter is the most necessary instrument used in all most all the industries for measurement of accurate pH.

    pH measurement is the basic requirement in pharmacy, it plays a definite role in all the titrations like - acid base titration, precipitation titration etc.

Condition for the use of Indicator : pH at the equivalent point or end point and pH range of inductor should be same.

Titration error is zero : i.e., end point = equivalent point, while visual titration, slight excess of titrant required for end point.

So, titration error = end point – equivalent point.

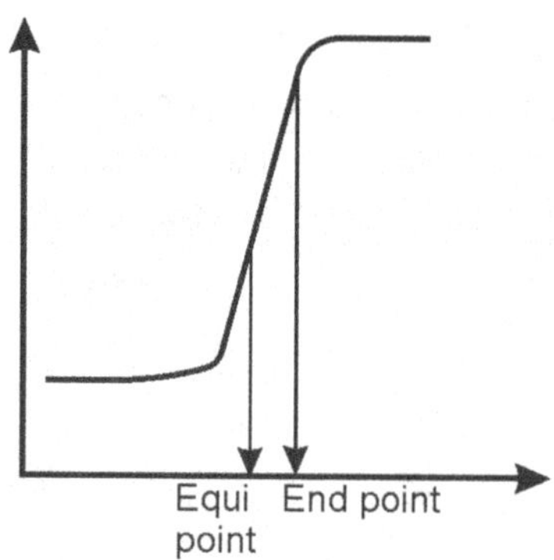

Fig. 13.15

pH affects stability, bio-availability of drug etc., so Pharmacopoeia states perfect pH for different formulations and injections. If there is change in pH then that injection or sample can't be used because it may cause severe problems.

Eg :   **pH**

Sodium thiosulphate $\rightarrow$ 7 to 9

injection

(antidote for CN^- poisoning)

- Sodium lactate injection $\rightarrow$ 5 to 7

Sodium diatrizoate injection $\rightarrow$ 6.6 to 7.6

- pH meter requires standardization / Calibration / validation.

- Due to no. of factors if instruments show wrong pH, so pharmacopoeia tells that it is required to validate them.

  [For standardization, we require standard buffer solution of known pH.

  As per B.P.

  0.5 M KHP (Potassium hydrogen pthalite) has pH – 4 if pH meter shows pH other than this, then we can set it.

- In market, buffer tablet is available dissolve it in water and measure the pH.

- Setting correct pH in pH meter by using known pH buffer solution is called standardization or validation or calibration.

(ii) End Point Detection

(pH metric titration)

Advantages over visual Indicator method

(i) pH meter is versatile as compared to indicator because each indicator has certain pH range. So, same indicator can't be used for all types of acid-base titrations but same pH meter can be used for all types of acid-base titration.

(ii) pH meter doesn't require any indicator.

Condition for the use of Indicator

(i)   pH at the equivalence point or end point and pH range of indicator should be same.

(ii) Titration error is zero i.e., (end point or equivalence point) while in visual titrations excess of titrant is requied for end point.

So, titration error = end point – equi. Point

- To get sharp end point means one drop gives drastic change in colour and pH.
- While sluggish end point gives gradual colour change.
- In case of other instruments or in case of visual titrations, at the end point only indicator undergoes changes].

(iii)   Coloured solution can be easily determined by pH meter eg : Paracetamol syrup.

(iv)   We can use pH meter both in aqueous and non-aqueous system.

(v)   All types of acids and bases can be titrated very easily.

   Eg : weak acid, very weak acid, weak base, very weak base etc.)

(i) Strong acid Vs strong base

(HCl V/s NaOH)

Q – Describe methods of locating end point

Ans : All the 3 techniques are to be written. I, II and III.

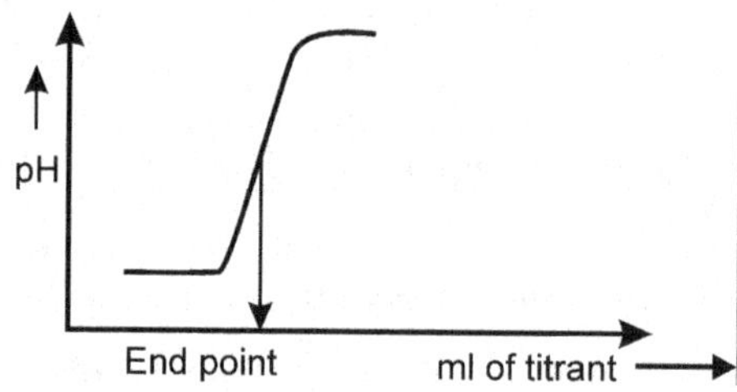

Fig. 13.16

End point location is very easy here because at equivalence point, there is a drastic change in pH.

(ii) Weak acid Vs strong base

(HAc Vs NaOH)

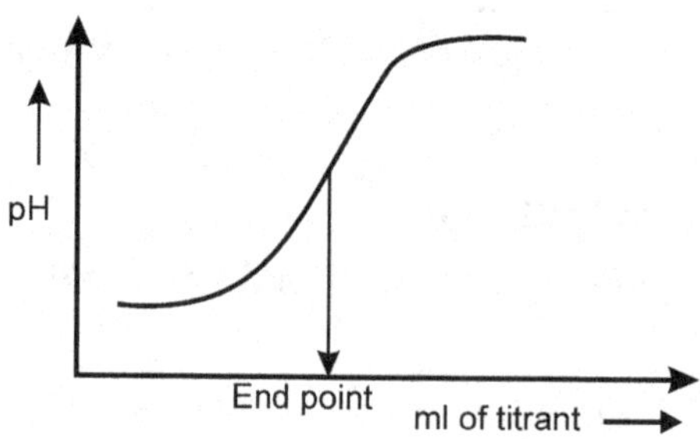

Fig. 13.17

Here end-point location is different because slope is bit less.

(iii) Very weak acid Vs strong base

$(H_3Bo_3$ Vs NaOH$)$

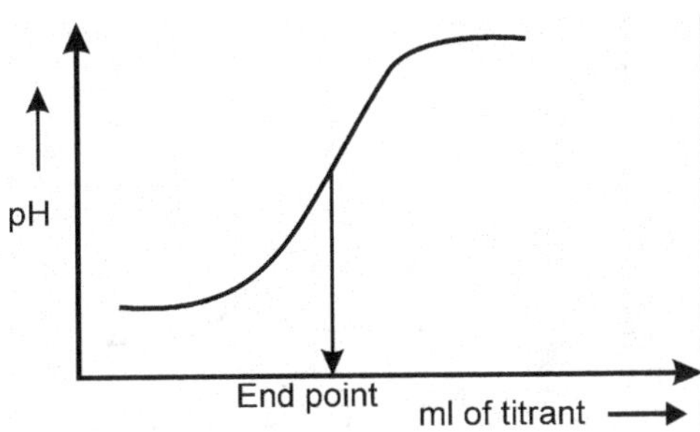

Fig. 13.18

- Here, end point location is very difficult (sluggish end point) because slope is negligible.

- So, for more accuracy in detection of end point location, scientists have found out other techniques also.

II First Derivative Graph

- It indicates change in pH per ml of titrant addition.

- Here, change in pH for the volume of titrant added is polotted as ordinate Vs the volume of titrant (v) added as abscissa.

- From the shape of graph, it becomes clear that maximum change in pH occurs at equivalence point.

- The end point can be readily recorded by drawing perpendicular from the peak of the graph on volume axis (abscissa).

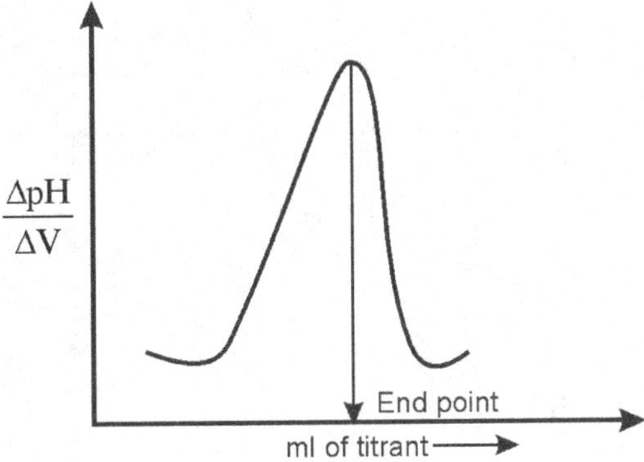

Fig. 13.19

III.   Second Derivative Graph

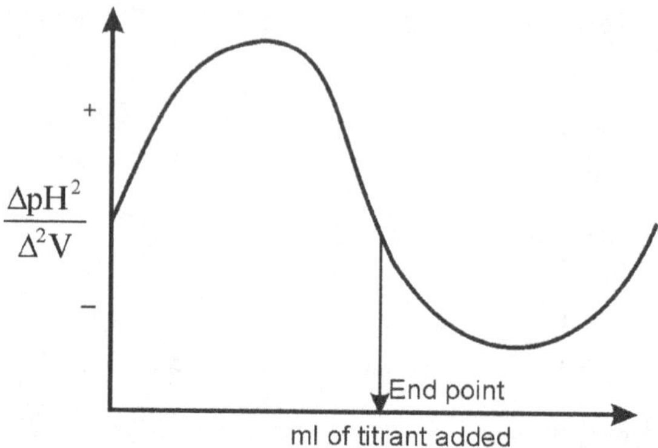

Fig. 13.20

The end point is shown as a zero point where the slope or curve of $\dfrac{\Delta^2 pH}{\Delta^2 V}$ is maximum)

Determination pka or pkb of Weak Acids or Weak Bases

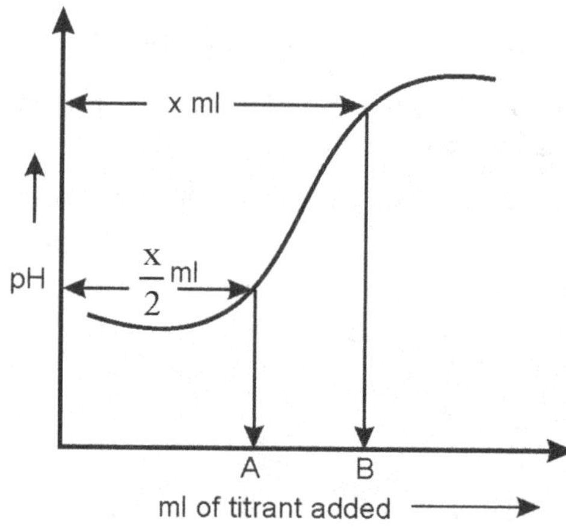

Fig. 13.21

B = equivalence point

A = half neutralization point

Handerson Hasselbalch's Equation

$$pH = pka + \log \left[\dfrac{\text{Salt}}{\text{Free acid}} \right]$$

At half neutralization point,

[salt] = [Free acid]

$\therefore$ pH = pka

- Thus, this is practically useful technique for finding out pka and pkb.

IV Pharmacopoeial Assays

- Pharmacopoeial assays are determined by general electrometric end point detection method.

- It can be either pH or potentiometry using glass or platinum or saturated) calomel electrode etc.

- Generally two types of analysis carried out by the same system.

    (i) Aqueous titration

    (ii) Non–ayucous titration

       (water free condition)

- Non-aqueous titration is much more common.

- More than 60% of drugs are estimated by the non-aqueous method using pH metry.

[But in non-aqueous method, calomel electrode requires some modification because in calomel (reference) electrode, water is used in plenty.

Modification : Water is removed and methanol is used for dissolving substances of electrode]

Examples of Pharmacopoeial Assays

- Acetazolamide tablet assayed by non-aqueous titration using titrant Tetra Butyl Ammonium Hydroxide (TBAH). It is strong base even stronger than NaOH, KOH

Drug	**Titrant**
- Allopurinol	TBAH
- Amiloride Hcl (pure powder)	$HClO_4$ (strongest acid)
- Benzathicin penicillin	$HClO_4$
- Bromhexidine Hcl	$HClO_4$

[Other examples of non aqueous titrations]

1. Amoxicillin   2. Caffiene

3. Quinine HCl   4. Thrimethoprene

5. Thiamine HCl

Applications of Potentiometry

Stability of Drugs

- Major cause of unstability of drug is oxidation.

- More than 80% of drugs decompose by oxidation.

- Oxidation is a chain reaction and even a trace of O_2 is required to start reaction.

- So, for protecting drug against oxidation, we require measurement of drug by adding antioxidant.

Mechanism of Action of an Antioxidant

Its mechanism of action is based on simple principle. Any compound which has a standard reduction potential less than that of drug can be used as stabilizer or antioxidant for that drug.

- For this, we require to measure standard reduction potential of drug by potentiometer.

  E.g: Riboflavin has standard reduction potential 0.2 volt and it is oxidized first in comparison to Vitamin C having potential + 0.136 v.

- In tablets, there are some gaps between particles. i.e., there is air or O_2 to decompose because most oxidation processes are chain reaction. So, there can be thousands of reactions with the help of a small quantity of O_2 initiating the process.

- Most popular antioxidant is Na-metabisulphite i.e., $NaHSO_3$ having potential - 0.92 volt.

- This anti oxidant itself undergoes oxidation by consuming oxygen of bottle or tablet. So, O_2 is not available for the drugs to react.

(ii) End–point Determination

(Potentiometric titration)

Here, measurement of potential during course of titration.

Principle : During course of titration. pH or potential goes on changing and at equivalence point, there is a drastic change in potential or pH.

- Those compounds which have different potential or pH after end point and before end point can be titrated by using potentiometer.

- Suppose both the compounds i.e., (titrant + sample) are having same potential, then titration is not possible.

- Generally, potentiometry is used for redox titrations.

Advantages of Potentiometry over Visual Redox Titration

(i) Versatile : In all the titration, same potentiometer can be used.

- All iodometric – iodimetric titrations are scientifically redox titrations.

- In different redox titrations, different indicators are used because potential at equivalence point is different in different types of titrations.

  e.g : 2, 6 dichlorophenol indophenol indicator for ascorbic acid titrations

- Redox indicators have different colours in oxidizing state and reducing state. So, they also undergo colour change depending upon potential.

  E.g : $KMnO_4$ $\rightarrow$ in oxidizing state gives pink colour

                           $\rightarrow$ in reducing state it becomes colourless

  Ferroin $\rightarrow$ in oxidizing state gives pink colour

                           $\rightarrow$ in reducing state becomes red coloured.

Condition for Selection of Indicator

(i) Potential at equivalence point and potential of indicator should be very closer.

- So, same indicator can't be used for all redox titrations but same potentiometer can be used for all redox titrations.

(ii) Titration error is zero

- While in visual titration, end point is little higher than equivalence point.

- In potentiometric titration, end point and equivalence point is same.

(iii) All the types of compounds can be easily detected by potentiometry and compounds having less potential can also be detected and analysed).

- While in case of redox titration

  E.g : if $KMnO_4$ is indicator, then

  $$KMNO_4 \rightarrow Mn^{+2}$$

  Pink   colourless

  + 1.5 V (if this potential of 1.5V is obtained then only the conversion is possible)

(iv) Coloured solution can be easily titrated by potentiometry but not by visual titration.

Eg : Paracetamol syrup (very coloured) solution.

(v) We can carry out potentiometry very easily in both aqueous and non-aqueous system.

I. End Point Location Methods

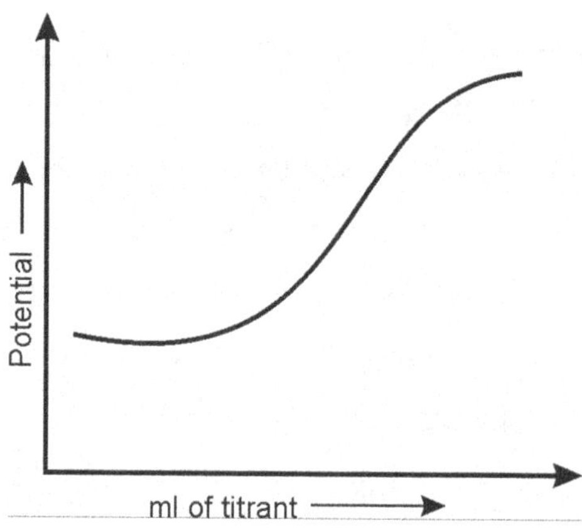

Fig. 13.22

OR

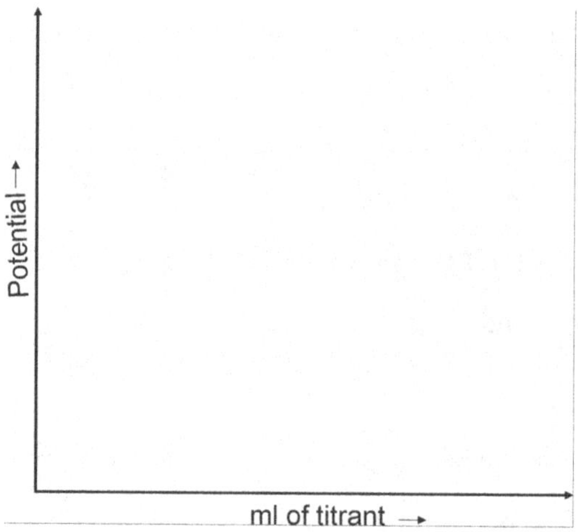

Fig. 13.23

II First Derivative Method

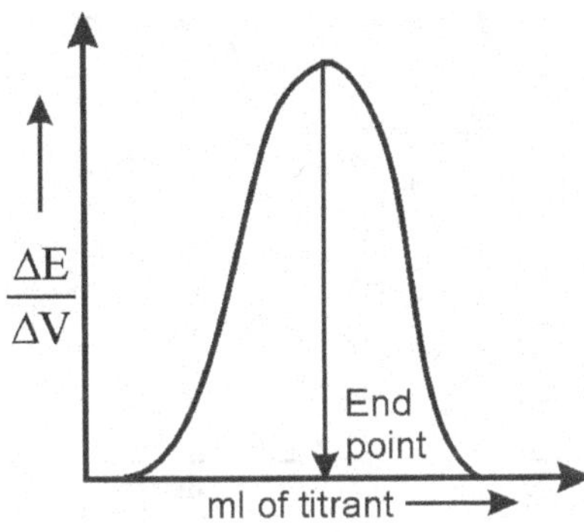

Fig. 13.24

III. Second Derivative Method

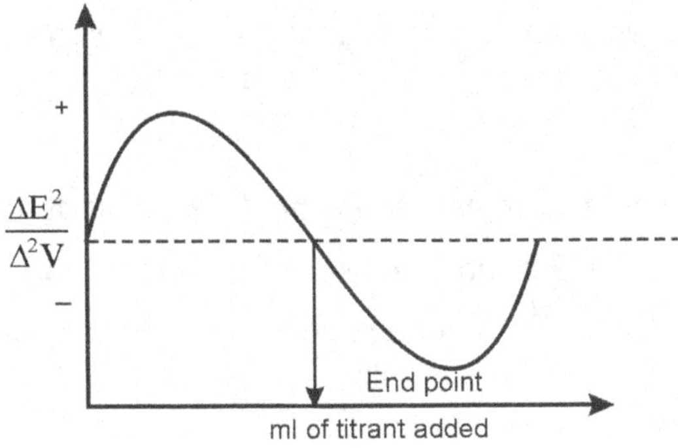

Fig. 13.25

Amperometric Titration

- Potential is applied between two electrodes externally and current is measured in ampere during course of titration and end point is detected by measuring the change in current.

Basic Principles

1. Here we use two electrodes :

    (i) working electrode (platinum electrode)

    (ii) Reference electrode (saturated calomel electrode)

- Oxidation–reduction are simultaneous processes but we have to counter balance the other process in which we are not interested.

- Here, we apply constant potential which is little higher than $E_{1/2}$ of the particular substance.

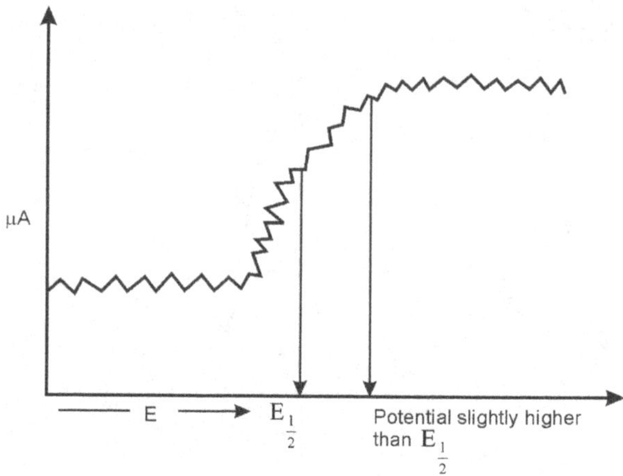

Fig. 13.26

- When all the sample (which is responsible for current production) is converted to final product, then a little addition of titrant i.e T_r causes current production and if we add more titrant, then current goes on increasing.

(ii) $S_r + T_r \rightarrow S_t$

where, $S_r =$ Sample responsible for current production

$T_r =$ Titrant responsible for current production

$S_t =$ Final product, not producing current.

So,

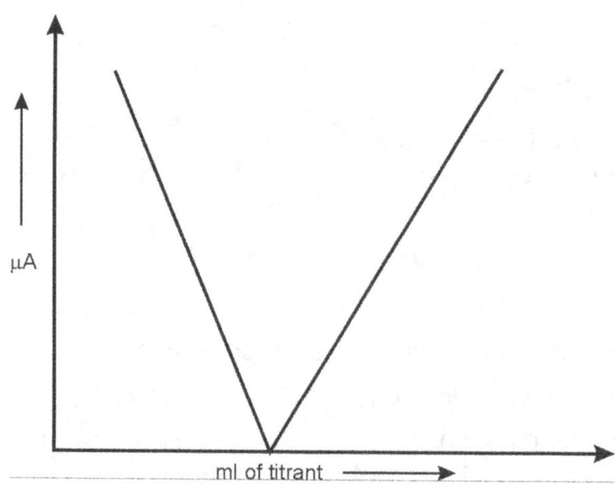

Fig. 13.27

- Initially maximum concentration of sample is present, which is undergoing reduction and produces maximum current.
- As we go on adding titrant, S_r will be converted to S_T, which is not reducing and not producing current and as long as S_r is present T_r cannot exist.
- so, current will be only due to S_r, whose concentration goes on decreasing as we go on adding titrant and so current also decreases.
- At the end point, all S_r is converted to S_T and so S_r is also not present and T_r is also not present, so there is no current production.
- After end point, as we go on adding titrant i.e. T_r, there is current production only due to T_r, because now S_r is not present and S_T is present but it is not producing current.

So, as the T_r increases, current also increases.

Method of Detecting End–Point in pH Potentiometry

- There are different methods adopted to locate end point.
- The critical problem in location of end point is to know the point at which the quantities of reacting species are present in equivalent amounts at the equivalence point.
- It is generally found graphically, there are three methods used for this purpose.
1. In the first method values of (E) or pH are recorded on graph paper as ordinate and the volume of titrant (v) added as abscissa. (Figure A).
   - A smoothe line is drawn for all the points and a point which gives the volume (V) corresponding to the maximum slope of curve is found out.
   - It is necessary to small increments of titrants near the equivalence point for accurate results, since it involves drawing the best curve through the experimental observations.
2 In the second method, difference of emf or pH for the volume of titrant added as abscissa.
   - From the shape of graph it becomes clear that maximum change in emf (E) or pH occurs at the equivalence point.
   - The end point can be readily recorded by drawing perpendicular from the peak of the graph on volume axis (abscissa figure B).
3. The third method uses second derivative i.e., $\Delta^2 E \big/ \Delta V^2$ where in the square of difference in potential or pH of the volume added Vs the square of volume added is plotted. (Figure C).

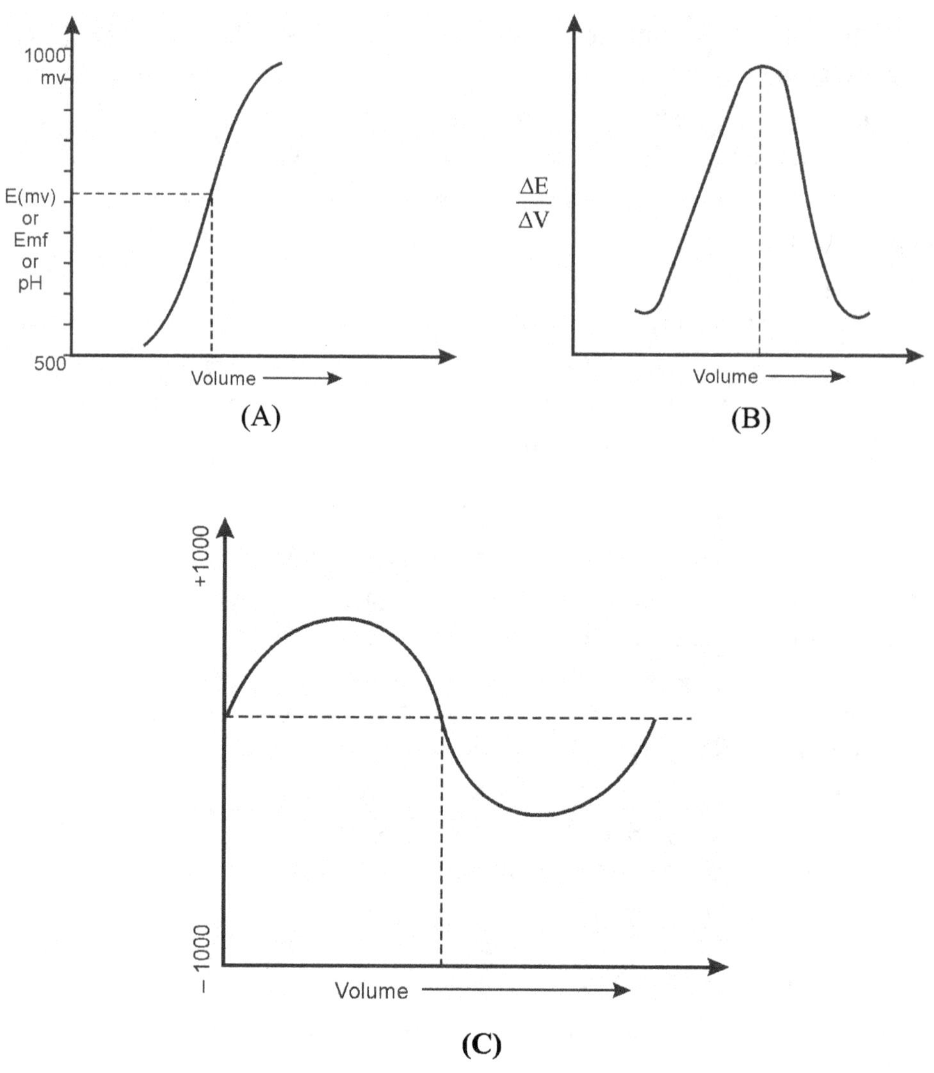

Fig. 13.28

Types of Reactions by Potentiometer

- Various types of titrations involving different chemical reactions are possible to be covered and followed using potentiometer with appropriate electrode systems.

Some such chemical reactions are given below:

1. Neutralization Reactions

- In this type of reaction acid can be titrated against alkali and vice-versa.

- The indicator electrodes used may be hydrogen, glass or antimony and colomel as a reference electrode.
- The accuracy or end-point depends upon the magnitude in the change of emf (e) in neighbourhood of equivalence point.
- This depends upon the concentration (amount) and the strength of acid and alkali used.
- Less accurate results occur when acid or alkali are very weak and dilute.
- Dibasic, tribasic and polybasic acids can be titrated with alkali to intermediate or full point.
- This possible provided that the dissociational constant for each stage in the titration is sufficiently apart.
- In the titration of mixture of acids the first inflation in the titration curve occurs when the strong acid is completely neutralised and the second when neutralization is complete.

2. **Redox Reactions:** Many redox titrations are possible using potentiometer provided no heating or cooling in the chemical reaction.

- Indicator electrode most commonly employed is platinum.
- The potential of the indicator electrode is a function of the ratio of oxidized and reduced forms of an ion.
- The potential of indicator electrode is given by the expression.

$$E = E_o + \frac{0.0591}{n} \log \frac{[oxi]}{[Red]};$$

Where E_o is the standard oxidation potential (or reduced potential) of the system.

- The equivalence point is indicated by sudden influction in the titration curve.
- From the standard value of reduction potential and the observed values of the ratios of concentrations [oxi]/ [Red] can be determined.

3. **Precipitation Reaction**

- Potentiometric titrations are possible for certain types of reactions involving precipitations.
- The solubility product of the almost insoluble material formed during a precipitational reaction determines the ionic concentration at the equivalence or end point.
- The indicator electrode must rapidly come into equilibrium with one of the ions.

- Silver electrode is used in the titration of halides against silver nitrate.
- The potential of the electrode is given by the expression.

$$E = E_o + \frac{0.0591}{n} \log [M^{n+}]$$

Where $[M^{n+}]$ is the ionic concentration present during the titration and in equilibrium with slightly soluble precipitate.

4. Complex formation and EDTA Reactions

- When a particular metal ion forms a complex with ligand, its determination is possible using appropriate indicator electrode.
- In determination of mercury ions mercury–mercurous chloride electrode can be used.

  Similarly, EDTA titrations can be followed for determination of metal ions like Fe, Cu, Cd etc.

Dead Stop End-Point Method

- Determination of moisture or water by Karl–fischer reagent method is most commonly carried out by dead stop end point technique.
- This technique can be adopted for many chemical reactions.
- The principle of this technique is as follows.
- In a uniformly stirred solution of an analyte two small but similar platinum electrode are dipped and a small potential (1-100 mv) is applied, current flows as long as electrods remain depolarised.
- When one component gets consumed or removed by the addition of the titrant current ceases to flow.
- For the method to be applicable, only requirement is that a reversible rev-ox, system be present either before or after the end-point.
- In the titration of iodine against thiosulphate, when two platinum electrodes are immersed in the iodine solution and ; connected to the battery appricible current flows through cell ($I_2 + 2\bar{e} \rightarrow 2I$).
- The amount of oxidised form reduced at cathod is equal to that formed at anode.
- Both electrodes remain depolarised (seen by current flowing through galvanometer) until the oxidised component on the reduced component of the system is consumed by the titrant.
- Current thus, flow until end point.
- At or after point the current becomes zero.

  <u>In the titration of iodine against thiosulphate</u>

- At or after the end-point the current becomes zero.
- In the iodine against thiosulphate titrations a rapid decrease in current is observed near the vicinity of the end point.
- Such titrations are given the name as "Dead stop end point".
- Other examples include titrations of thiosulphate with iodine, nitrate ion by stron sulphuric acid medium, ion or salt with ferric sulphate, etc.
- A circuit diagram of dead stop end-point method is shown in figure.

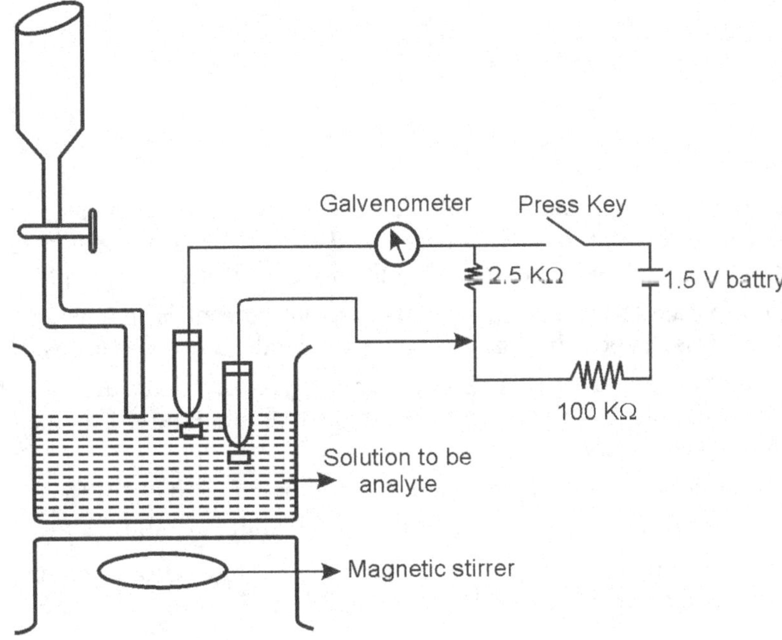

Fig. 13.29 The assembly of "Dead Stop End Point Method".

- The assembly consists of a beaker (vessels) of suitable size mounted on magnetic stirrer containing a solution to be titrated.
- Immersed in this solution are two bright platinum electrodes which are connected to a suitable potentiometer (shown in circuit) which is in turn is connected to the 1.5 volts battery.
- A microammeter galvanometer is incorporated in the circuit.

  Small volume of titrant is added through microburette and current flowing through galvanometer is noted.
- When current stops, the volume corresponding to it, is recorded.

CHAPTER 14

AMPEROMETRIC TITRATIONS

Introduction

- In amperometric titrations, the voltage applied across the indicator electrode and the reference electrode is kept constant and the diffusion current passing through the cell is measured and plotted against the volume of the reagent added.
- From polarographic technique, it is known that current is independent of applied voltage impressed upon dropping mercury electrode or any other electrode.
- Now if we take an excess of supporting electrolyte the factors affecting the limiting current is the rate of diffusion of electroactive material from the bulk of the solution to the electrode surface.
- This is because migration current is eliminated under such conditions.
- Thus id $\propto$ concentration of electro active material in the solution.
- If by any method, the electro active material is removed by interaction with any reagent the diffusion current will naturally decrease.
- The diffusion current is because of polarisation at a micro electrode.

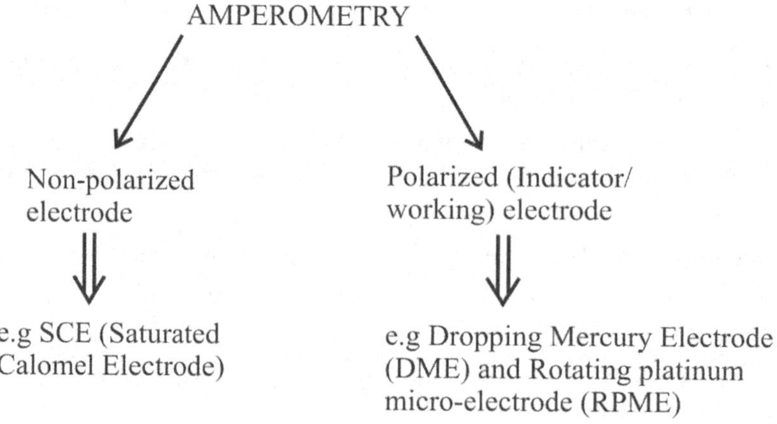

Dropping Hg-Electrode

Construction

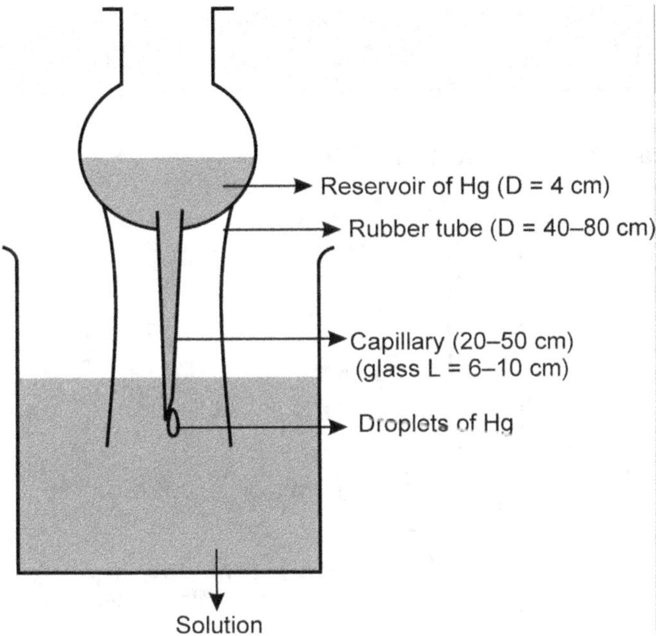

Fig. 14.1

Drop Time : Time taken for formation of droplet of Hg from capillary.
- Drop time is adjusted by adjusting height of Hg.
- Size of droplets depends on pore size.

Advantages
- Reproducible S.A
- Hg forms amalgous with Metal ion.
- Alkali metal ion which are reducible, so they have lower reduction potential.
- Constant removal of electrode surface which eliminate the poisonous surface.
- H^+ high over voltage of Hg, make deposition of ion and is difficult to reduce.
- Used from range of 0.4 to -1.8 v.

Disadvantages
- This electrode not used above 0.4 volt because, the Hg dissolves and anodic wave is recorded.
- Change in potential

- Anodic – 0 to +ve side
- Cathodic – 0 to –ve side
- If less than – 1.8 V the H^+ is liberated.
- Surface Area of drop changed by changing size of drop.
- Capillary may be easily blocked and care must be taken to avoid touching of tip of capillary with foreign material.

Rotating Platinum Micro Electrode (RPME)

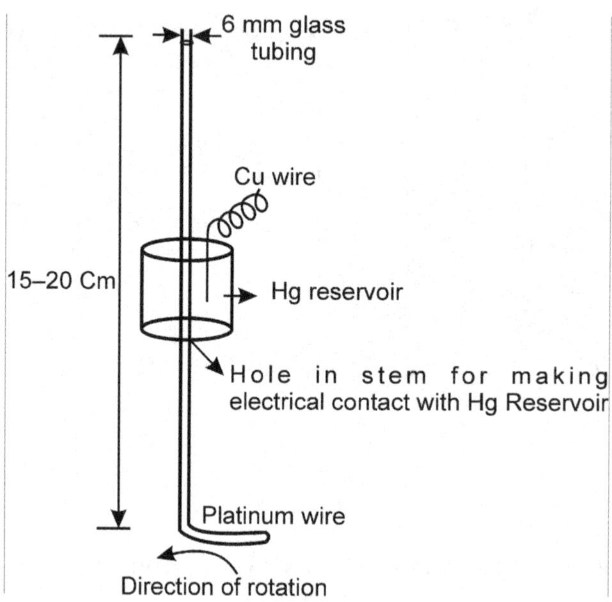

Fig. 14.2

Advantages over Dropping Mercury Electrode

(i)   Simple to construct.

(ii) Increase the mark able range to +ve voltage side upto 0.9 V. This can be used at +ve potentials whereas DME may not be used.

(iii) Technique is more sensitive because the rotation of electrode increases the value of I_D as much as 20 times.

- It consists of glass tube 15-20 cm
$$D = 6 \text{ mm}$$
- Short length point wire extends 5-10 mm from wall of glass tube.
- Electrode mounted in the shaft of a motor and rotated of about 600 RPM.

Amperometric Titrations

- Removal of O_2 is necessary.
- It is done by bubbling purified N_2 before commencement of titration.
- Supporting electrolyte is KCl.
- maximum suppresors – gelatine, dye, surfactant are added before titration.
- Potential can be applied and is determined by recording the polarogram of substance.

Different Types

1. Electrode reducible Vs non-reducible ions

   Eg : pb and sulphate ions

2. Electro non-reducible Vs electro reduce ions

   Eg : Cl^- and Ag^+ Both are reducible

   Pb and chromate dichromate

3. Redox titration

4. DEAD stop end point technique.

1. Reducible and Non-Reducible Ions

Eg : Pb sulphate ions

- Flask – pb and titrant $\rightarrow$ sulphate ions
- pb ions being reducible at cathode, give I_D whereas the sulphate ion being non-reducible show no diffusion current.
- The concentration of pb^{+2} ions is decreases as SO_4^{-2} ions remove some pb^{+2} ions.

  Here, thus, from graph. We can conclude $\rightarrow$ decrease in current with decrease in concentration.

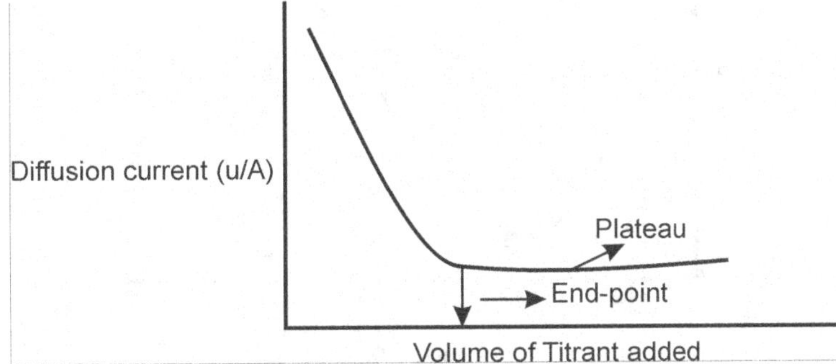

Fig. 14.3 Graph of I_D against volume of titrant.

- When all pb used, I_d is minimum. When add more SO_4^{-2}, no change in I_D and plateau reached.

2. Non-Reducible and Reducible Ions

eg : Cl^- and Ag^+

- when titrated ion is non-reducible and titrant is reducible, the curve is as shown.

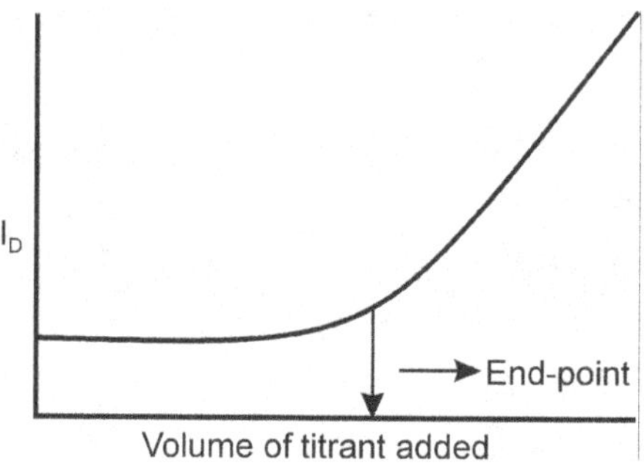

Fig. 14.4.

- In this case, the titration curve is horizontal line and starts to rise after end-point. Cl^- gives no change in I_D.
- Addition of Ag^+ gives precipitation of AgCl and doesn't affect I_D.
- After end-point more Ag^+ added. Ag^+ is electro reducible and thus increases in I_D.

3. Electro-Reducible

Eg : Lead ions and dichromate ions.

- When both the titrated ions are reducible at cathode, the current will drop to end point and there will be increase again to give a "V" shape titration curve as shown.

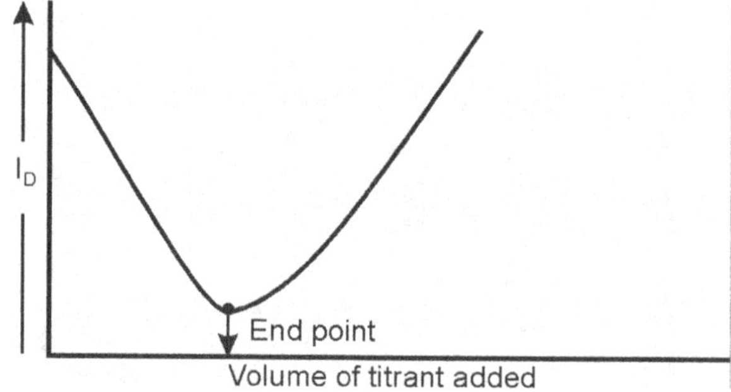

Fig. 14.5

- Then lead ions are removed from the solution, the current decreases then increase after end-point because of increase in concentration of dichromate ions.
- Precipitation of pb dichromate $\rightarrow$ decrease of I_d add more titrant $\rightarrow$ increase of I_d.

4. Redox Titration

- In Oxi-Red system, where both oxidising and reducing agent give I_D, the titration curve is as shown.

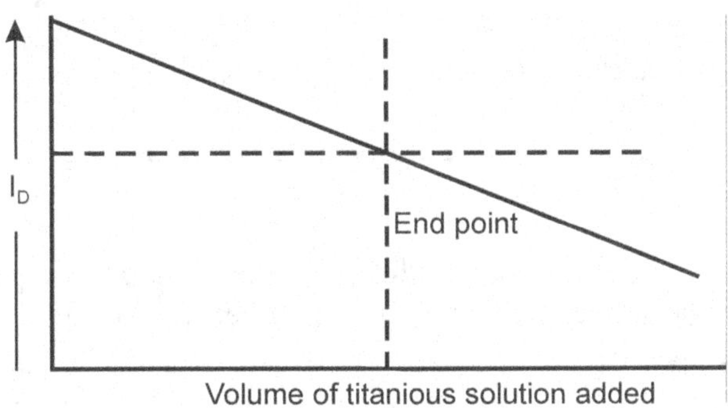

Fig. 14.6

Eg : Fe^{+3} ions titrated agains Titaneous ions

- The I_D decrease linearly with addition of titrant to ferric ions until obtains zero value at end point.
- At this point ferric completely reacted.
- when more addition of titrant, I_D caused by the oxidation of titaneous ions is set up.
- A change in slope caused by difference in diffusion coefficient.
- point of intersection of 2 lines gives end-point.

5. Dead Stop End Point Method

- This technique is modification of the classical amperometic titration.
- Method applicable only when oxi-red system involved before and after the end-point.
- 2 point electrodes are immersed in the titration cell.
- Small and constant voltage is applied to these two electrodes.

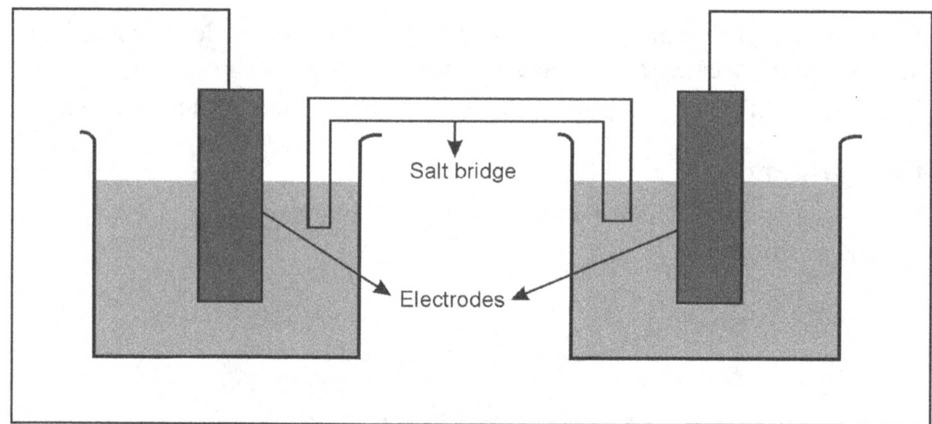

Fig. 14.7

- The amount of oxidized form reduced at the cathode is equal to that formed by oxidation of the reduced form at anode, when the reactant involves a reversible system.

- At this stage electrodes are depolarized.

- After end point electrode remains depolarised as the titrant does not involve reversible system.

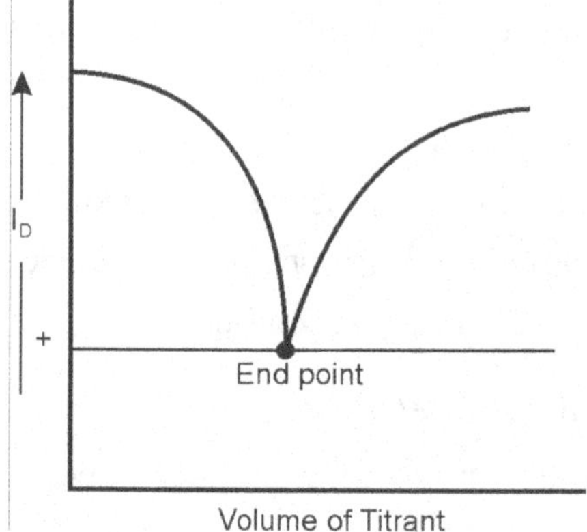

Fig. 14.8

- Thus current becomes zero at end-point and shoots up then.

- **Uses :** Applied for oxi–red systems. Involves titrations of iodine, bromine, $^{+}3$ titanium, $^{+}4$ cerium etc.

- Important use is titration of water with Karl Fisher reagent.

  Advantages : simple

Advantages of Amp. Titration

- Apparatus is simple
- Accuracy is higher than polarography.
- Temperature need not to be constant.
- Used and best for traces of elements with good precisions (μg to ng).
- Not necessary to maintain constant current.
- End-point is found graphically.
- Dilute solution can be titrated with accurate substance which can't be determined by palorography can be determined by it.
- More sensitive than conducto and potentiometric titration.
- Presence of salts act as supporting electrolytes.

Disadvantages

- Inaccurate results due to co-precipitation.
- Foreign substances should not be present in large concentration than substance to be titrated, as relative current becomes smaller.
- Used as microdetector in HPLC.
- Quantification of mixture of ion is possible.

Chapter 15

SOLVENT EXTRACTION

"Extraction is removal of desired components from the solid mix by contact with a suitable solvent.

Or

"The transfer of desired component from one liquid phase to another liquid immiscible with the first."

"Extraction technique involves solubilizing the active constituents and removing it with a suitable extracting solvent."

The extraction method using extracting liquid can be classified into 2 categories.

   (i) Solid-Liquid extraction

   (ii) Liquid-Liquid extraction

Solid-Liquid Extraction

- The separation and isolation of desired constituents is based on solubility phenomena.
- Extracting solvent is chosen with highest solubilizing power of desired constituents.
- Since active material present in solid is extracted out by using liquid phase it is called solid-liquid extraction.

Different Techniques

   (i)   maceration

   (ii) percolation

   (iii) Continuous percolation

   (iv) Soxhelt extraction

- Depending upon the nature of solid material and active constituent, method is adopted.
- Generally, soxhelt apparatus using continuous extraction method is employed.

Soxhelt Apparatus

- The soxhelt apparatus is made up of glass consisting of three parts.
- A suitable size round bottom flask (Part A).
- Main body (Part B) has a siphon glass tube and side arm.
- This holds a thimble for sample material.
- Condenser (Part C).
- Extracting solvent is placed in flask (A) heated on water bath or hot plate.

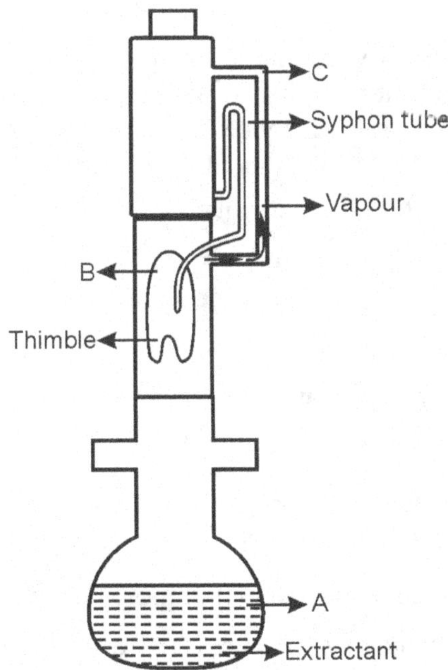

Fig. 15.1

- Vapours of solvent pass through side arm of body to condenser.
- On condensation, the droplets of solvent fall on the sample placed in thumble and extracts the constituent.
- Continuous extraction of material is accomplished using very less volume of extracting solvent.

Advantages :- simple, economical

Disadvantages :- Not used for thermo labile constituents.

Liquid-Liquid Extraction

- Solvent extraction technique is basically liquid-liquid extraction method in which a solution is brought in contact with another solvent, (usually organic) essentially immiscible with each other.

- By extraction and separation of phases one or more solutes are transferred into second solvent.

- The separation is generally effected using separating funnels bringing 2 or 3 extractions with fresh charge of extracting solvent.

- Separation by this method is rapid, simple and quantitative.

- Liquid-Liquid extraction method is based on Nernst law.

- "The ratio of activities of salute material in a pair of 2 immiscible liquid at an equilibrium is a constant".

- If 2 solvents are in contact with each other and a solute substance that is soluble in both solvents is added to it then that substance will distribute itself in both solvents in such a way that the ratio of concentration of two solutions remains constant. This is called as Distribution Coefficient or Partition Coefficient.

Partition Coefficient = K

$$K = \frac{ce}{cr} = \frac{ae}{ar}$$

where,

ae = activity of solute in extractant

ar = activity of solute in reffinate

ce = concentration of solute in extractant

cr = concentration of solute in reffinate

Extractant : Solvent used to take out desired compound from the mixture.

Reffinate : Solution which contains desired solute from which the desired solute is to be removed.

$K' = K_{app}$ (apparent partition coefficient)

$$U = \frac{Ve}{Vr}$$

where,

U = Ratio of phase volume

Ve = Volume of extractant

Vr = Volume of reffinate

Different Types of Extraction

1. Single extraction
   One time efficient
2. Multiple extraction
   double efficient
3. CCD – counter current distribution
   four times efficient
4. Continuous extraction
   triple efficient

Single Extraction

- If K, for the solute between the solvents is known, it is possible to calculate the fraction of that solute present in each of the phases.

Here,

P = Fraction of solute in extractant (upper phase at equilibrium.)

Q = fraction of solute in reffinate (lower phase)

$$P = \frac{\text{amount of solute in extractant}}{\text{Total amount of solute}}$$

Now $\qquad P = Ce. \ Ve$

where, $\quad Ce$ = concentration of solutea in extractant

$\qquad Ve$ = Volume of extractant

Similarly, Cr and Vr for reffinate

We know $\qquad$ Total amount = concentration × volume

$\therefore \qquad\qquad P = \dfrac{Ce.Ve}{Ce.Ve + Cr.Vr}$

Now, we know, $\qquad \dfrac{Ce}{Cr} = K$ (partition coefficient)

and $\qquad\qquad U$ = ratio of phase volume = $\dfrac{Ve}{Vr}$

Now $\qquad\qquad P = \dfrac{Ce.Ve}{Cr.Vr\left(\dfrac{Ce}{Cr}.\dfrac{Ve}{Vr}\right)+1}$

$$P = \frac{\dfrac{Ce}{Cr} \cdot \dfrac{Ve}{Vr}}{\left(\dfrac{Ce}{Cr} \cdot \dfrac{Ve}{Vr} + 1\right)}$$

$\therefore$
$$P = \frac{K.U}{K.V + 1}$$

Now,   % of $P = \dfrac{K.U}{K.U + 1} \times 100$

Also, $P + Q = 1$

$\therefore$ $Q = 1 - P$

$$Q = 1 - \frac{KU}{KU + 1}$$

$$= \frac{KU + 1 - kU}{KU + 1}$$

$$Q = \frac{1}{k.U + 1}$$

Examples

1. K of aspirin is 4 between ether water system. Calculate the quantity of aspirin that is extracted in 100 ml of aq. solution and is extracted with 30 ml of ether.

    $Ve = 30$ ml (ether – upper phase-extractant)

    $Vr = 100$ ml (H_2O – lower phase-Reffinate)

Now, $U = \dfrac{Ve}{Vr} = \dfrac{30}{100} = 0.3$

Now, $p = \dfrac{KU}{Ku + 1} = \dfrac{0.3 \times 4}{0.3 \times 4 + 1} = \dfrac{1.2}{2.2} = \dfrac{6}{11} = 0.555$

$\therefore$ $P = 0.555$

Now,   % of $p = 55.5\%$

$Q = 1 - P$

$Q = 1 - 0.555$

$Q = 0.44.5$

% of $Q = 44.5\%$

2. If given, Aspirin = 200mg and AMT Extracted

   Now, 200 mg = 100%

$$\therefore \qquad 55.5\% = \frac{200 \times 55.5}{100} = 111.0$$

   $\therefore$ 111 mg of drug extracted in upper phase.

3. What if K = 8, then find fractions P and Q.

$$P = \frac{8 \times 0.3}{8 \times 0.3 + 1} = \frac{2.4}{3.4} = \frac{12}{17} = 0.7058$$

$$Q = 1 - P = 1 - 0.7058$$

$$= 0.2942$$

$$\therefore \quad P = 70.58\% \quad \text{and} \quad \% \text{ of } Q = 29.42\%$$

3. What if K = 16 then p and Q ?

$$P = \frac{16 \times 0.3}{16 \times 0.3 + 1} = \frac{4.8}{5.8} = 0.8275$$

$$\% P = 82.75\%$$

Thus, we can conclude that if K increases P increases and if V increases then also P increase thus efficiency is single time.

So, by using single extraction we can't achieve 100% of extraction as we add only once.

Example

The solute is known to have K = 4 between water ether. If 15 ml of Ag solution of compound is extracted with 20 ml portion of ether, what is % of original solute in ether layer.

   K = 4, Ve = 20 ml, Vr = 15 ml

$$\therefore \qquad U = \frac{Ve}{Vr} = \frac{20}{15} = 1.33$$

$$P = \frac{4 \times 1.33}{4 \times 1.33 + 1} = \frac{5.32}{6.32} = 0.8417$$

$$\% \text{ of } P = 84.17\% \quad \therefore \quad Q = 15.82\%$$

Multiple Extraction

Compound dissolved in aq. solution

Extractant – 50% extracted

Add again extractant and again repeat the process.

Here, multiple time extractant is added.

- It is possible to calculate the fraction extracted of the any no. of extraction or to calculate the no. of extractions necessary to achieve any desired extent of extraction.

- If partition isotherm is linear then the same fraction of the solute remaining in the reffinate is extracted into the upper layer (phase) each time. Then the fraction of total extracted in the nth extraction is equal to, the fraction of the total in the extraction remaining (q) × the fraction of total extracted in single extraction (p) = q.p

- Thus for completeness of extraction, by employing small volumes of solvents by adopting repeated extractions is called as "multiple extraction analysis".

η	Fraction extracted in n^{th} extraction	Fraction in Total extraction	Fraction remaining in reffinate
1.	P	P	$Q = (1–P)$
2.	$P \times Q$	$P + P \times Q$	$1–(P+PQ) = Q^2$
3.	$P \times Q^2$	$P + PQ + PQ^2$	$1–(P + PQ + PQ^2) = Q^3$
4.	$P \times Q^3$	$P + PQ + PQ^2 + PQ^3$	$1– (P + PQ + PQ^2+PQ^3) = Q^4$
5.	$P \times Q^4$	$P+ PQ + PQ^2 + PQ^3 + PQ^4$	Q^5

$\therefore$ Total fraction extracted $= 1 – Q^n$ after n^{th} extraction.

Example

Paracetamol, $K = 5$ if 100 ml aq. solution containing the paracetamol is extracted with

(A)   40 ml of ether

(B)   2 times 20 ml of ether

(C)   4 times 10 ml of ether

(D)   8 times 5 ml of ether.

What % gets extracted?

(A) $k = 5$, $Ve = 40$ ml, $Vr = 100$ ml

$$U = \frac{Ve}{Vr} = \frac{400}{100} = 0.4$$

Now, $P = \dfrac{KU}{KU+1}$ $\therefore$ $P = \dfrac{5 \times 0.4}{5 \times 0.4 + 1} = \dfrac{2}{3} = 0.666$

% of $P = 66.6\%$

(B) $n = 2$, $k = 5$, $U = \dfrac{Ve}{Vr} = \dfrac{20}{100} = 0.2$

$Q = \dfrac{1}{Ku+1}$ $Q = \dfrac{1}{1+1} = \dfrac{1}{2} = 0.5$

Now, Total extracted $= 1 - Q^n$

$$= 1 - Q^2$$
$$= 1 - (0.5)^2 = 1 - 0.25$$
$$= 0.75$$

% of Total extracted $= 75\%$

(C) $n = 4$, $Ve = 10$, $Vr = 100$, $K = 5$

$$\therefore U = \frac{10}{100} = 0.1$$

$$Q = \frac{1}{Ku+1} = \frac{1}{1.5} = \frac{10}{15} = 0.6666$$

Total extracted $= 1 - Q^n$

$$= 1 - Q^4$$
$$= 1 - (0.6666)^4$$
$$= 0.8102$$

% of extracted $= 81.02\%$

(D) $n = 8$, $Ve = 5$, $Vr = 100$ $\therefore U = \dfrac{5}{100} = 0.05$, $K = 5$

$$Q = \frac{1}{Ku+1} = \frac{1}{1.25} = \frac{4}{5} = 0.8$$

Total extracted $= 1 - Q^n$

$$= 1 - Q^8$$

$$= 1-(0.8)^8$$
$$= 0.8322$$

% of total extracted = 83.22%

Note that M.E is more efficient than S.E.

Why Multiple extraction is efficient than single extraction?

- If K = 4 in ether water system. Compare the efficiency of extraction of 10 ml aq. solution of compound with

(1) 40 ml ether

(2) 4 times 10 ml ether

(1)   K = 4, $U = \dfrac{40}{10} = 4$ and $p = \dfrac{ku}{ku+1}$

S.E $P = \dfrac{4\times 4}{4\times 4+1}$ $= \dfrac{16}{17} = 0.9411$

% of P = 94.11%

(2)   n = 4, k = 4, $U = \dfrac{10}{10} = 1$

∴ $Q = \dfrac{1}{KU+1}$ $= \dfrac{1}{5} = 0.2$

M.E   Total extracted $= 1 - Q^n$

$$= 1 - (0.2)^4$$
$$= 1 - 0.0016$$
$$= 0.9984$$

% of Total extracted = 99.84%

∴ ME is more efficient than SE

Seperability Factor

Different compounds have different k values. If they have same k, separation is impossible since, $\alpha = \beta$ where, α and β seperability factors.

Factors affecting L-L extraction (seperability factor)

1. Choice of solvent
2. Control of ionic strength
3. Control of pH
4. Control of ion hydrophobicity

1. Choice of Solvent

E.g : Diethyl ether, chloroform, Hydrocarbons

Selection of solvent depends on   → Density of solvent

→ Boiling point

→ Vapour phase

→ low toxicity and inflammability

→ High distribution co-efficient

E.g : If we want to separate mixture of caffeine + sodium oxalate.

- First dissolve in aqueous solution and extract with $CHCl_3$. Caffeine is soluble in H_2O as it is salt. Sodium oxalate remains in aq. layer as it is insoluble in water.

    Solubility → Petroleum ether used for fats, oils and waxes.

    → Diethyl ether – for aspirin

    → $CHCl_3$ and ethanol (2:1) – for morphine and related alkaloids.

2. Control of Ionic Strength

- If the salt concentration increases the solubility decreases and the solubility decreases by increase in ionic strength, is called as Salting Out Effect, which effects k_{app} (apparent partition coefficient).

- If a salt concentration of aq. phase is raised very high and the solubility of non-electrolyte in aq. phase will be reduced. This helps in more complete extraction of a solute having greater solubility in aqueous phase.

- The reduction of solubility by increasing the ionic strength is known as salt out effect.

    Eg : NaCl in aqueous phase the solute will be salted out into organic extracting phase.

    Amm. Sulfate → protein will be precipitated by salting out method.

3. Control of pH : (Important Factor)

- Solubility of a substance is greatly influenced by pH or hydrogen ion concentration of a system.

- The polarity of solvent and solute play a great role.

- A polar solute would be more soluble in polar solvent and non polar solute in non-polar solvent.

- Generally, ionized species are more soluble in polar solvents and unionized in non-polar solvents.

- These forms can be readily interchanged by adjusting pH of a medium.

- 80% drug are basic in nature, while 10-15% are acidic and 5-10% are amphoteric in nature.

  Eg : Mixture of acetyl salicylic acid and antihistamine. Dissolve in H_2O and then acid HCl and extracted with ether.

  Antihistamine remains in aq. phase as salt, antihistamine hydrochloride.

  Make it basic and extract the drug.

Example

Acetaminophine, pka = 10 at pH = 10. What is % of acetaminophenone in aqueous system and organic system.

Now,

$$pH = pka + \log \frac{[salt]}{[acid]}$$

$$10 = 10 + \log \frac{[salt]}{[acid]}$$

$$\text{Log } \frac{[salt]}{[acid]} = 0$$

$$[Salt] = [acid]$$

50% of drug in aqueous phase and 50% of drug in solvent.

- So, if pH and pka is equal, drug will be 50% in organic and 50% in aqueous phase.

- When pH is one unit higher than pka then 90.9% of drug in aqueous solution.

  pH = 11 and pka = 10

$$\therefore \log \frac{[salt]}{[acid]} = 1 \therefore \frac{[salt]}{[acid]} = \frac{10}{1}$$

  PH = 12 and pka = 10

$$\frac{[salt]}{[acid]} = \frac{100}{1}$$

  pH = 13 and pka = 10

$$\frac{[salt]}{[acid]} = \frac{1000}{1}$$

$\therefore$ 99.9%, of drug in aq. solution (salt formation)

- If pH is 3 unit higher than pka, 100% drug in aq. phase in form of salt and if pH is 3 units lower than pka, 100% drug in organic phase.

- If pH is 3 unit higher than Pk_b is then 100% of drug in organic solvent and if pH is 3 unit lower than Pk_b then 100% in aqueous solvent phase (salt form).

4. Control of Hydrophobicity

1. Acid Dye Method

- If drug (W-B).

- adjust pH to acidic and we obtain salt and salt has the charge.

- Addition of counter ions of –ve charge.

  $\therefore$ Complex are formed.

$$D^+ \qquad \bar{e} \qquad \rightarrow D^+ \text{-e} \qquad \text{Drug counter ion complex}$$

$$\downarrow \qquad\qquad \downarrow$$

Extracted   Counter ion can't be

in org. solvent   extracted in org. solvent

- So by adding of counter ion we can control hydrophobicity.

- It is mainly applied for determination of quarternary ammonium compound.

- Use of spectrophotometry is done for measurement of (λ max).

  Eg : Procaine, Thiamine, Elthambutol.

2. Base Dye method

Here drug is weak acid

Eg : Glycyrrhiza $\rightarrow$ (WA)

Dye $\rightarrow$ (methylene blue) (W/B)

Continuous Extraction

- This method of extraction is carried out when the distribution ratio is low. The method makes use of continuous flow of immiscible solvent through the solution to be extracted.

- Although a distribution equilibrium is never reached during the time of contact of two liquids. Solute do get removed by passing or flowing of solvent.

For this method special type liquid-liquid extraction apparatus is used.

3 Types

(i)   The extractant lighter than reffinite

    Eg : ether, benzene, petroleum ether, hexane

(ii)   The extractant heavier than reffinate

    Eg : $CHCl_3$

(iii)   For solid powder

    Eg : soxlet Extraction

(i) Extractant Lighter than Raffinate

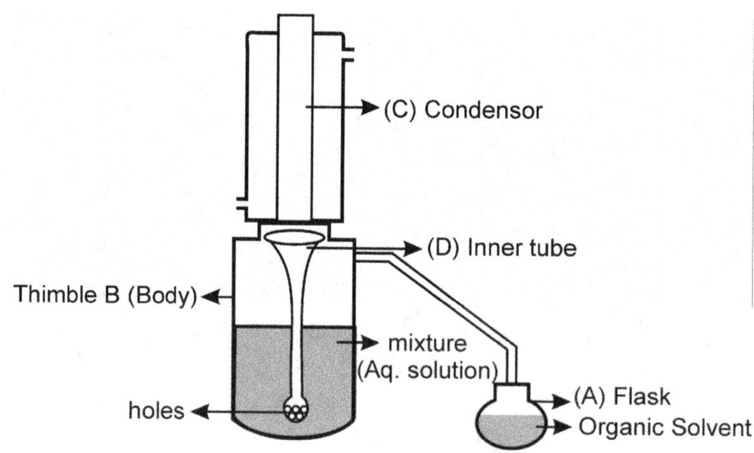

Fig. 15.2

- as extractant is lighter it is upper phase and aq. solution is lower phase.
- In the process a suitable solvent is placed in flask A. (lighter than sample solution).
- It is connected to body B which holds sample solution. In this is placed glass funnel D. Condenser C is connected to main body.
- Solvent placed in flask is heated.
- The vapour of which pass to condenser and fall as droplets into funnel of glass tube.
- They pass through holes of bulb and enter solution. In the process it extracts solute.
- The solvent collected over sample flows back into flask. Process continued till complete extraction obtained.

(ii) Extractant Heavier than Raffinate

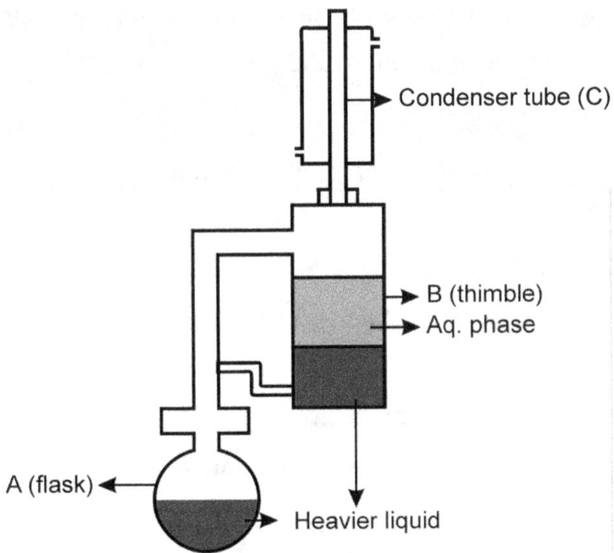

Fig. 15.3

- The extracting solvent is (heavier than sample solution) is placed in flask (A) and heated.
- The vapours pass from side tube of body of apparatus B to condenser C.
- On cooling droplets of solvent pass through sample solution and gets accumulated at bottom of body, from where it flows into the flask. Process continued till complete extraction obtained.

CCD (Counter Current Displacement)

- If a sample solution contains two or more substances having similar distribution coefficients then more extractions using large number of separating funnels is required. This process is inconvenient.

- So, a technique called CCD is used.

- In this method, a special apparatus (Craig apparatus) is used which can bring out multiple extractions simultaneously.

- Two immiscible solvents move in opposite direction, 1 in upper phase and 1 in lower phase.

- Now, $P = \dfrac{KU}{KU+1}$ and $Q = \dfrac{1}{KU+1}$ and $P + Q = 1$

- If KU increases and increase P of solute in upper phase and thus higher concentration of drug in extraction.

- Assume, $P = Q = 0.5$ and suppose 16 part of solute is added in lower phase.

- After shaking 8 parts in upper phase and 8 in lower phase.

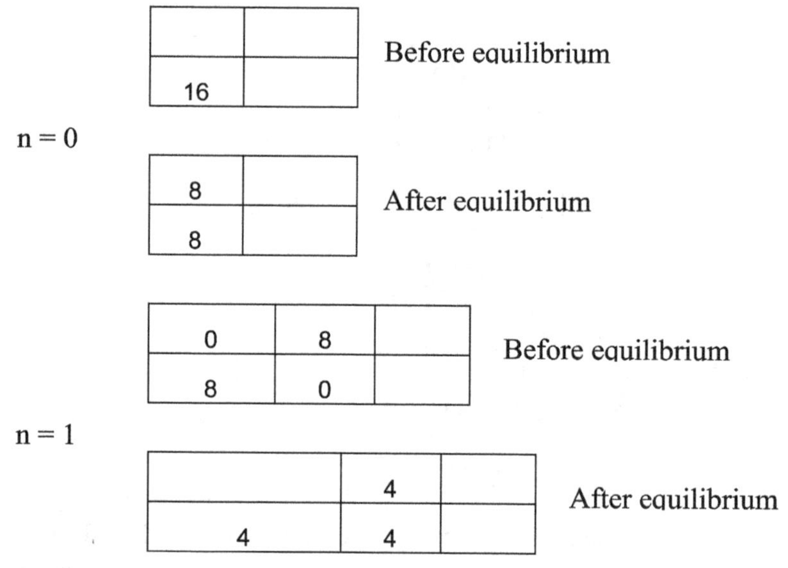

And so on.

If no. of transfer $= n$; no. of tube $= r$

Then,

F_{nr} = fraction of the total solute containing in both layer of rth no. tube and n^{th} no. of transfer.

1. $f_{nr} = T_{nr} = \dfrac{n!}{r!(n-r)!}\, p^r\, q^{n-r}$

But if value of and n and r is very high then,

2. $r_{max} = np$

r_{max} = tubes containing max fraction.

3. Adjacent tube fraction

$$\frac{tnr}{tn(r-1)} = \frac{p(n-r+1)}{(qr)}$$

4. $Tnr_{max} = \dfrac{1}{\sqrt{2\pi rpq}}$

where, Tnr_{max} = fraction of solute in max tube.

Example

After 120 transfer in CCD the 2 components they have their max at tube no. 27 and tube no. 83.

The distribution was carried out with 10 ml aq. buffer 5 ml of ether in each phase.

Calculate

1. Partition coefficient of component.

2. Calculate the fraction in both the max tube.

3. Calculate the fraction of slow moving extraction in tube no 25 and 86.

Here, n = 120, Ve = 5 ml, Vr = 10 ml $\therefore$ U = 0.5

r max$_{(a)}$ = 27   r max$_{(b)}$ = 83

r max = nP $\therefore P = \dfrac{r\,max}{n}$

$P(a) = \dfrac{27}{120}$ and $P(b) = \dfrac{83}{120}$

$P(a) = 0.225$ and $P(b) = 0.691$

$Q(a) = 0.775$ and $Q(b) = 0.309$

Now,
$$Q = \frac{1}{KU + 1}$$

$$\therefore \quad Q(a) = \frac{1}{KaU + 1}$$

$$0.75 = \frac{1}{Ka(o.5) + 1}$$

$$0.3875\,Ka + 0.775 = 1$$

$$Ka = \frac{0.225}{0.3875}$$

$$Ka = 0.5806 \qquad\qquad \text{.... (1)}$$

$$Q(b) = \frac{1}{kbU + 1}$$

$$0.309 = \frac{1}{kb(0.5) + 1}$$

$$0.1545\,Kb + 0.309 = 1$$

$$Kb = \frac{0.691}{0.1545}$$

$$Kb = 4.472 \qquad\qquad \text{.... (2)}$$

2.
$$Tnr_{max} = \frac{1}{\sqrt{2\pi npq}}$$

$$Tnr_{max(a)} = \frac{1}{\sqrt{2 \times 3.14 \times 0.225 \times 120 \times 0.775}}$$

$$Tnr_{(27)} = 0.087 \qquad\qquad \text{.... (1)}$$

$$Tnr\ max\ (b) = \frac{1}{\sqrt{2 \times 3.14 \times 0.309 \times 0.691 \times 120}}$$

$$Tnr_{(83)} = 0.078 \qquad\qquad \text{.... (2)}$$

3.

$$\frac{Tnr}{Tn(r-1)} = \frac{Tn(27)}{Tn(26)} = \frac{p(n-r+1)}{qr}$$

$$\frac{Tn(27)}{Tn(26)} = \frac{0.225(120-27+1)}{0.775 \times 27}$$

$$Tn(26) = \frac{0.087}{0.02} = 0.085$$

Similarly, $$\frac{Tn26}{Tn25} = \frac{0.225(120-26+1)}{0.775 \times 26}$$

$$Tn\,25 = 0.08$$

Similarly, $Tn\,86 = 0.066$

Determination of Alkaloids in Crude Drug and Chemicals

- Alkaloids contains various impurities.

- Impurities present in alkaloids are :

1. Water soluble matter:

- Sugar, glycosides, starch, protein, gums, mucilage, Tannins and Saponins.

    They are insoluble in $CHCl_3$ and ether but soluble in $Al - OH$

    Make it alkaline and extract with $CHCl_3$ ether

    White solution matter

    Alkaloid converted to free base.

2. Water insoluble matter

Resin, fats, oil, colouring matter

Insoluble in acid/alkaline/neutral solution but soluble in organic solution.

Make solution acidic and extract with $CHCl_3$

Aq. Phase $\rightarrow$ alkaloid

organic Phase $\rightarrow$ impurities

3. Organic Acids

Water soluble ammonia Salts

$\downarrow$

Treated with Ammonia and extracted with organic solvent

$\downarrow$

Organic phase – alkaloid

Aq phase – Acid

4. Organic Base

Difficult to separate so special technique required.

E.g : Solanasia drug contains no. of non alkaloidal bases which are volatile in nature.

$\rightarrow$ Heat for 100°C for ½ hour $\rightarrow$ impurity volatilises

E.g : Nux vomica $\rightarrow$ it contains brucin and strychinin

- Treated with HNO_3 make solution acidic. Brucin oxidized to carboxylic function present in Aq. Phase.

- **Strychnin** extracted in $CHCl_3$

Eg : Opium

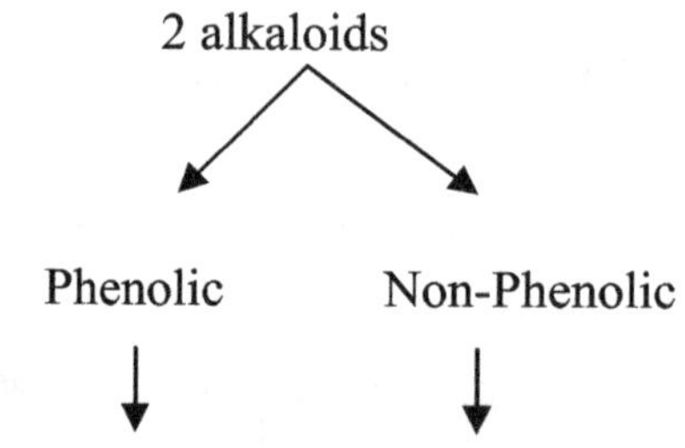

$Ca(OH)_2 \rightarrow$ Phenolic alkaloids converted to Ca-salt   (aq.phase)

And Non-phencolic extracted out in organic solvent.

CHAPTER 16

KJELDAHL METHOD

In 1883 Kjeldahl introduced analytical method for organically bound nitrogen.

Basic Concept

The digestion of organic material e.g. Protein, using H_2SO_4 and a catalyst to convert any organic nitrogen to ammonium sulphate in solution. By making the mixture alkaline any ammonia can be steam distilled off and resulting alkaline distillate titrated with standard acid.

Construction : (H_2SO_4, Potassium sulphate, catalyst ammonia sulphate)

- Digestion flask $\rightarrow$ kjeldahl flask
- Sprary trap $\rightarrow$ to prevent droplets of NaOH being driven during distillation. Condenser end dipped into a known volume std. acid in conical flask (Erlenmeyer adsorption)
- Apparatus $\rightarrow$ alkali resistant glass
- Digestion flask $\rightarrow$ 200 ml (round bottom)
- Steam generator $\rightarrow$ 100 ml
- Distillation Head $\rightarrow$ Conducts steam from generator
- Evolved Vapours $\rightarrow$ Collect in spray trap to condenser (30-40 cm length)
- Funnel $\rightarrow$ for addition of alkali to digestion flask.
- Delivery tube has hole $\rightarrow$ to prevent clogging by condenser.
- Absorption flask $\rightarrow$ 15 ml 4% boric acid +3 drops methyl red indicator and water to cover condenser end.

Apparatus

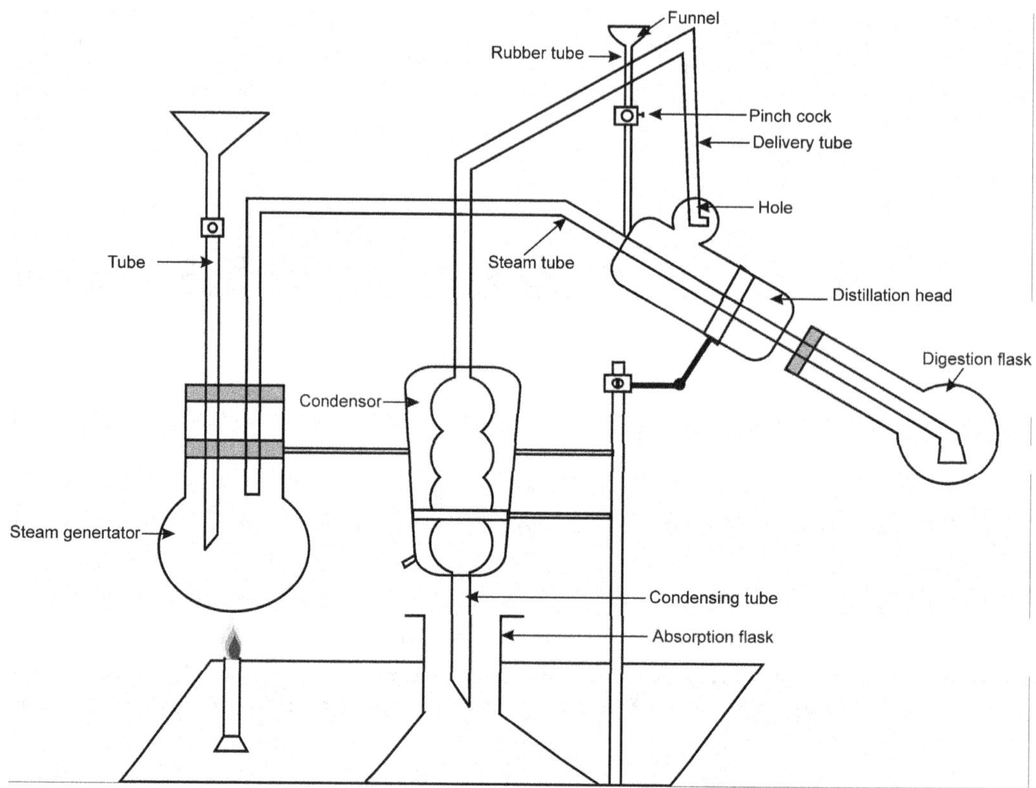

Fig. 16.1

Few Important Points

1. Potassium sulphate is added to H_2SO_4 digestion mixture in order to raise boiling point. Reduce the digestion time.

2. It has been found that ratio of salt to acid is too high the excessive temperature attained may result in loss of ammonia.

   $\therefore$ Optimum salt conc. $\rightarrow$ 1.0-1.5 gm potassium sulphate ml of sulphuric acid

   Boiling point $\rightarrow$ 365–388°C

3. Action of catalyst is required to achieve quantitative decomposition of most organic compounds in a reasonable time.

   Catalyst $\rightarrow$ salts of Hg, selenium and copper. Mostly Hg oxide or Hg sulphate used.

4. Early digestion of many substances the mixture discolours in some cases charring to dark brown. Frothing may occur. As heating is continued colour disappear, the solution colourless, this is known as "clearing".

5. Clearing – a sign of conversion of carbonaceous material to carbon dioxide and other small molecules doesn't coincide with complete conversion of N_2 into ammonia.

   $\therefore$ Necessary to prolong digestion after clearing precipitation.

6. Easily decomposed substances, such as unsubstituted amides, release all N_2 even before clearing has occurred.

7. Kjeldahl $\rightarrow$ determination of N_2 such as amides and amines.

   Azo compounds, some Heterocyclic rings, nitroso, nitro groups $\rightarrow$ resistant to complete decomposition under kjeldahl conditions.

   $\therefore$ sp. Treatment $\rightarrow$ primary reduction of nitro groups and then analysed.

General Method

- After digestion $\rightarrow$ neutralization of H_2 with NaOH.
- This frees ammonia which is removed from mixture by steam distillation.
  Steam $\rightarrow$ externally generated current of steam fed to solution.
- Steam passes out and carrying ammonia (volatile) and is condensed and collected.
- Distillate received in standard HCl solution of known volume.
- Excess acid back–titrated with standard alkali to know ammonia content.
- For each ammonia molecule found in distillate, one N_2 atom was present in sample.

Variations

Boric acid used to receive ammonia from steam distillation. The ammonia is fixed as ammonium borate, which can be titrated directly as base with a standard HCl. Displacement of weak acid basic by strong acid HCl.

Advantages : used of only one standard solution instead of two.

Analysis of Ammonia $\rightarrow$ Colorimetry or Acid base titration.

- For micro samples $\rightarrow$ colorimetry used.

  Colorimetric analysis $\rightarrow$ formation of yellow to brownish colloidal dispersion upon addition with Nessler's reagent. (potassium mercuric iodide).

- Standard solution of Ammonia + reagent $\rightarrow$ absorbance measured at 410 nm and compared to standard.

  Colorimetric analysis $\rightarrow$ Phenol – sodium hypochlorite reagent.

- colour $\rightarrow$ blue and absorbance $\propto$ ammonia concentration

  Acid base titration

- not used because of excess of H_2SO_4 in mixture.

  Redox titration of ammonia with hypobromite or Na-Ca hypo chloride + excess hypo bromite

  $$\rightarrow NH_3 + 3OBr \rightarrow N_2 + 3H_2O + 3Br^-$$

Procedure

1. Weight accurate part of organic sample $\rightarrow$ 0.04 g of N_2 and place it in kjeldahl flask.
2. Add 0.7 g of Hg-oxide + 15 g of potassium sulphate + 40 ml H_2SO_4.
3. Heat flask in inclined position.
4. Frothing occurs and can be controlled by adding antifoaming agent.
5. Boil reactants for 2 hours.
6. After cooling add 200 ml H_2O + 25 ml 0.5 M sodium thiosulfate and mix well.
7. Add 11 M NaOH and down the inside of flask to make the mix strongly alkaline (approx $\rightarrow$ 115 ml).
8. Before the mixing, connect the flask to a distillation apparatus, in which tip of delivery tube is submerged just below surface of a measured volume of 0.1 M HCl.
9. Boil until 150 ml of liquid have been distilled out into receiver.
10. Add methyl red indicator to HCl solution and titrate with 0.1 M NaOH (a ml).
11. Carry out blank titration on an equal volume of 0.1 M HCl. (b ml)

    The % of Nitrogen in sample is given by,

    $$= \frac{(b-a) \times 0.1 \times 14 \times 100}{\text{wt.of sample}_{(gm)}}$$

Application

- Industrial research, microbiological experiments, Pharma industries for estimation of free N_2.
- For Protein hydrolysates, amino acids, serum amides and amines.

  Drugs like $\rightarrow$ isoprenaline sulphate, primidone, Amino acetic acid, Tyrosine, Dried Human plasma, Dried Human serum, Pentamide, Human fibrinogen.

Diazotisation Titration (Sodium Nitrite Titration)

Diazotisation of Aromatic Amines

Primary aromatic amines, which may be $Ar^- NH_2$, undergo reaction with an acid, nitrous acid solution to $\rightarrow$ give diazonium salts used in synthesis of organic dyestuffs.

Reaction

$$A_r - NH_2 + HNO_2 + HCl \rightarrow Ar + N_2 + Cl^- + H_2O$$

1. Nitrosation of amine

$$Ar - NH_2 + HNO_2 + HCl \rightarrow Ar - NH - N = O + H_2O$$

2. Tantomerization of nitrosamine

$$Ar - NH - N = 0 \rightleftharpoons Ar - N = N - OH$$

3. Decomposition of Diazohydroxide

$$Ar - N = N - OH + HCl \rightarrow [\, Ar - N \equiv N \,]^+ \, Cl^- + H_2O$$

Coupling of Diazonium Salts

- The highly reactive $Ar - N_2 + Cl^-$ (Diazonium salt) reacts with second organic compound $\rightarrow$ to yield Diazo compound with elimination of HCl. The Phenol is reactant. This Reaction is called "Coupling Reaction".

$$Ar - N_2 + Cl^- + \bigcirc\!\!-OH \longrightarrow Ar - N \equiv N - \bigcirc\!\!-OH + HCl$$

- Diazo product $\rightarrow$ highly conjugated and therefore absorb radiation of long wavelengths. Therefore most of them coloured.

Determination of Sulfonamides

- Diazo formed by coupling.
- concentration of Diazo measured by spectrophotometry.
- coupling reagent $\rightarrow$ Bratton–Marshall Reagent [N–(1–naphthyl) ethylenediamine.]

Procedure

- Diazotization of amine in acid solution, excess nitrous acid destroyed by reaction with sulfamic acid.

$$HNO_2 + H_2NSO_3H \rightarrow H_2SO_4 + N_2 + H_2O$$

- Coupling reagent added → colour produced due to coupled diazo product.
- Absorption of solution measured.

Important Note

- The addition of Sodium Nitrite to HCl causes the formation of Nitrous acid. This nitrous acid diazotises the aromatic amino group. At end point, excess nitrous acid formed is shown by immediate formation of deep blue colour with starch iodide paper.

$$NaNO_2 + HCl \rightarrow HNO_2 + NaCl$$

End point Detection

1. External Indicator Method

- Detection of end point depends on excess of HNO_2 using starch-iodide paper/paste.
- The starch iodide paper is prepared by immersing a filter paper in starch mucilage and kI solution. The iodide reacts with starch mucilage to give the blue colour.

2. Amperometric End Point Detection Method

- a pair of platinum electrodes are immersed in titration liquid.
- Electro polarization occurs when a small voltage (30-50 mv) is applied across the electrodes and no current flows through the sensitive galvanometer included in the circuit.
- Liberation of excess nitrous acid at end point depolarizes the electrode and current flows in the galvanometer.
- This is known as the dead stop end point. The electrodes must be clean, otherwise, the end point is delayed.

Procedure

Specified amount of drug is dissolved in about 50 ml of water and 20 ml of HCl.

- Solution is stirred and cooled to about 15°C. The mixture is titrated against 0.1 M $NaNO_2$ solution and end point is detected.

Types of Diazotisation Titration

1. Direct titration
2. Reverse method
3. Special method

1. Direct Titration

- One mole of drug + 3 moles of concentric HCl $\rightarrow$ Temp 4°C by ice $\rightarrow$ Titrated with 0.1 N $NaNO_2$ $\rightarrow$ end point by standard iodide paper.

2. Reverse Method

- Used when the resulting diazonium salt is insoluble like napthylamine sulphonic acid.
- zwitter ions are formed which are difficult to solubilize.
- Hence, solution of amine is treated with sodium Na-nitrite and resulting solution is run into solution of HCl.

3. Special Method

- For amino phenols : as they can't be titrated by direct method, when treated sodium nitrite they form quinines which are highly unstable.
- Reaction carried out in the presence of copper sulphate which forms stable diazo oxide and diazo coupling reaction can be carried out.

Applications

- Direct Titration – Benzocaine, Dapsone, Procaine HCl, Sulfa drug.
- Conversion to amino groups by chemical Reactions

  (a) By reduction $\rightarrow$ e.g. metronidazole, Chloramphenicol

  (b) Hydrolysis $\rightarrow$ e.g. Paracetamol etc.

CHAPTER 17

KARL FISCHER TITRATION

Introduction

Drugs and pharmaceutical aids may contain varying amount of water, in the form of water of hydration (or) water absorbed superficially by the substance during the storage, manufacturing, transportation, when it is exposed to the atmosphere.

The presence of water generally deteriorates the activity of the drug and also decreases the life time of the drug if present beyond the specific limits, so care has to be taken during the storage and manufacturing of the drug so that the water content does not exceed beyond the limit. Therefore pharmacopocias all over the world prescribe limit of the content of the water.

Methods

There are several methods for the determination of moisture content. These are classified as :

1. Drying Method
2. Distillation with immiscible organic solvent
3. Karl Fischer Method for determination of water.
4. Karl Fischer Titration

1. Drying Method

This method is based on removal of moisture and volatile matter by drying in vacuum oven so that water content gets evaporated or by using a absorbent in desiccators so that the moisture gets absorbed.

2. Distillation with Immiscible Organic Solvent

This method is based on distillation of sample with immiscible organic solvent like benzene or toluene and the distillate is collected and from that water content can be calculated. This method is mainly useful for vegetable oil drugs.

3. Karl Fischer Method

This is the most important method proposed by Karl Fischer in 1935 which is considered to be specific for water. In this method the titrations were done by Karl Fischer reagent along with the sample, by which the water content can be known by the difference between the two titrations which gives the volume of Karl Fischer reagent consumed by sample. The water percentage can be known by the formula.

$$\text{Water \% (w/w)} = \frac{V \times \text{minimum water equlent of water per ml of Karl Fischer reagent}}{\text{Wt. of sample in (mg)}} \times 100$$

Composition of Karl Fischer Reagent

The Karl Fischer Reagent is composed of Iodine, sulphur dioxide, pyridine and methanol.

According to stoichometric equations the composition of the reagent should be on molar basis, $1I_2 : ISO_2 : ICH_3OH : 3C_5H_5N$. The Karl Fischer reagent is usually prepared as a solution of I_2, SO_2 and pyridine in methanol; the approximate molar ratio being $1I_2 : 3SO_2 : 10C_5H_5N$.

Strength of Karl Fischer Reagent: Numerous side reactions occur among the substances and the reactants are depleted. The observed strength of the reagent is always less than that of theoretical strength because of the consumption of Iodine by the side reactions.

Strength of freshly prepared Karl Fischer reagent = 80% of theoretical value.

But this rapidly falls to 50% in 1 month and 40% in 3 months.

The typical strength of Karl Fischer reagent for micro scale titration is in the range of 3-6 Mg H_2O/ml reagents.

Theory

Step (1) : $3C_5H_5N + SO_2 + I_2 + H_2O \rightarrow 2C_5H_5NHI + C_5$

Step (2) :

From step-1 it is clear that the oxidation of sulphur dioxide takes place by the Iodine to yield sulphur trioxide and hydrogen iodine there by consuming one mole of water i.e., each one molecule of I_2 disappears against each molecule of water present in the sample, and the sulphur tri-oxide so formed reacts with methyl alcohol to form a complex.

From both of reactions it is pertinent that in the presence of large excess of pyridine, all reactants as well as products of reaction mostly exist as complexes.

Importance of Pyridine: The first reaction is reversible and pyridine forces the position of equilibrium to the right by combining with the hydrogen iodide produced.

It also increases the stability of the reagent by forming change transfer complexes with iodine and sulphur-di-oxide, thus reducing the vapour pressure of these volatile substances.

Stability of the Reagent: The stability of the reagent could be improved significantly by the replacement of methanol with 2- methoxy–ethanol. The following precautions have to be taken so as to prevent the deterioration of the reagent, namely.

1. Always prepare the reagent a day or two before it is to be used.

2. Great care must be taken to present and check any possible contamination either of the reagent or sample by atmospheric moisture.

3. All glasswares must be thoroughly dried before use.

4. Standard solution should be stored out of contact with air.

5. It is essential to minimise contact between the atmosphere and the solution during the course of titration.

Interference of Reagent: Most classes of organic compounds do not interfere. Therefore water can be titrated in the presence of :

1. Acids

2. Alcohols

3. Phenols

4. Ethers

5. Hydrocarbons

6. Anhydrides

7. Amines, amides

8. Halides

9. Sulphides

Material that consume iodine interfere. Thiols and ascorbic acid are examples of substances that interfere quantitatively, so a separate analysis is made that permits a correction to be applied.

Carbonyl compounds interfere by forming acetals and ketals with methanol, releasing water in the process.

Remedy: This interference is eliminated by converting the carbonyl compounds to cynohydrin by addition of hydrogen cyanide.

Carboxylic acids are capable of esterification with methanol, this condensation reaction produces water and may invalidate the determinations, and such condensation reactions are promoted by excess Karl Fischer reagent.

Remedy: The usage of pyridine (or) dioxane as titration medium will limit esterification reactions.

Substitute

Methanol can be eliminated from the reagent. It was found that a karl Fischer reagent prepared with 40% formamide and 60% pyridine reacts 100 times faster with water than does the conventional reagent containing methanol.

Instrumentation

The Apparatus consists of a pair of identical platinum electrodes, a mechanical stirrer with adjustable speed and a burette.

Principle

This method consists of titration of sample in methanol in Karl Fischer reagent which incorporates I_2, SO_2, pyridine methanol. The reactions involved are:

$$I_2 + SO_2 + H_2O \rightarrow 2HI\ SO_3$$

$$SO_3 + C_5H_5N \rightarrow C_5H_5NSO_3\ (\text{pyridine -5})$$

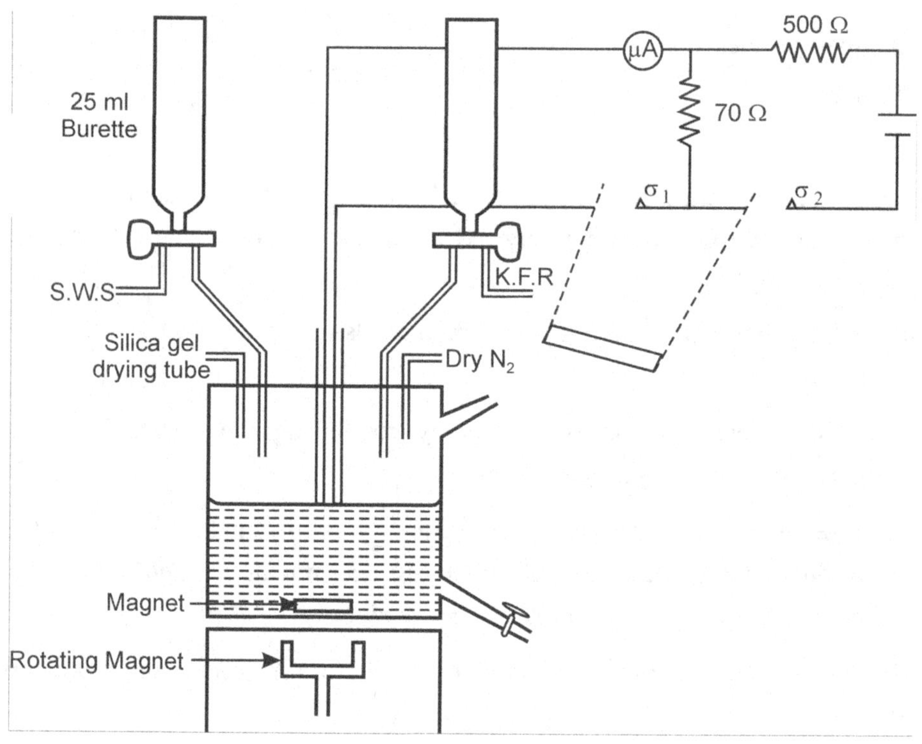

Fig. 17.1

$$HI + C_5H_5N \rightarrow C_5H_5N.\ HI$$

$$C_5H_5N.SO_3 + CH_3OH \rightarrow C_5H_5N.HSO_4CH_3$$

$$H_2O + I_2 + SO_2 + 3C_5H_5N + CH_3OH \rightarrow 2C_5H_5NHI + C_5H_5NH.SO_4.CH_3$$

The basis for analysis is on the quantitative relationship existing between charge passed and I_2 produced by the reagent according to reaction.

Therefore generation of I_2 is automatically stopped when excess of it is detected by indicator electrode.

It essentially consists of two electrodes across which an AC is applied and subsequently a marked drop in voltage between the electrodes takes place as soon as excess of I_2 is present.

Advantage

1. No calibration is required as the method is absolute and is entirely based on the stoichiometry of the above said equation.

2. It allows the detection of amounts of water ranging between 0.1 mg and 10 mg in solid as well as liquid samples.

Limitation of Karl Fischer Titration

The Karl Fischer titration has a number of serious limitations due to the possible interferences with the agents namely :

1. Oxidizing Agents

e.g. Chromates, Cu(II), Fe(III), $Cr_2O_7^{2-}$, peroxides, salts and higher oxides.

e.g. $MNO_2 + 4C_2H_5NH^+ + 2I^- \rightarrow MN^2 + 4C_5H_5N + I_2 + H_2O$

2. Reducing Agents

e.g. Sn(II) salts, sulphides, $S_2O_3^{2-}$ and

3. Compound that have tendency to form water with ingredients of Karl Fischer reagent.

e.g.

(a) Basic oxides ; e.g. ZnO

$$ZnO + 2C_5H_5NH^+ \rightarrow Zn^{2+} + C_5H_5N + H_2O$$

(b) Salts of weak acids; e.g. $NaHCO_3$;

$$NaHCO_3 + C_5H_5NH^+ \rightarrow Na^+ + H_2O + CO_2 + C_5H_5N$$

Standardization of Karl Fischer Reagent

Karl Fischer reagent is standardized by titrating known quantities of water.

Crystalline hydrates have been proposed as primary standards because they have high equivalent weights and are non-volatile. Such a standard should meet the following criteria :

1. It should be commercially available in reagent–grade purity and should contain the theoretical water content.

2. It must release its water quantitatively for reaction with KF reagent in methanolic solution, and must not undergo side reactions with the reagent.

3. It should be stable and should not absorb atmospheric moisture under ordinary conditions.

4. Its water content should be accurately determinable by any independent method.

    Many substances have been tested and found unsatisfactory.

    e.g. Sodium acetate trihydrate is hygroscopic at high humidity and efflorescent at low humidity.

5. Sodium tartarate dehydrate appears to be a satisfactory primary standard; the theoretical water content of this substance is 15.66%. Its only disadvantage is that it is not soluble in methanol so the titration must be carried out slowly enough to ensure that all of the water is released before the end point.

Standard Water Solution

Weigh about 100 ml volumetric flask and its stopper, pipette about 1 ml of water into the flask, put the stopper in place, and reweigh. Dilute to volume with reagent grade absolute methanol.

The same lot of methanol must be used in titration, because the water content of methanol may vary from lot to lot.

The reagent was standardized against the standard water solution.

Pipette 25 ml of absolute methanol in to a dry 100 ml flask. Titrate with Karl Fischer reagent, contained in a 25 ml burette and protected with a drying tube, until the appearance of the characteristic colour of active reagent. From the reactions it is clear that 1 mole of water $\cong$ 1 mole of I_2.

Pyridine reacts with SO_3 forming a complex which neutralises HI thereby presents its oxidation to I_2.

Methanol reacts with pyridine–sulphur trioxide.

In the absence of methanol water reacts with the complex and 2 moles of water is then equivalent of 1 mole of iodine.

$$C_5H_5NSO_3 + H_2O \rightarrow C_5H_5N\,H_2SO_4$$

Procedure

It was observed that absolutely little or no current flows unless and until the solution is totally free from any polarizing substances. This is due to absorbed layers of O_2 and H_2 on anode and cathode. The current flows only when two electrodes get depolarized.

- The Karl Fischer reagent is pumped into burette by means of hand bellows.
- The excess of moisture is presented by employing an appropriate – arrangement of desiccant tubes.
- The stirring is accomplished with the help of a magnetic stirrer.
- The End point is achieved by employing an electrical circuit comprising of a microammeter (A), platinum electrodes, together with 1.5 V to 2.0 V battery connected across a variable resistance of about $2.5\,\Omega$.

- First of all the resistance is adjusted in such a manner that an initial current passes through the platinum electrodes in series with a micrometer (A). After each addition of a reagent, the pointer of the micrometer gets deflected but quickly returns to its original position. At the end of the reaction a deflection is obtained which persists for 10-15 seconds.

Precaution

The air in the system must be kept dry with P_2O_5, anhydrous $CaCl_2$ or silica gel.

Advantage

This method is widely applied for moisture determination of drug substances because it is very rapid, specific and requires very small amounts of sample.

Photometric Karl Fischer Titration

This method can be carried by measuring the absorbance of the titration solution at 525 nm; at which wavelength active reagent absorbs light, but spent reagent does not, as titrant is added to the solution.

A plot is made of absorbance vs volume of titrant. Before the end point the absorbance remains closer to zero, but after the end point it increases, linearly with volume. The end point is marked by the intersection of the two straight lines.

Advantage

This titration provides greater sensitively and precision than can be achieved with visual detection of end point.

Automated Electro-Chemical Karl Fischer Analysis

- Modern KF-titrators are equipped with specially designed titrations vessels that are exclusively meant to check and prevent the contact with atmospheric moisture.
- These devices are armed with microprocessors that will perform the requisite operations sequentially in a programmed manner automatically and also gives out a printout of desired results including the percentage moisture content.
- The modern KF-titrators not only afford greater accuracy and precision in results but also offer much ease and convenience, as compared to classical techniques based on caulometry (a) controlled current potentiometry using two indicator electrodes.
- In this procedure the I_2 needed to react with water is normally generated within the titration vessel. The end point is marked by a definite and permanent reddish

colour. Stopper the flask and retain it for end point colour comparisons. This is the blank titration. It indicates the volume of reagent equivalent to the water contained in 25 ml of absolute methanol.

- Pipette 15 ml of absolute methanol and 10 ml of standard water solution in to another dry 100 ml volumetric flask. Titrate to the end point with Karl Fischer reagent.

The colour was matched closely with that of blank titration.

Note: The titrations should be carried out quickly to avoid the introduction of significant amounts of moisture from the air.

Subtract the blank titration volume from the standardization volume and calculate the titration of the KF-reagent. The result must be expressed as milligrams of water equivalent to 1 ml of reagent.

The Karl Fischer reagent should be restandardized daily.

Applications of Karl Fischer Method

1. Predinsolone Sodium Phosphate

Materials Required: Karl Fischer reagent 100 ml, predinsolone sodium phosphate 0.2 gm and anhydrous methanol 20 ml.

Procedure: Add 20 ml anhydrous methanol to the titration vessel and titrate to amperometric end-point with the KF- reagent. Quickly add 0.2 gm of predinsolone sodium phosphate sample, stir for 1 min. and again titrate to the amperometric end-point with the KF-reagent. The difference between the two titrations gives the volume of Karl Fischer reagent consumed by the sample.

The maximum water equivalent is 3.5 mg of water per ml of KF-reagent.

Hence the % of water $\dfrac{W}{W}$ in the given sample may be calculated by the following equation.

$$\text{Water \%} \left(\dfrac{W}{W} \right) = \dfrac{V \times 3.5}{\text{Wt. of sample (mg)}} \times 100$$

Precautions

1. The reagents and solutions used must be kept anhydrous and necessary care should be taken throughout to prevent exposure to atmosphereic moisture.

2. The KF-reagent should be protected from light and preferably stored in a bottle fitted with an automatic burette.

3. The water equivalent of KF-reagent should always be determined before use.

Assays

A number of other official pharmaceutical substances may be assayed for the water content by the Karl Fischer method as summarized in the following Table.

S.No.	Name of Substance	Quantity	Prescribed Limit Of water % $\left(\dfrac{W}{W}\right)$
1.	Rifamycin solution	0.2 gms	12 – 17
2.	Sodium, methyl Hydroxy benzoate	1 gm	NMT 5
3.	Triamcinolone Acetonide	0.2 gm	NMT 2

NMT = Not more than

Finally we can conclude that the use of commercially available Karl Fischer reagent must be validated in order to verify in each case the stoichiometry and the absence of incompatibility between the substance being examined and the reagent.

CHAPTER 18

OXYGEN FLASK COMBUSTION METHOD

In 1955, Schoniger devloped this method for analysis for organically combined halogens.

Basic Concept

- When complete combustion of organic compound takes place, organic matter gets destroyed and halogen is released.
- The halogen released is absorbed in the combustion flask into NaOH solution to yield mixture of iodide and iodate.
- Subsequent oxidation and then acidification in the presence of iodide give iodine (free) which is determined by titration with a standard solution of sodium thiosulfate.
- Sulfur is also determined by oxygen flask combustion method besides Fl, Cl, Br

Advantages

- Simple rapid and accurate
- Applied to pharm. formulations such as tablets, capsules, creams and ointments.

Apparatus

- Conical iodine flask – 500 ml – stopper attached.
- platinum wire $\rightarrow$ 13 cm long or 11 platinum gauze. (specified dimensions) and 1 mm diameter.

General Method

- Sample 5-10 mg on to a shaped piece of paper, which is folded in such a way that tail (wick) is free.

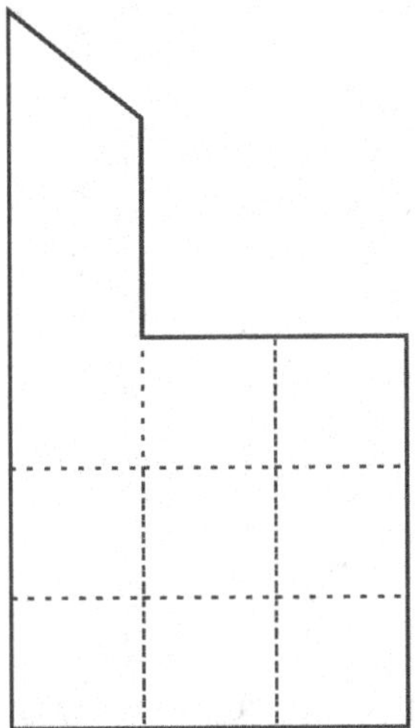

Paper shape for wrapping sample

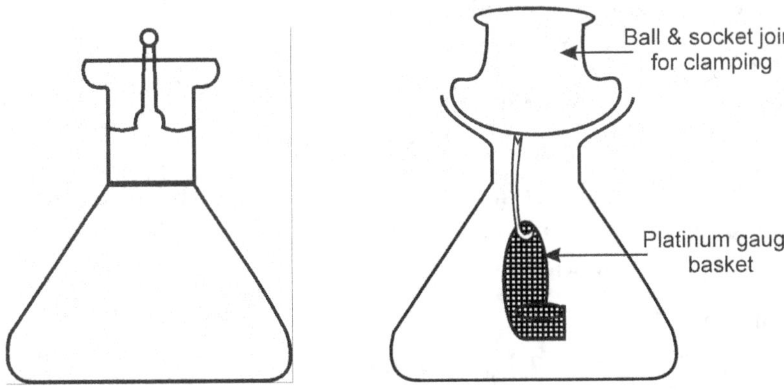

Fig. 18.1 Oxygen flask combustion apparatus.

- Placed in platinum basket suspended from ground glass stopper.
- The flask contains few ml of absorbing solution (aq. NaOH) is filled with oxygen then sealed using stopper with platinum basket attached.
- The wick of paper is ignited before the stopper is placed or ignited by remote electrical control or an infrared lamp.
- Combustion is rapid and completes in 5-10 seconds.

- After standing for a few minutes until any combustion cloud has disappeared, the flask is shaken for 2-3 minutes to ensure complete absorption has taken place.

- The solution can then be treated by a method appropriate to the element being determined.

Procedure for Iodine

- Absorbing liquid $\rightarrow$ 10 ml H_2O + 2ml 1N NaOH.

- After completion of combustion process add excess Br_2 solution (5-10 ml) and allow to stand for 2 minutes.

- Remove excess Br_2 using 1 ml formic acid.

- Sweep out any Br_2 vapour from flask with a current of air.

- Add 1 gm of KI and titrate with 0.02 N sodium thiosulfate solution using starch mucilage as indicator.

  Each ml of 0.02 N $Na_2S_2O_3 \cong$ 0.000423 gm of I_2.

  R×n $3I_2 + 6NaOH \rightarrow 5\ NaI + NaIO_3 + 3H_2O$

  $\qquad 2NaI + 15\ Br_2 + 15\ H_2O \rightarrow 5\ NaIO_3 + 3OHBr$

  $\qquad 6\ NaIO_3 + 30\ KI + 36\ HBr \rightarrow 18\ I_2 + 6\ NaBr + 30\ KBr$

  $\qquad I_2 + 2\ Na_2S_2O_3 \rightarrow Na_2S_4O_6 + 2\ NaI$

Procedure for Chlorine

- Absorbing liquid $\rightarrow$ 20 ml of 1N NaOH solution

  $\qquad\qquad$ + 2.5 ml Nitric acid + 10 ml N/10 $AgNO_3$

- After completion of combustion, titrate excess $AgNO_3$ with 0.05 M ammonium thiocyanate using ferric ammonia sulphate as indicator.

- Perform blank titration with sample.

- Difference $\rightarrow$ volume of N/10 $AgNO_3$

  Each ml of 0.1 N $AgNO_3 \cong$ 0.001773 gm of chlorine.

- Organically combined chlorine is converted to free chlorine by flask combustion method and halogen is absorbed into NaOH.

- This yields mixture of chloride and hypochlorite.

- Addition of $AgNO_3$ precipitates chloride as AgCl.

- Excess unreacted $AgNO_3$ is back titrated with ammonia thiocynate solution with help of ferric alum as indicator.

  Reaction : $\qquad Cl_2 + 2NaOH + NaCl + NaOCl$

  $\qquad\qquad\qquad Cl_2 \equiv 2AgNO_3$

$$0.001773 \text{ gm} = 1 \text{ ml of } 0.05 \text{ N AgNO}_3$$

$$NaCl + AgNO_3 \rightarrow NaNO_3 + AgCl \downarrow$$

Procedure for Bromine

- Absorbing liquid $\rightarrow$ 15 ml mixture of 1 volume 30% H_2O_2 and 9 volume 1N H_2SO_4.
- After complete combustion, Add 5 ml of 2N HNO_3 + 10 ml 0.1 N $AgNO_3$.
- Titrate the unconsumed $AgNO_3$ with 0.05 N NH_4 SCN using ferric acid as indicator.
- Blank determination is carried out.
- Difference $\rightarrow$ ml of $AgNO_3$ consumed by sample.
- Each ml of 0.1N $AgNO_3$ $\equiv$ 0.003995 gm of Br_2.

Procedure for Fluorine

- Absorbing liquid $\rightarrow$ 20 ml water.
- After combustion add H_2O to produce 50 ml.
- Take 2 ml and add 20 ml H_2O + 10 ml alizarine fluorine blue solution + 3 ml 2% of Na-acetate + 6% w/v HAC (glacial) + 10 ml cerous nitrate. H_2O to produce 50 ml.
- Allow to stand in dark for 1 hour and measure.
- Organically combined F is converted to free F by combustion in oxygen in Silica flask.
- Boro Silicate glass avoided as F reacts with boron.
- F absorbed in to H_2O and determined by calorimetry 610 nm using alizarine flourine blue and cerous nitrate in acetate buffer.

Procedure for Sulfur

There are two methods available

Method I - estimation of sulfur in absence of halogens and phosphorus.

Method II - in presence of halogens or phosphorous.

Method I

- Burn specified quantity of sample material in flask $\rightarrow$10 ml H_2O + 0.1 ml H_2O_2 (30 %) (Absorbing liquid)
- After combustion, cool solution in ice for 15 minutes.
- Boil for 2 minutes $\rightarrow$ cool + 50 ml ethanolic acetic ammonia buffer (pH 3.7).
- Titrate with 0.05 M Barium perchlorate (Alizarin red indicator)

  color $\rightarrow$ orange pink.

Method II

- Absorbing fluid $\rightarrow$ 15 ml H_2O + 1 ml H_2O_2 (10%).

- After completion $\rightarrow$ boil for 10 min $\rightarrow$ cool + 60 ml.

- Titrate solution 0.01M Barium perchlorate as titrant using 0.1 ml of 0.2% thoron and 0.1 ml of 0.0125% methylene blue as indicator until color changes from yellow to pink.

- Each ml 0.01 M Barium perchlorate $\equiv$ 0.00032 gm of S.

$$Vc = v\,[1 + 0.0008\,(t_1 - t_2)]$$

where V_c = Corrected volume of titrant

V = the volume of titrant used

t_1 = temperature of titrant during standardization

t_2 = temperature of titrant during determination

Reaction : $S + O_2 \rightarrow SO_2$

$SO_2 + H_2O \rightarrow H_2SO_3$

$H_2SO_3 \xrightarrow{\;H_2O\;} H_2SO_4$

- Sulfuric acid generated is titrated against a std. solution of alkali using methyl red or other suitable acid-base indicator.

Applications

- Diazepam, Diodone inj, flurouracil, Niclosamide and Thyroxine sodium.

CHAPTER 19

ERRORS AND STATISTICS

Introduction

In Analysis, there are two values for a result, true result and practical result. The degree of success of an experiment is determined by the concurrence of true value and practical value of the experiment. The accuracy and the precision of the method are the determining the factors and help us in finding out the sources of error which may be introduced into the experiment. Quantitative analysis involves estimating the sample, also the knowledge of the chemistry involved and also the possibilities of interferences and statistical evaluation of experimental values.

Bio-Statistics has been defined as the application of statistical methods to biological, physical and chemical sciences. The use of statistical methods is constantly increasing in analytical chemistry. A good understanding of biostatistics is essential because it is an indispensable tool for the design and analysis of experimental analytical data and in the interpretation of experimental results for dependable conclusions. A preliminary acquaintance will help not only in applying biostatistical methods but also in a better appreciation of their potential value.

Accuracy: It is defined as the agreement between the observed value and the true value. The absolute error is a measure of the accuracy of the measurement. Accuracy defines the correction of a measurement.

Precision: It is defined as the agreement between a number of measurements taken for the same quantity. Precision expresses the reproducibility of a measurement. The mean deviation is the measure of precision.

Classification of Errors: Errors in an experiment are inherent. The Errors may be broadly classified into two types.

1. Determinate Errors or Constant Errors and

2. Indeterminate Errors or Accidental Errors.

1. Determinate Errors

These are the errors which occur frequently and which can be determined and avoided. The following are the various errors under this category.

(a) Operational and personal errors

(b) Instrumental and Reagent Errors.

(c) Errors of Method

(d) Additive and proportional errors.

(a) Operational and Personal Errors: These errors arise due to the individual analyst and no way connected to the method or procedure of the experiment. Personal errors occur due to the constitutional inability of an individual to make observations correctly.

(b) Instrumental and Reagent Errors: These are the errors due to the instruments and the reagents not being pure or which contain impurities.

(c) Errors of Method: This is due to the errors in experimental procedure, incorrect sampling, occurrence of side reactions and a difference between the observed end point and stoichiometric end point of a reaction.

(d) Additive and Proportional Errors: The absolute value of an additive error is independent of the amount of constituent present in the determination. Proportional errors arise for taking incorrect values for calculating the experimental values.

2. Indeterminate Errors or Accidental Errors

These are the minute errors which cannot be determined. They are due to reasons over which the analyst has no control. They are called as intangible errors because they cannot be predicted and therefore cannot be eliminated.

Minimization of Errors: The determinate errors can be minimized by adopting any of the following methods.

Calibration of Apparatus and Application of Corrections: All instruments (weight, flasks, burettes, pipettes, spectrophotometers etc.) should be calibrated and the appropriate corrections applied to the original measurements.

Running a Blank Determination: This consists in carrying out a separate determination, the sample being omitted under exactly the same experimental conditions as are employed in the actual analysis of the sample. The object is to find out the effect of the impurities introduced through the reagents, vessels and solvents.

Running a Control Determination: This consists in carrying out a determination under as nearly as possible identical experimental conditions upon a quantity of a standard substance which contains the same weight of the constituent as is contained in the unknown sample. The weight of the constituent in the unknown can then be calculated from the relation.

$$\frac{\text{Result for the standard}}{\text{Result for the unknown}} \times \frac{\text{Weight of constituent in standard}}{X}$$

where 'X' is the weight of the constituent in the unknown.

Running of Parallel Determinations: In some cases the accuracy of a result may be established by carrying out the analysis in an entirely different manner. For example iron may be first determined gravimetrically by ignition of the precipitate to iron (III) oxide. It may be then determined titrimetrically by reduction to the iron (II) state, and titration with standard solution of an oxidizing agent like potassium permanganate. If the results obtained by the two radically different methods are concordant, it is highly probable that the values are correct within small limits of error.

Running of Parallel Determinations: These serve as a check on the result of singly determination and indicate only the precision of the analysis. In titrimetry, performing duplicate or triplicate titration is a typical example.

Standard Addition: A known amount of the constituent being determined is added to the sample, which is then analysed for the total amount of constituent present. The difference between the analytical results for samples with and without the added constituent gives the recovery of the amount of added constituent. If the recovery is satisfactory, our confidence in the accuracy of the procedure is enhanced. Standard addition method is usually applied to physico-chemical procedures such as spectrophotometry and polarography.

Internal Standards: Internal standard procedure is of particular value in spectroscopic and chromatographic determinations. It involves adding a fixed amount of a reference material (the internal standard) to a series of known concentrations of the material to be measured. The ratios of the physical value (absorbance or peak area) of the internal standard and the series of known concentrations is plotted against the concentration values. This should give a straight line. Any unknown concentration can then be determined by adding the same quantity of internal standard and finding where the ratio obtained falls on the concentration scale.

Amplification Methods: In determinations in which very small amount of material is to be measured this may be beyond the limits of the apparatus available. In such cases, if the small amount of material can be reacted in such a way that every molecule produces two or more molecules of some other measurable material.

Isotopic Dilution: A known amount of the element being determined, containing a radioactive isotope, is mixed with the sample and the element is isolated in a pure form (usually as a compound), which is weighed or otherwise determined. The radio-activity of the isolated element is measured and compared with that of the added element. Then the weight of the element in the sample can be determined.

Statistical Treatment of Data

Important Statistical terms which can be applied for statistical treatment to observations and readings in analytical chemistry are:

Analysis of Variance (ANOVA): A Statistical technique used to test the equality of three or more sample means and thus make inferences as to whether the samples come from populations having the same mean.

Average: A single value that describe the characteristic of the entire mass of data.

Biased Errors: Biased errors are those which arise because of bias in selection, estimation etc.

Coefficient of Variation: A relative measure of dispersion which expresses the standard deviation as a percentage of mean.

Correlation: It is a statistical tool which measures the closeness of the relationship between two variables.

Data: A collection of any number of related observations on one or more variables.

Dependable Variable: The variable which is to be predicted in regression analysis.

Experiment: The activity that result in an event.

Experimental Error: The variation in responses caused by the extraneous factors is termed as experimental error.

Graph: A graph is a visual form of representation of statistical data.

Linear Relationship: A particular type of association between two variables that can be described statistically by a straight line.

Mean: A central tendency measure representing the arithmetic average of a set of observations.

Parameter: A measure which describes the characteristics of a population.

Population: The total number of individual observations from which inferences are to be made at a particular time.

Range: The difference between the largest and the smallest value of the distribution of data.

Raw Data: Information before it is arranged or analysed by statistical methods.

Regression: The statistical method which helps us to estimate the unknown value of one variable from the known value of the related variable.

Regression Analysis: This technique is concerned in measuring the probable form of the relationship between the two variables.

Regression Equations: The two equations based on two regression lines are called regression equations.

Regression Line: A line fitted to a set of data points to estimate the relationship between two variable.

Representative Sample: A sample that contains the relevant characteristics of the population in the same proportion as they are included in that population.

Sample: Selection of a part of a population to represent the whole population.

Sampling Errors: Errors that arise due to drawing inferences about the population on the basis of a sample are termed sampling errors.

Standard Error of Estimate: A measure of the reliability of the estimating equation, indicating the variability of the observed points around the regression line, i.e., the extent to which observed values differ from their predicated values on the regression line.

Statistics: A measure computed from the data of sample. (Numerical measures describing the characteristics of a sample, commonly represented by Roman letters).

Test of Significance: A statistical test used to determine whether observed frequencies between two samples draws from the same population are actually due to chance or whether they are really significant.

Variable: Any quantity or quality liable to show variation from one individual to the next in the same population.

Variance: It is defined as the means of squares of deviations.

Absolute Error: The absolute error of a determination is the difference between the observed or measured value and the true or most probable value of the quantity measured. It is generally a measure of the 'accuracy' of the measurement.

Relative Error: The relative error is the absolute error divided by true or most probable value. It is usually expressed in terms of percentage or parts per thousand.

Mean (Average) Deviation: It is evaluated by determining the arithmetical mean of the results, then calculating the deviation of each individual measurement from the mean and finally dividing the some of the deviations (regardless of sign) by the number of measurements. It is denoted by "d".

$$d = \Sigma \frac{(X_i - X)}{n}$$

where

X = average

X_i = Individual reading

Σ = Summation

n = number of measurements

Relative Mean Deviation: It is the mean deviation divided by the mean. This may be expressed in terms of percentage or in parts per thousand.

$$\text{Relative mean deviation} = \frac{\text{Mean deviation}}{\text{Mean}} \times 100$$

Standard Deviation: Standard deviation is the most commonly used absolute measure of dispersion. The concept of standard deviation was first introduced by Karl Pearson in 1893. It is expressed in the same units of measurement as the observations, whereas, variance is expressed in squared units. The term "standard" is assigned to this measure of variation is probably because it is the most commonly used and is the most flexible in terms of variety of applications of all the measures of dispersion. It is clear that standard deviation is a measure of the spread in a set of observations. In this method, the drawback of ignoring the algebraic sum as in mean deviation is overcome by taking the square of deviations, thereby, making all the deviations positive. Standard deviation is defined as the square root of the variance. Thus, the sample standard deviation(s) would be

$$s = \sqrt{\frac{\Sigma(x_i - x)2}{n-1}}$$

As it measures the dispersion or variability of a distribution, the larger the standard deviation mean, the greater is the value of variability. On the other hand, there will be homogeneity in a series when the standard deviation is small.

Merits and Demerits of the Standard Deviation

Merits

(a) It is rigidly defined

(b) It is based on all the observations.

(c) It is less affected by sampling fluctuations.

(d) For comparing two or more samples or varieties or distributions, the coefficient of variation is useful as it is based on the standard deviation and arithmetic mean. These important points indicate that the standard deviation is the best measure of dispersion. It is the most extensively used measure in statistical analysis of the agricultural as well as the biological and the medical sciences.

Demerits

(a) It is difficult to calculate as compared to the other measures of dispersion.

(b) It gives more weightage to extreme values and less to the values which are near to the mean.

Variance: Variance is also called Mean Square Deviation. This term was first introduced by R.A. Fisher in 1913. The term "Variance" is used to describe the square of the standard deviation. This is an important measure in the quantitative analysis of the data in the biological, agricultural and medical sciences. Therefore, the analysis of variance helps us in isolating the effects of various factors. The variance is very important statistic because of some mathematical properties that can be used in developing statistical theories. To calculate the variance, the deviations of the variables from the mean are squared and then added. The sum of the squares of deviations is divided by the number of observations to get the variance of the sample. This measure has an advantage over the mean deviation because the sum of squares of deviations is always positive. The variance is defined as the mean of squares of deviations. Symbolically;

$$F^2 = \frac{\Sigma (X_i - \overline{X})^2}{n}$$

where,   X = arithmetic mean and N = number of observations

Comparison of Results: Statistical figures obtained from a set of results are of limited value by themselves. It is only comparing them with the true value of with other sets of data then it is possible to determine whether its analytical procedure has been accurate or precise or if it is superior to another method. There are three common methods for testing results

1. Student's t-test

2. The variance ratio test (F – test) and

3. Chi square (x^2) test.

These methods of test require a knowledge of what is known as the number of degrees of freedom (statistical term, this is the number of independent values necessary to determine the statistical quantity). Then a sample of 'n' value has n degrees of freedom, whilst the sum $\Sigma(x_i - x)^2$ is considered to have (n – 1) degrees of freedom.

(i) Student's t-test: This t-test concept was introduced by an English chemist, W.S. Gosset. It is a term used for small samples; its purpose is to compare the mean from a sample with some standard value and express some level of confidence in the significance of the comparison. It is also used to test the difference between the means of two sets of data X_1 and X_2.

The value of 't' is obtained from the equation

$$t = \frac{\sqrt{n} - X\,(\overline{X} - \mu)}{S}$$

Where, $\overline{X}$ is sample mean, n is sample size, μ is the true value and S is the standard deviation of the sample given.

It is then related to a set of t-tables in which the probability (P) of the t-value falling within certain limit is expressed, either as a percentage osr as a function of unit, relative to the number of degrees of freedom.

Chi-square Test: The X^2 test (Pronounced as chi-square test) is particularly useful as a means of testing whether the recorded data are in agreement or not with the "null hypothesis". The chi-square test gives a yes or no answer to the correctness of the null hypothesis.

The symbol X^2 is the Greek letter, Chi. The X^2 test was first used by Karl Pearson in the year 1890. The quantity X^2 describes the magnitude of differences between the observed and the expected frequencies. This test is helpful to find out whether such differences are significant or not. It is defined as :

$$X^2 = \Sigma \frac{(f_0 - f_e)^2}{f_e}$$

where f_0 = observed frequency,

f_e = expected frequency

If the observed frequencies and the expected frequencies are identical, the computed X^2 value will be zero. Therefore, the possible value of X^2 ranges upwards from zero. To determine the value of X^2, the steps required are :

Calculate the expected frequencies (f_e)

Find out the difference between the observed frequencies (f_o) and the expected frequencies (f_e). If the deviation $(f_0 - f_e)$ is large, the square deviation $(f_0 - f_e)^2$ is also large.

Square the values of $(f_0 - f_e)^2$ and divide each value by respective value of f_e and obtain the total $\Sigma(f_0 - f_e)^2 / f_e$. This will be the value of X^2 which ranges from zero to infinity.

The calculated value of X^2 is compared with the table value for the given degrees of freedom at either 5% or 1% level of significance. If the calculated value of X^2 is less than the tabulated value at a particular level of significance, the difference between the observed and the expected frequencies is not significant, and could have arisen due to fluctuations of sampling. On the other hand, when the calculated value is more than the tabulated value, the difference between the observed and the expected values is significant.

Characteristics of Chi-Square Test: The Chi-square distribution has some important characteristics :

- This test is base on frequencies, whereas, in theoretical distribution the test is based on mean and standard deviation.
- The other distribution can be used for testing the significance of the difference between a single expected value and observed proportion. However, this test can be used for testing difference between the entire set of the expected and the observed frequencies.
- A new chi-square distribution is formed for every increase in the number of degrees of freedom.
- This test is applied for testing the hypothesis but is not useful for estimation.

Assumptions for Validity of Chi-Square Test: There are a few assumptions for the validity of chi-square test :

- All the observations must be independent. No individual item should be included twice or a number of times in the sample.
- The total number of observations should be large. The chi-square test should not be used if n > 50.
- All the events must be mutually exclusive.
- For comparison purpose, the data must be in original units.
- If the theoretical frequency is less than 5, then we pool it with the preceding or the succeeding frequency, so that the resulting sum is greater than 5.

Applications of Chi-Square Test: The chi-square test is applicable to varied problems in agriculture, biology and medical sciences besides other statistical analyses. They are :

- To test the goodness of fit.
- To test the independence of attributes.
- To test the homogeneity of independent estimates of the population variances.

CHAPTER 20

MISCELLANEOUS METHODS

Introduction

Ethyl alcohol is commonly known as alcohol. It is very widely used in pharmacy for various purposes. It serves as vehicle in pharmaceutical preparations and manufacture of various formulations. The amount and strength of alcohol used varies from preparation to preparation. In some preparations different strength of alcohol is used, while in others industrial methylated spirit is used. The denatured spirit or industrial methylated spirit contains upto 5% methyl alcohol in alcohol. Detection of it is usually recommended in pharmacopoeias, since it is toxic and harmful to the health.

Determination of alcohol content is very routinely carried out in pharmaceutical industry. Different methods are used for its determination. The methods adopted by pharmacopoeia of India are discussed below.

Traditionally determination of alcohol in galenicals is carried out by distillation method followed by physical measurements of the distillate. During the distillation following steps are carried out which decides particular method to be used.

1. Distillation of all the ethyl alcohol from the sample.
2. Remove of volatile impurities and interfering materials.
3. Test on the distillate for identification of methyl alcohol or isopropyl alcohol; and dilution of distillate to record specific gravity to be is measurable range.

Amongst distillation methods, the following methods are followed:

Method I is a general method and is applied for normal samples containing sufficient alcohol, while *Method II* is mainly for the samples containing volatile substances. *Method III* is similar to Method II but is mainly for the complex solutions containing other volatile substances.

Distillation Methods

The basic principle of this method is the distillation of the liquid sample using an appropriate distillation assembly. The distillate is then analysed either by determining specific gravity of distillate at specified temperature or by refractive index. In distillation method care is to be taken to minimise the loss of alcohol by evaporation. Three methods are used in distillation depending upon the nature of the sample. An appropriate treatment is given to the sample before placing it in distillation assembly. The distillation apparatus used in alcohol determination is described below.

Apparatus

The apparatus (Fig. 20.1) consists of four parts. Part A is a 500 ml capacity round bottom flask. To this is fitted distillation head (B) with a steam trap. A vertical condenser (C) is fitted to the distillation head. The distillate is collected in 100 to 200 ml capacity volumetric flask (D). This flask is generally immersed in a ice-water mixture during distillation.

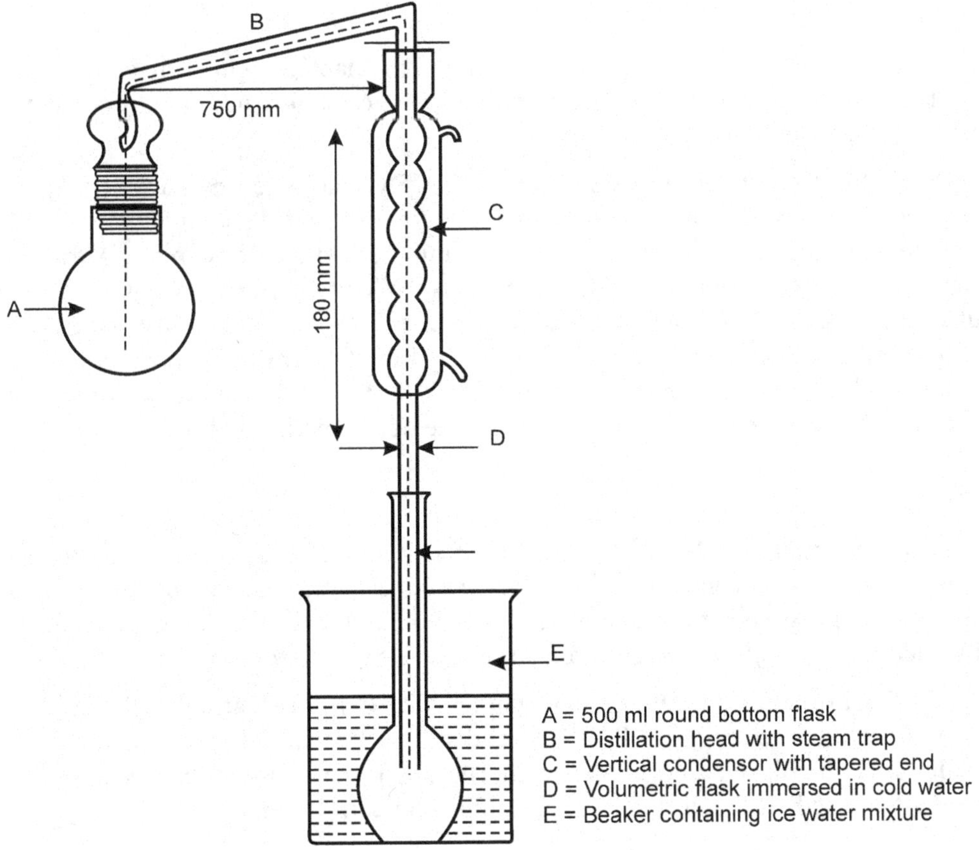

Fig. 20.1 Apparatus for alcohol determination.

Method I

This general method is used for normal samples which do not need any special treatment. For working, place 25 ml of an accurately measured sample at 25^0C into distillation flask.

Add about 150 ml of water, little pumic powder and distill. Collect not less than 90 ml of distillate in 100 ml volumetric flask placed in a beaker containing ice-water mixture. Adjust the temperature of distillate to 25°C and make up the volume to 100 ml with distilled water. Determine the specific gravity at 25°C and referring to the table given in standard books find the corresponding percent of alcohol. Multiply the volume by four to get alcohol content in the sample. If the sample gives frothing during distillation add few drops of liquid paraffin or silicon oil to prevent frothing. If the distillate appears turbid, follow Method III. Turbidity usually occurs due to the presence of steam volatile acids during distillation.

Method II

This method is used for the samples containing appreciable amounts of volatile matter. The volatile matter gets into distillate during distillation and hence requires removal by extraction with suitable solvent.

Place 25 ml of accurately measured sample at 25°C into a 250 ml capacity separating funnel, add about 100 ml water. Saturate this mixture with solid sodium chloride and add 100 ml of hexane. Shake vigorously for 2-3 minutes, allow to stand- till two layers separate and run the lower into distillation flask. When the hexane (upper layer) with about 25 ml of sodium chloride solution and place it into the flask. Make the mixture in distillation flask just alkaline with 1 N sodium hydroxide using solid phenolphthalein as indicator. Add little piece of pumic and distill till 90 ml is collected in volumetric flask. Determine the alcohol content as per the procedure described in Method I.

Method III

This method is similar to Method II in certain respects. If the sample contains methyl alcohol or isopropyl alcohol, test for their presence or absence in distillate is made. Sometimes sample preparations contain industrial methylated spirit (containing about 5% methyl alcohol). This gives colour to oxidation of methyl alcohol into formaldehyde.

Place 25 ml of accurately measured sample at 25°C in distillation flask, and 150 ml water, little pumic powder and collect 100 ml distillate. Transfer this to separating funnel, add solid sodium chloride and extract with 100 ml hexane. Using the lower layer now proceed as per Method II and find out the alcohol content.

Since many preparations containing alcohol are made using industrial methylated spirit or denatured spirit, detection for methyl alcohol and/or isopropyl alcohol is done on the distillate. For this two tests are carried out as follows:

1. For Methyl Alcohol

Take 5 ml of distillate, add 1 drop of dilute phosphoric acid, 1 drop of potassium permanganate solution, mix and allow to stand for one minute. Then add drop wise sufficient sodium bisulphite solution till permanganate colour is discharged. If slight brown colour is there then add one drop of dilute phosphoric acid. Now add 5 ml of freshly prepared chromotropic acid solution and heat on water bath at 60°C for ten minutes; no violet colour is produced.

This test is based upon the oxidation of methyl alcohol to formaldehyde which forms Schiffs base with chromotropic acid to give violet colour.

2. For Isopropyl Alcohol

To 1 ml of distillate add 2 ml mercuric sulphate solution and heat on water bath. No precipitate is formed (indicates absence of isoprophyl alcohol.).

In the earlier editions of pharmacopoeia there was method IV which involved preliminary extraction of 25 ml of sample with 25 ml of sulphuric acid water by 100 ml light petroleum ether. After the petroleum ether extraction, the aqueous phase is transferred to the distillation flask and distillate collected. Now-a-days this method is no longer adopted.

Gas-Liquid Chromatographic Methods

Now-a-days gas chromatography is widely used in pharmaceutical analysis. This method is adopted for certain specified samples containing alcohol. It gives accurate results rapidly.

A gas-liquid chromatography apparatus as described in pharmacopoeia or standard text books is used. Two methods are followed.

In method I, solutions used are (a) solution containing 5% v/v ethylalcohol and 5% v/v propyl alcohol as internal standard. (b) Sample solution is diluted such that it contain between 4.0-6.0% alcohol: (c) 5% propyl alcohol is added to the dilute sample.

For GLC, porapak Q or chromosorb 101 column maintained at 150°C, nitrogen as carrier gas, flame ionization detector is used.

Method II is for samples containing methyl alcohol. Since many preparations are made using industrial methylated spirit which contains upto 5% methyl alcohol, detection and determination of methyl alcohol peak is done using GLC.

Determination of alcohol containing volatile oils, sample needs to be analysed carefully. The preparation containing alcohol if it is acidic, it should be neutralised with sodium hydroxide solution and if it is alkaline with sulphuric acid before distillation. Furthermore if preparations contain chloroform besides ethyl alcohol then separation of chloroform during distillation need to be carried out using modified apparatus which is described in pharmacopeias and pharmaceutical codex.

Table 1

Specific gravity at 25°	Ethanol* content	Specific gravity at 25°	Ethanol* content
1,0000	0	0.9826	13
0.9985	1	0.9814	14
0.9970	2	0.9802	15
0.9956	3	0.9790	16
0.9941	4	0.9778	17
0.9927	5	0.9767	18
0.9914	6	0.9756	19
0.9901	7	0.9744	20
0.9888	8	0.9733	21
0.9875	9	0.9721	22
0.9862	10	0.9710	23
0.9850	11	0.9698	24
0.9838	12	0.9685	25

* % v/v at 15.36°

(Reproduced from "Text Book of Pharmaceutical Analysis" by Mahadik and Dr. H.N. More with permission from Dr. K.R. Mahadik).

CHAPTER 21

GASOMETRY

Introduction

Gasometry or gasometric analysis is the analysis on the estimation of various gas constituents present in a gas mixture. This analytical method is widely employed for the analysis of different gases like oxygen, carbondioxide, nitrous oxide etc. The gasometric methods are divided into three different groups :

- Volumetric or absorptiometric methods.
- Titrimetric methods
- Physical or instrumental methods.

Volumetric Methods

- The basic principle is that a measured volume of the sample at a specific temperature and pressure is exposed in a closed container or vessel to a suitable solid or liquid reagent.
- When the reaction is over, the change in volume is measured.
- The decrease in the volume is due to the absorption of gas constituent by a specific absorbent.
- The difference is equal to the proportion of a particular constituent to be determined i.e., $V_a - V_b$ where 'V_a' is the volume of gas mixture before absorption and 'V_b' is the volume of gas mixture after the absorption of one constituent.

Titrimetric Methods

- The unreacted alkali is estimated by titration with a standard solution of acid by passing the sample through a standard solution containing excess Barium hydroxide.

- Generally carbondioxide i.e., an acidic gas is estimated by this volumetric method.

- From the volume of standard alkali consumed, the amount of the carbondioxide can be calculated.

$$CO_2 + Ba\,(OH)_2 \rightarrow BaCO_3 \downarrow + H_2O$$

Physical or Instrumental Methods

- The gases can be estimated by making use of physical properties like thermal conductivity, refractive index, density etc.

- In gasometry, the choice of a particular method depends upon several factors. They are :

  1. Sample size.
  2. Concentration of the gas in the mixture.
  3. Availability of the equipment.
  4. Availability of reagents.
  5. Accuracy desired.

- The amount of gas constituents in the mixture is expressed in terms of present volume.

- All measurements should be made at Standard Temperature and Pressure i.e. at S.T.P.

Absorbing Reagents (Absorbents) For Various Gases

1. *Absorbents for Oxygen*

   (a) Alkaline pyrogallol solution

   (b) Sodium hyposulphite solution

   (c) Yellow phosphorous (solid)

   (d) Chromous Chloride solution

   (e) Ammonium Chloride-ammonium hydroxide solution.

2. *Absorbents for Carbondioxide*

- Carbondioxide is an acidic gas so the absorbents for CO_2 are invariably basic or alkaline in nature. They are :

  (a) Potassium hydroxide solution (36%).

  (b) Sodium hydroxide solution (32%).

  (c) Barium hydroxide solution (1N).

3. ***Absorbents for Carbon Monoxide***

   (a) Human or animal blood.

   (b) Cuprous chloride solution.

   (c) Cuprous sulphate solution.

   (d) Solid reagents – hoolamite and hypocalite.

   - Hoolamite is a mixture of pumice and iodine pentoxide in fuming H_2SO_4.

   - Hypocalite is a mixture of oxides of cobalt, silver, copper and magnesium.

4. ***Absorbents for Hydrogen***

   (a) Palladium metal or colloidal palladium.

   (b) Palladous chloride solution (1% W/V)

5. ***Absorbents for Paraffin hydrocarbons (Alkanes)***

   - No satisfactory absorbents are available for alkanes.

   - Hence a technique known as combustion analysis is used where the gases are oxidised to carbon dioxide and water vapour by means of thermal oxidation.

   $$CH_4 + 2O_2 \rightarrow CO_2 \uparrow + 2H_2O$$
   $$C_2H_6 + 3O_2 \rightarrow 2CO_2 \uparrow + 3H_2O$$

   - The volume of carbon dioxide formed is proportional to the volume of methane in the mixture.

6. ***Absorbents for Olefinic Hydrocarbons i.e. Alkenes***

   (a) Solution of $HgSO_4$ in sulphuric acid.

   (b) 5% KBr solution saturated with bromine.

   (c) Palladous chloride solution.

   (d) Solution of silver salts in concentrated H_2SO_4.

7. ***Absorbents for Acetylenic Compounds (Alkynes)***

   (a) 0.1 N bromine solution.

   (b) Ammonical cuprous chloride solution.

   (c) Ammonical silver chloride solution.

Apparatus used in Gas Analysis

The equipment used in gas analysis are divided into two types.

   1. Precise or exact equipment

   2. Technical Equipment

      - The difference between precise and technical equipment is that the first category of equipment is a permanent setup of laboratory while the technical equipment is portable one.

      In gasometry, the following apparatus are generally used.

- Bunte burette.
- The hempel apparatus.
- The orsat apparatus.
- The Nitrometer.

Nitrometer

- It is most widely used equipment in the laboratory.
- It is used for the official assay of medicinal gases like oxygen and carbondioxide.
- Nitrometer consists of a graduated measuring tube and a levelling tube connected by means of a rubber tubing.
- Into the graduated measuring tube, the absorbent is taken and the gas to be determined is introduced from the inlet situated at the top of the tube.
- By moving the levelling tube, the level of the absorbent solution is adjusted.
- This equipment is widely used for the assay of oxygen and carbondioxide.

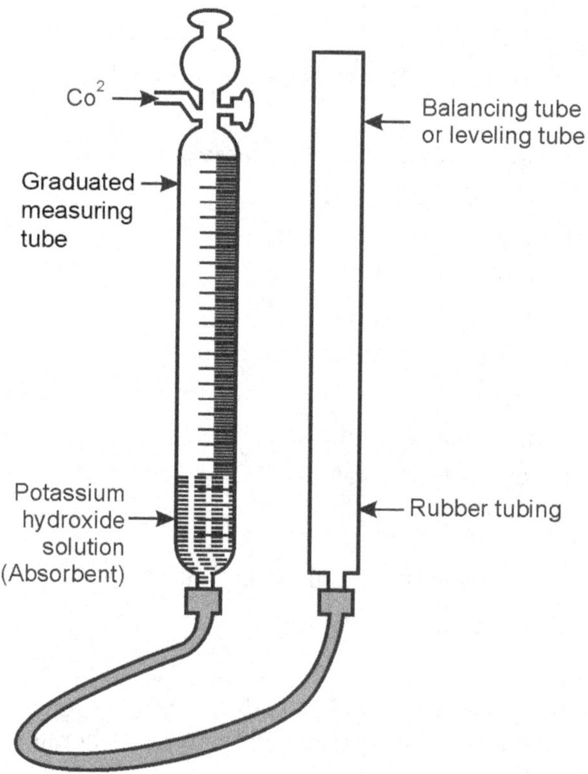

Fig. 21.1 Nitrometer.

Assay of Oxygen I.P. using Nitrometer

- According to I.P, oxygen should contain 99% v/v of oxygen.
- It is usually supplied in metallic cylinders.
- It is an example of medicinal gas, widely used in conditions of hypoxia.

Principle

- The decrease in the volume of oxygen gas, when a suitable absorbent is used, and measured.
- The decrease in volume is equal to the amount of oxygen gas present in the given sample.
- The absorbent used is a solution of ammonium chloride NH_4OH.
- When the gas is assayed by nitrometer method, the volume of the residual gas should not exceed 1 ml.

Procedure

- Place a sufficient quantity of Hg in 100 ml calibrated nitrometer, provided with a two-way stopcock and a two way outlet, and properly connected with a balancing tube.
- Connect one of the outlet tubes of the nitrometer with a gas pipette of suitable capacity.
- Place in the pipette a coil of copper wire which extends to the uppermost portion of the bulb and add about 125 ml of solution of $NH_4Cl - NH_4OH$.
- Draw the liquid free from air bubbles through the capillary opening connection and stopcock opening in the nitrometer by reducing the pressure in the nitrometer tube and opening the stopcock controlling the connection with the gas pipette and then close.
- Having completely filled the nitrometer, the other stop cock opening, and the other intake tube with mercury, draw into the nitrometer exactly 100 ml of oxygen by reducing the pressure in the tube.
- Close the stopcock, increase the pressure on the oxygen in the nitrometer tube and open the stopcock controlling the connection with the gas pipette.
- Force the entire volume of gas into the pipette.
- Close the stopcock and rock the pipette gently, providing frequent contact of the liquid, gas and copper spiral.
- At the end of fifteen minutes, most of the gas will have been absorbed by the liquid.

- To facilitate the absorption of the last portion of the oxygen, draw some of the liquid into the nitrometer tube and force the residual gas back uoon the surface of the liquid in the gas pipette.
- Again rock the pipette until no further diminution in the volume of the gas occurs.
- Draw the residual gas, if any, into the nitrometer tube and measure its volume.
- The volume of the gas remained unabsorbed does not exceed 1 ml.

Assay of Carbon Dioxide I.P. using Nitrometer

- According to I. P. CO_2 should contain 99% v/v of CO_2.
- It is usually supplied in metallic cylinders.
- It is an example of respiratory stimulant.

Principle

- The decrease in the volume of carbon dioxide when a suitable absorbent is used is measured.
- The decrease in the volume is equal to the amount of CO_2 present in the given sample.
- The absorbent used is 50% w/v potassium hydroxide solution.
- When the gas is assayed by the nitrometer method, the volume of the residual gas should not exceed 1 ml.

Procedure

- Place sufficient quantity of mercury in 100 ml nitrometer or a gas burette provided with a two-way sropcock and a two-way outlet and properly connected with a balancing tube.
- Connect one of the outlet tubes of the nitrometer with a gas pipette of suitable capacity and place in the pipette about 125 ml of a 50% w/v solution of KOH.
- Draw the liquid free from air bubbles through the capillary opening, connection and stopcock opening in the nitrometer by reducing the pressure in the nitrometer tube and opening the stopcock controlling the connection with the gas pipette and close.
- Having completely filled the nitrometer, the other stopcock opening and the other intake tube with Hg, draw into the nitrometer, by reducing the pressure in the tube, exactly 100 ml of CO_2 at NTP.
- Close the stopcock.
- Increase the pressure on the gas in the nitrometer tube, and open the stopcock controlling the connection with the gas pipette.

- Force the entire volume of gas into the pipette.
- Close the stopcock and rock the pipette gently providing frequent contact of the liquid and the gas.
- At the end of 5 minutes when most of the gas has been absorbed by the liquid, facilitate the absorption of the remainder by drawing some of the liquid into nitrometer tube and forcing the residual gas back upon the surface of the liquid in the gas pipette.
- Again rock the pipette until no further diminution in the volume of gas occurs.
- Draw the residual gas if any in nitrometer tube and measure its volume; not more than 1 ml of gas remains.

Analysis of Mixture of $CO_2 + O_2 + N_2O$

Nitrometer is generally employed in order to determine the various constituents in this mixture.

Procedure

- The given gas mixture ($CO_2 + O_2 + N_2O$) is introduced into a nitrometer containing 50% w/v KOH solution.
- After the complete absorption of one constituent (CO_2), the volume of the residual gas is measured.
- Let V_1 = Volume of gas mixture ($CO_2 + O_2 + N_2O$) before absorption and V_2 = Volume of gas mixture ($O_2 + N_2O$) after the absorption of one constituent (CO_2).
- $\therefore$ The difference $V_1 - V_2$ is equal to the volume of CO_2 present in the given mixture.
- Now, the gas mixture ($O_2 + N_2O$) is introduced into another nitrometer containing a solution of $NH_4Cl - NH_4OH$.
- After the complete absorption of one more constituent (O_2), the volume of the remaining gas is measured.
- Let V_2 = Volume of gas mixture ($O_2 + N_2O$) before absorption and V_3 = volume of gas sample after the absorption of oxygen.
- $\therefore$ The difference $V_2 - V_3$ is equal to the volume of oxygen present in the given gas mixture.
- Finally, the volume of the gas left unabsorbed in both the absorbents is equal to the volume of nitrous oxide present in the given sample.

The Orsat's Apparatus

It is an example of precise equipment.

1. ***Water cooled gas reservoir or gas burette "G"***
   - It is a graduated bulb of 50 to 100 ml capacity.
   - On the other side it is connected to a water reservoir bottle "W" with a rubber tube and on the other side to a manifold of "MM" of gas pipettes A, B, C etc.

2. ***Water bottle "W"***
   - It contains enough water to push out the whole of the gas in "G".
   - The water is coloured with some dye to make level visibility easier.
   - Methyl organic or Methyl red may be used as dyes.

3. ***Capillary Manifold MM***
   - The capillary tube carries a number of gas pipettes linked to it through independent stopcock.
   - At the end of the capillary tube there is a three-way stopcock "S" which can connect the manifold to atmosphere or to the source of gas through a U-tube filled with glass wool for filtering the gas free of solid particles.

4. ***Gas pipettes A, B, C***
   - Each pipette consists of two bulbs of almost equal volume connected by a U-bend tube at the bottom.
   - In one of the bulbs, absorbing solution is taken.
   - The free-ends of pipettes are closed with rubber stoppers.

The above four are the essential parts of Orsat's apparatus.

Analysis of Gas Mixture Containing CO_2 + CO + O_2 + N_2

The various constituents present in the above mixture can be estimated by Orsat's apparatus.

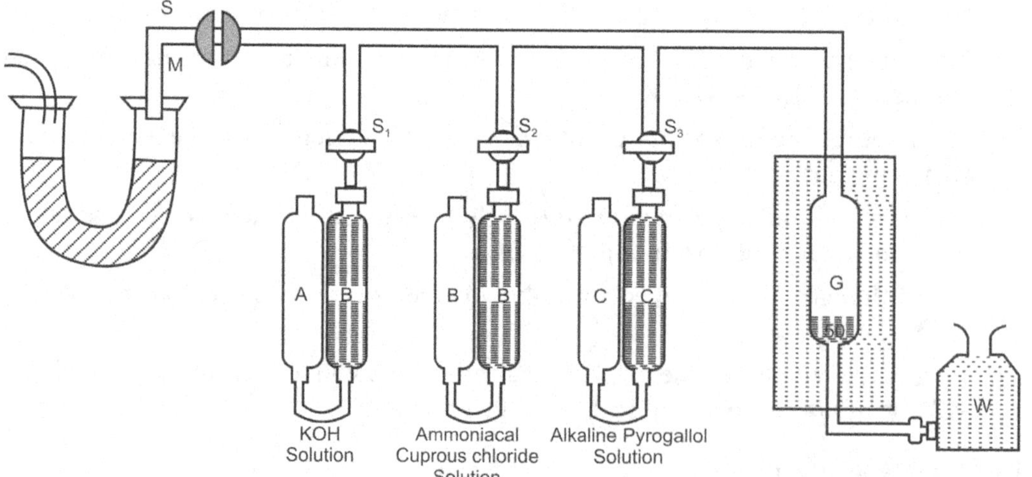

Fig. 21.2 Orsat's apparatus.

Principle

- The various gas constituents present in the gas mixture can be separately absorbed in different absorbents.
- For quantitative measurements, a known volume of the gas mixture is taken. Its volume at STP is measured.
- After absorption of each constituent, the volume of the residual gas is measured.

  The absorbents used are :

Pipette A : KOH solution (Absorbent for CO_2).

Pipette B : Ammonical Cuprous Chloride solution (Absorbent for CO).

Pipette C : Alkaline Pyrogallol solution (Absorbent for O_2)

Nitrogen gas is left behind, as it does not react with any of the absorbing solutions.

Procedure

- Open the stop-cock "S_1", lift the water-bottle to remove the gas from "G" to "A".
- When the bulb of "A" is filled with gas, start lowering the bottle "W" to take the gas back into "G".
- The to and fro slow movements of gas between "G" and "A" should be repeated six times or more.
- This helps in the absorption of CO_2 in the sample completely.
- In the end, allow the solution in "A" to rise back to its initial level. Allow the gas in "G" to acquire the temperature of water in the jacket.
- Equalise the water level in "G" and "W" and read the gas volume and record it.
- Let V_1 = Volume of gas mixture (CO_2 + CO +O_2 +N_2) before absorption and V_2 = Volume of gas mixture after the absorption of CO_2.

  $\therefore$ (V_1–V_2) ml is equal to the volume of CO_2 in the given gas mixture.

Repeat the experiment for absorption of carbon monoxide in Ammonical cuprous chloride solution in gas pipette 'B'.

Let V_2 = Volume of gas mixture (CO_2 + O_2 + N_2) and

V_3 = Volume of gas mixture after the absorption of CO.

(V_2 – V_3) ml is equal to the volume of CO in the given gas mixture.

Similarly repeat the experiment for absorption of oxygen gas in alkaline pyrogallol solution, in gas pipette 'C'.

Let V_3 = Volume of gas mixture $(O_2 + N_2)$

V_4 = Volume of residual gas after the absorption of O_2.

$\therefore$ $(V_3 - V_4)$ ml of equal to the volume of O_2 gas in the given gas mixture.

Finally the volume of gas, V_4 ml, unabsorbed is equal to the volume of nitrogen (N_2) gas present in the given sample.

Report the analysis as :

Initial volume of gas mixture	$= V_1$ ml.
Volume of carbon dioxide	$= (V_1 - V_2)$ ml.
Volume of carbon monoxide	$= (V_2 - V_3)$ ml.
Volume of oxygen	$= (V_3 - V_4)$ ml.
Volume of nitrogen gas	$= V_4$ ml.

CHAPTER 22

SAFETY MEASURES, PREVENTION & FIRST AID IN LABORATORY

Introduction

Every person in his life should more or less have to face even a small accident at some time or the other. The students who enter a laboratory must know the rules of a laboratory. It is important that each student must be well acquainted with the safety rules in the laboratory. He should also be ready to render medical aid to himself and his friends in accidents. Each and every student should be well versed with the rules, various types of accidents, safety measures and precautions to be taken in a laboratory.

First aid is a safety treatment given to a person before consulting a doctor to save his life from danger. So, each and every person should be aware of the first aid.

Appearance of a Laboratory

A laboratory and its surrounding environment should be kept clean. It contains different racks in which various types of chemicals are placed. It also contains different types of glass ware and burners. "Cleanliness is next to godliness". This proverb should be followed in a laboratory.

Materials in a Laboratory

All the materials in a pharmaceuticpals lab are made up of glass.

Different types of glass wares are found in the laboratory such as Test tubes, conical flask, volumetric flasks, Round bottomed flasks, pipettes, Burettes and various type of other materials.

Materials to be carried into a Laboratory

Every person who enters the laboratory or pharmacist should possess the following items while entering the laboratory

- Napkin — To clean the glass ware after washing with water or to wipe the hands.

- Hand kerchief — To hold the hot vessels or hot flasks.
- Match box (or) lighter — To light the burner.
- White chart — To be placed before the student so that stains on the tiles can be prevented.

Arrangement of Chemicals in the Laboratory

There are definite racks to place the chemicals in the laboratory.

Sodium metal, Bromine, Acids and Inflammable organic solvents such as Benzene, Ether, etc., should not be kept in the laboratory in larger amounts.

Residual quantities of metallic sodium should not be discarded into the water sink but collected in special bottles containing liquid paraffin or kerosene oil.

Ether, Benzene, lower alcohols, acetone and other inflammable liquids should be kept away from the open flame.

Solution like chloroform should be stored in tightly fitted amber coloured bottles.

All substances in the organic laboratory especially the organic compounds such as Phenyl hydrazine, Aniline, Nitrous compounds, aromatic hydro carbons and other noxious substances should be kept in tightly closed containers.

Appearance of a Person in the Laboratory

The student or a pharmacist should wear a white coloured thick coat before entering the laboratory called as lab. coat or Apron. Stains on the dresses and slight burn can be prevented by wearing the lab. coat.

Dressing and Hair Style

A student should be very alert in the laboratory. If any laziness is showed, it will be dangerous to the student only. One should not be panicky. Report each accident, even a small incident to the instructor. Consult the Doctor in case of danger.

Safety Measures to Prevent Accidents

Handling of Vessels

Handle smaller bottles with solutions and substances holding the entire bottle in your hand rather than the neck only.

Large bottles are usually handled by their necks. These bottles are carried on the palm of the other hand.

A microscope is also a microbe seeing instrument seen in the laboratory which must be handled carefully.

The test tubes should always be held with the help of a test tube holder.

All the glass wares should be handled carefully.

The test tubes and other glass containers should be heated carefully and gradually. It should be noted that the test tube or glass containers should be wiped dry before putting them over a naked flame or on a gauge.

Ether, Benzene, lower alcohols, Acetone and other inflammable liquids should be carefully handled away from the open flame.

All substances in the organic lab, especially the organic compounds such as Phenyl hydrazine, Aniline, Nitrous compounds, and aromatic hydro carbons should be handled with great care trying not to inhale their vapour. If some substance gets on the hands, wash it thoroughly with soap and brush.

First Aid

First aid is defined as the immediate treatment given to the accident victim or to treat sudden illness, quickly and correctly before medical help is made available.

As a result of ever increasing population and complexities of day-to-day routine life, the chances of a person to meet with accidental injuries are increasing. Anything that happens unexpectedly and by chance, affecting health of a person can be called as an accident. Accidents can occur at any time and at any place, usually at odd times and at odd places where a doctor is generally not available. The severity of accident may vary from skin abrasions which may be associated with increased heart beating due to fear up to sudden death of the patient. The accidents require immediate attention and prompt treatment. If the person does not get medical help in time, the condition may get worse and his life may be in danger. In such cases the first aid is the kind of treatment which is given to the victim till the medical aid by a doctor is available. First aid is only a step in treating an injured person in case of an accident or sudden illness. It does not mean a complete care and cure of the injuries. After first aid, the victim must be taken to a doctor or a hospital.

Objects of First-Aid

The pharmacist must know the objects of first aid.

1. To prevent any danger to life.
2. To prevent further injury and deterioration of the condition of the patient.
3. To give relief from pain.
4. To make medical care available at the earliest.

First-Aid Kit

A laboratory should always contain a first-aid kit. The first-aid kit should contain the following materials :

1. Sterile gauge.
2. Bandages of different sizes.
3. Triangular Bandages.
4. Adhesive Bandages.
5. A pair of scissors and forceps.
6. Aromatic spirit of ammonia.
7. Antiseptic solution like dettol, mercurochrome etc.
8. Burn ointments.
9. Emergency drugs like pain killers, antibiotics and packets of O.R.S. etc.

All the articles should be properly arranged and well preserved in the kit so as to prevent contamination or spoilage. These items should be periodically examined. Spoiled or contaminated articles as well as expired medicines should be replaced with new ones. The first aid kit should be always kept in the laboratory in ready to use form because emergency may arise at any time.

Types of Accidents in Laboratory

Anything that happens unexpected and by chance which affects the health of a person can be called as an accident. Accident can happen at any time in the laboratory, the intensity of which may vary from minor skin abrasions up to sudden death of the victim.

Accidents do not just happen, they are caused. Many of the accidents are the results of carelessness, thoughtlessness, neglect and momentary lack of concentration on the part of human beings. Many of the accidents are caused due to tiredness, stress, worry, anger, illness, bad news or even good news. Let us study about different kinds of accidents which the pharmacists are facing in the laboratories.

1. Fainting

Any student can faint at any time in the laboratory due to weakness, or various types of odours of the chemicals etc. Fainting can happen suddenly when the brain's blood flow is interrupted. Numerous reasons cause blood interruption. Examples include: Emotional distress and standing too long without moving in the laboratory.

What to look for

- Victims reports
- Dizziness, seeing spots and nausea

- Sweating
- Pale Skin

What to do?

If a person appears to faint.

Safety Measures, First-Aid

When the person is about to fall.

- Prevent the person from falling.
- Have the person lie down and raise the legs 8-12 inches.
- Loosen tight clothing, especially from around the neck.
- Place a cool wet cloth on fore head

If fainting has happened.

- Lay the victim down and raise the legs 8-12 inches unless a head injury is suspected from victim falling.
- Loosen tight clothing and belts.
- If the victim falls, check the injuries.
- Place a cool, wet cloth on the victim's fore head.

Precautions

1. Do not come to the laboratory without taking breakfast or light food.
2. Stand a way from the allergic chemicals.

2. Severe Allergic Reactions

In laboratory, due to chemical inhalation, some type of allergic reactions occur. Allergic reactions range from mild to severe. When allergic reactions are sudden and massive it is known as Anaphylaxis. Such reactions can be caused by an insect sting, a particular food or food additive or a particular drug. It is a life threaten situation. If untreated, anaphylaxis can be fatal within 5-30 min. About 60-80% of the anaphylactic deaths are caused by an inability to breathe because swollen air way passages obstruct air flow to the lungs. Another main cause that results in death is when blood vessels dilate so blood is deficient in the body.

Symptoms

- Sneezing, coughing or wheezing.
- Shortness of breath.
- Tightness and swelling in the throat.

- Severe itching, burning, rash or hives on the skin.
- Swelling of face, tongue, mouth.
- Blue around lips and mouth.
- Dizziness.
- Nausea and vomiting.
- Unconsciousness.

First-Aid

1. Check the pulse.
2. Seek medical attention immediately.
3. Epinephrine is the only life saving treatment for anaphylaxis. If the victim has his or her own physician prescribed epinephrine kit, help the victim in using it. First aiders do not have access to epinephrine except through a victim kit. Follow the kit instruction. It is the only thing that can save the life of a person in anaphylactic shock. It works by opening up the air way, causes blood vessels to constrict and stimulate the heart to beat more forcefully.
4. These emergency kits no longer require refrigeration but must be stored in dark room at room temperature.

Precautions

Stand away from the allergic chemicals.

3. Putting off Fire in Laboratory

It is a common danger that occurs in any laboratory. If an inflammable liquid takes flame inside a vessel, it should be tightly closed with a glass plate, porcelain or metallic object or a wet towel or even with a wooden plate. In this way, the flame is expected to be extinguished.

Safety Measures

- Never try to blow off the flame or extinguish it with water.
- If the burning liquid is spilt on the floor, extinguish the flame with dry sand.
- If the fire is in the hood, first close the shutter or the door and then proceed as already mentioned.
- If fire happens to be in the laboratory turn off the burners and electric heaters and use fire extinguishers to control the fire. Fire extinguishers should be regularly checked.
- Use a woollen blanket to fight fire on a man. Wrap the victim tightly and hold for 1-2 min. The time is sufficient to extinguish the flame.

- Heat test tubes and other glass containers very carefully and gradually. It should be noted that the test tube or glass containers should be wiped dry before putting them over a naked flame or on a gauge.

  First degree burn

  Second degree burn

  Third degree burn

First Degree Burn

These are not severe burns. In this burn only the skin surface is burnt.

First-AID

- Treat slight burn with glycerol or with cotton wool soaked in alcohol.
- Keep immediately an ointment on that burn.

  This is not dangerous. Only the surface skin is burnt.

Second Degree Burn

This is another type of burn. This is sometimes severe. The inner flesh is burnt.

First-Aid

- Put off the fire by throwing a blanket.
- In case of strong burns place cotton, wool or gauge soaked with saturated aqueous solution of picric acid or 1-2% $KMnO_4$ or tannin solution. The treatment removes pain and prevents vescication.
- Now treat the affected areas with Vaseline.
- It should be noted that never clean wet, burnt skin with water.
- If pain is strong, give the victim a tablet of Aspirin before advising or carrying him to the doctor.

Third Degree Burn

These burns are very dangerous and very severe. Infection due to burns of the burnt body part contamination and is another serious condition.

First-Aid

1. Put off the fire by throwing water, covering the flames with blanket or coat.
2. Without wasting time, put plenty of cold water or any other non-inflammable liquid over the burnt area. If possible immerse the affected part in cold water for 15-20 minutes, or until the pain disappears (In case of extensive burns do not immerse the part for a long time, as it may intensify the shock). If that is not

possible, soak clean cloth in cold water and put it over burnt area. It needs to be changed frequently. This treatment with cold water will remove residual heat from tissues and prevent further damage.

3. Do not try to remove the clothing from the burnt area rather cut them around.

4. Keep the victim calm and in lie down position to avoid shock.

5. Give him reassurance.

6. If the burning is extensive, wrap the victim in a clean cloth and shift the patient immediately to a nearby hospital.

*In case of chemical burns, wash them thoroughly with water until all chemicals has been washed away.

4. Inhaled Poisoning

Most of the people get poisoned by the inhalation of most of the chemicals in the laboratory. Victims of inhaled poisons are often unaware of the presence of toxic gas. It is difficult to tell if a person is a victim of inhaled poison. Sometimes, a complaint of having the flu is really a symptom of inhaled poisoning. Although many symptoms resemble flu, there are differences. For example, inhaled poisoning does not produce low grade fever, generalised aching or lymph node involvement.

Symptoms

Inhaled poisoning signs and symptoms are :

- Headache.
- Ringing in the ears (tinnitus).
- Angina (chest pain).
- Muscle weakness.
- Nausea and vomiting.
- Dizziness and visual changes (blurred or double vision).
- Unconsciousness.
- Breathing and cardiac arrest.

Precautions

Organic solvents like Ether, Benzene, lower alcohols, acetone and other inflammable liquids should be carefully handled away from the open flame. Try also not to inhale their vapours. Heat them on water bath with closed heater elements.

First-Aid

1. Remove the victim from toxic environment and bring into fresh air immediately.

2. Get the victim to 100 percent oxygen immediately. Call the EMS.

3. Check the $ABCH_s$.

4. Seek medical attention for all suspected victims of inhaled poisoning.

5. Infections due to Acids & Alkalies

Some acids and alkalies in the laboratories cause certain type of infections. If acid or alkali gets on the skin or clothes, wash them immediately with excess of water and then with 3% sodium carbonate solution (in case of acid) or 1% acetic acid (in case of alkali). In case of severe burn, place a pad of cotton, wool and gauze soaked with solution used for heat burns on the affected part. In case eye is affected, wash the eye with plenty of water, then with 2% sodium bicarbonate solution or saturated Boric acid solution. Wash the eye for at least 15 minutes and then consult a doctor.

First-Aid

- Wash the infected area with water.

- Apply an ointment on the affected part.

- If the skin is injured with broken glass, remove its fragments with forceps, treat the wound with dettol (1:500) and apply a bandage. Fasten it with adhesive tape.

- Go for fresh air in case of a noxious gas is inhaled. To breathe in dilute solution of ammonia is also useful in this case.

Conclusion

Every person should follow the instructions of the laboratory. Then only a person will be safe till the end of the lab work.

Do not be panicky. Report each accident, even very slight one to the instructor. Consult the doctor in severe cases.

CHAPTER 23

CALIBRATION OF VOLUMETRIC GLASSWARE

Introduction

For volumetric analysis, we commonly employ graduated conical flasks, burettes and pipettes. For weighing the substances, we use weights of different denominations. The accuracy of a weighing of volumetric estimation depends upon the accuracy with which the weighing are done or the accuracy with which the volumes of different solutions are measured.

Any article or substance should be weighed at room temperature only. Similarly the volume measuring devices should be used at 27°C to give correct measurements. But in India, the laboratory temperatures usually vary between 30°C to 45°C. As the glassware and weights undergo expansion therefore errors creep in volume and weights. These reduce the precision. Hence corrections have to be done to suit the laboratory conditions. This process is called 'calibration'. Distilled water is generally used as the reference material in the calibration of the volumetric glassware. Calibration process pertaining to glassware consists in determining the weight of water contained or delivered by a particular glassware and converting weights of water into volume with the help of density.

Calibration of Weights

Method of substitution is used to calibrate the individual weights against the standards to eliminate the possible error due to inequality of the length of the balance arms.

Procedure

1. Put the standard weights on the left pan and put a base on the right pan.
2. See that the balance swings exactly on both the sides using a rider.
3. It is convenient to use the rider in the middle of the arm by placing an extra 0.005 g weight on the left pan during the whole operation.
4. Replace the standard weights with the weights to be calibrated and again determine the rest point (using a rider).
5. Repeat the above process with every piece in the weight box and determine a relation between the standard weight and the used weight in the form of a table showing the absolute error for each spent weight.
6. The correction can be applied.

Calibration of Volumetric Flasks

A volumetric flask is a flat bottomed pear shaped glass vessel with a long narrow neck. A thin line etched around the neck indicates the volume that it fills at 20°C. This flask is fitted with a ground glass stopper and it should be tied by a thread on its neck so that it is not lost or interchanged. A volumetric flask is used in the preparation of a standard solution. Hot liquids are never poured into the flask. The volumetric flasks are available in the capacities of 2,000, 1,000, 500, 250, 100, 50, 25, 10, 5, 2 and 1 ml (millilitre). The calibration of a volumetric flask will be useful only when highest accuracy is desired. Before calibration, the volumetric flask must be thoroughly cleaned and rinsed with the pure solvent.

Calibration Procedure

1. The volumetric flask is cleaned, rinsed and finally clamped in an inverted position to dry it completely.
2. Weight the dried volumetric flask.
3. Fill the flask with distilled water at room temperature until the meniscus stands on the graduation mark of the flask.
4. The water should have been standing for at least one hour prior to use so as to be certain that it has attained room temperature.
5. Any water sticking to the neck of the flask above the graduation level is wiped off carefully with the help of a filter paper.
6. Stopper the flask and reweigh to the nearest mg. The difference in the weight gives the volume contained in it.
7. The volume of water corresponding to this weight is calculated from the density of water at the given temperature and the error is worked out.
8. The temperature of the water is also measured.

9.   Add the correction to the apparent weight of water in grams to obtain the volume at 20°C.

10.   Make two or three determinations.

As per Indian pharmacopoeia, the tolerance on capacities for volumetric flasks are given below

Volumetric flask (Normal capacity)	Tolerence ($\pm$ ml)
10	0.02
25	0.03
50	0.04
100	0.06

Observation

Normal capacity of the volumetric flask   =

Temperature of water (t°C)   =

Weight of the flask   =

Weight of the flask filled with water   =

Apparent weight of water at t°C   =

Correction for 50 ml at t° C (from standard literature) =

Volume of the flask at 20°C   =

Calibration of Pipettes

A pipette consists of a long narrow tube with cylindrical bulb in the middle and a nozzle at its lower end. The upper part of the tube has a circular graduation. Pipettes are used to deliver a definite and accurate volume of a liquid. Pipettes can be classified into two categories, namely:

1. Those which have one mark and deliver a small, constant volume of a liquid under specific conditions (Transfer pipettes).

2. Those in which stems are graduated and are used to deliver various small volumes at discretion (graduated or measuring pipettes).

Transfer pipettes (one mark graduation pipettes) are not capable of high precision but are useful for delivering constant volumes of the liquid at 20°C. Normally 10 ml, 20 ml, 25 ml, and 50 ml capacities transfer pipettes are employed.

Before filling any solution, the pipette is rinsed 2 to 3 times with a small amount of the same solution. The pipette is then filled by dipping its tip under liquid and applying suction from mouth (corrosive and poisonous substances should not be sucked) to about 1-2 cm above the graduation mark. The extra liquid above the graduation mark is allowed to drain in an separate container until the bottom of the meniscus just coincides with the graduation mark removing the index finger. The jet is held just touching the side of the vessel for 15 seconds (draining period) to deliver the desired volume. Poisonous and corrosive substances like acids should be drawn using graduated pipettes with a provision of suction bulb attached at the open end of the pipette.

Calibration

1. Take sufficient distilled water in a beaker. The water should have been standing for at least one hour prior to use so as to be certain that it has acquired room temperature.
2. Record the temperature of the water.
3. The pipette must be thoroughly cleaned with a cleansing agent first and then with distilled water.
4. Take the clean pipette and fill it with water and drain. Repeat it two or three times until the temperature of the pipette is the same as that of water.
5. Fill the pipette with distilled water to a short distance above the mark and then run at until the meniscus is exactly on the mark.
6. Discharge the water of the pipette into a clean previously weighed weighing bottle. Allow the pipette to drain for 15 seconds after the outflow has ceased, keeping it in contact with the side of the bottle.
7. Weigh the weighing bottle and water.
8. Record the apparent weight of water.
9. Calculate the volume of water.
10. Make at least two or three determinations and record the observations.

Indian pharmacopoeia's tolerance on the capacity of the pipettes is as given below.

Transfer Pipettes

Normal capacity	Tolerence (±)
10 ml	0.02
25 ml	0.03
50 ml	0.05

Measuring or Graduated Pipettes

Normal capacity	Subdivision (ml)	Tolerance
1 ml	0.01	0.006
5 ml	0.05	0.03
10 ml	0.10	0.05

Observations

Temperature of water = ...°C

Capacity of the pipette = ...ml

Density of water at experimental temperature =............g/ml

No. of determinations	Empty bottle weight	Weight of weighing bottle + water	Apparent wt. of water	Volume of water at 20°C
				Average =

Volume of pipette at 20°C =

Calibration of Burette

Burettes are long cylindrical tubes of uniform bore throughout the graduated length. The tube is closed at the bottom by means of a glass stopcock or with a rubber tubing and carries a jet at the tip. Before filling it with any solution, it is rinsed 2-3 times with the small quantity (5-7 ml) of the same solution. Burettes are mainly used in titrations for the accurate delivery of a standard solution to the analyte until the end point is reached.

The rinsed burette is fixed into a suitable stand and clamped vertically. The burette is always filled upto zero mark. Air bubbles if present in the burette should be removed by speedily flowing the liquid through the jet into a receiver and again filled to zero mark.

Calibration

1. Clean the burette and lubricate the stop cock.
2. Fill the burette with water and adjust to zero mark and allow it to stand for 10 minutes (test for leakage).
3. Fill the burette with distilled water and note the temperature. Weigh a clean, dry stoppered flask of about 100 ml capacity.
4. Collect the water from burette into flask. Restopper it and reweigh the flask.
5. Note the temperature of water. The results are used by plotting a calibration curve.

Indian Pharmacopoeia-tolerance limits

Capacity	Tolerance
10 ml	0.01
25 ml	0.03
50 ml	0.05

Weight of 1 litre of water at different temperature

Temperature (°C)	Weight (g)	Temperature (°C)	Weight (g)
10	998.39	23	996.60
11	998.32	24	996.38
12	998.23	25	996.17
13	998.14	26	995.93
14	998.04	27	995.69
15	997.93	28	995.44
16	997.80	29	995.18
17	997.66	30	994.91
18	997.51	31	994.64
19	997.35	32	994.35
20	997.18	33	994.06
21	997.00	34	993.75
22	996.80	35	993.45

CHAPTER 24

RADIOIMMUNOASSAY

Definition

Radioimmunoassay (RIA) technique is developed between 1950-76 and used for the detection and measurement of trace quantities of drugs and metabolites in biological samples. This technique is mainly used when the determination of trace quantities are difficult by other standard analytical methods.

Principle

It involves competitive stream in which radioactive substrate (ligand) and non-radio active substrate compete with each other for a binding agent.

The basic principle involved in the immunoassay is mainly based on the ability of a given drug to inhibit the reaction between drug-specific antibodies and an appropriately labelled drug or drug derivatives.

The labelled drug should closely resemble the true drug structurally and should participate in the immuno chemical reaction with antibody as if it was the drug, however, it should have a unique feature that easily differentiates it from the drug.

In case of radioimmunoassay, the labelled drug may be tagged with a particular radioisotope.

The substrate (P) may be a vitamin, hormone, drug or other substance, the concentration of which is to be determined. To perform the assay same substance must be available with a radioactive tag. This is called as P^*. (I^{25} is the frequently used tag).

Binding agent used here is Q. It may be an ion-exchange resin, protein, or an antibody for the particular substrate. The concentration of binding agent used in all assays is also constant. The independent variable is P, whose concentration will vary.

It can be seen that an increase in the concentration of P will result in an increase in the concentration of non-radioactive bound substrate P^*Q and a decrease in the concentration of radioactive bound substrate PQ. The result will be an increase in free tagged substrate P*. Therefore the concentration of substrate P can be determined as some function of any two of the quantities B, P or T (The bound, free and total radio activity respectively) is

$$P = F (B, F), P = F^* (B, T) \text{ or } P = F^* (F, T)$$

$$P^* + Q \rightleftharpoons P^*Q$$

$$P + Q \rightleftharpoons PQ$$

One type of system which shows a very high degree of specificity for a particular substrate is an immune system. The assay is known as radioimmunoassay and uses as antigen-antibody reaction.

Procedure

In the typical IA procedure, known amounts to antibody, biological sample containing drug and labelled drug are mixed and incubated for a specific time period.

The interaction that occur is as follows :

$$\text{Antibody + Drug + } \quad \text{Labelled Drug} \rightleftharpoons \text{Antibody–Drug}$$

$$\begin{array}{ll} \text{(free drug)} & \text{(tagged with} \\ & \text{radioisotope)} \end{array} \quad \begin{array}{l} + \\ \text{Antibody–labelled drug} \\ \text{(Bound drug)} \end{array}$$

The reaction is allowed to reach equilibrium.

Increasing concentration of drug causes increased inhibition of binding of labelled drug to antibody. Quantitation of drug in a sample is achieved by comparing the analysis data from an unknown sample with those of a calibration curve performed concurrently using known concentration.

In case of RIA, which involves radio labelled drug or drug which is not active, it is essential that a physical separation of the fractions containing bound and free-labelled drug before the final measurement step. The separation can be done by various separation techniques such as electrophoresis, dialysis, gel filtration, selective adsorption of free labelled drug to inert solid particles, co-precipitation of labelled drug with antibody using a protein precipitant such as ammonium sulphate.

Increasing concentration of unlabelled drug reduces the amount of bound labelled drug-antibody complex. Therefore, the extent of binding between unlabelled and labelled molecules and antibody is a measure of the concentration of unlabelled drug in the sample.

RIA procedure depends on the following factors :

1. The production of an antisera with high affinity and specificity for the drug being assayed.

2. The synthesis of a labelled drug or derivative.

3. A convenient separation technique for bound and free labelled drug. To meet the ideal requirements the following criteria should be met :

   (a) The non-radioactive and radioactive antigens are indistinguishable chemically.

   (b) Both reactions go to completion.

   (c) Antibodies are specific and react only for the single antigen indicated in the reactions.

The major purpose of a RIA is to determine hormone drugs or any other substance of non-radioactive antigen. To conduct a RIA, first a standard curve must be constructed where the drug is plotted as some function of radioactivity. This is known as a dose response curve. It is constructed using data obtained by use of standard solutions.

Let the concentration of drug of radioactive antigen added to each of three test tubes be 6 picomoles PM/ml. To the first tube is added no non-radioactive antigen. To the second tube is added 3 PM/ml and to the third 2 PM/ml of non-radioactive antigen. Finally equal amounts of antibody (representing 3 PM of antibody binding sites/ml) are added to each of the three tubes and contents of each tube are well mixed. The tubes are then incubated until the reactions are completed.

Bound and free antigens are now separated by means of suitable physical separation methods for each of the three standards (*i.e.* radioactivity B of bound antigen and radio activity of F for free antigen).

The total radioactivity $(T) = (B + F)$ is the sum of the bound and free radioactivities.

Antigen	+	Antibody	→	Bound	+	Free
1. 6	0	6	3	3	1	2	1
2. 6	3	9	3	6	2	3	0.5
3. 6	12	18	3	15	5	6	0.2

The total concentration of antigen $C_T = (CB + C_F)$ is also equal to the sum of the concentration of radioactive and non-radioactive antigens.

Po – labelled drug *i.e.* radioactive

$C_T = P^o + P$

P – unlabelled drug *i.e.* non radioactive

Since radioactive and non-radioactive antigens are chemically indistinguishable, they are uniformly distributed in the system, thus

$$CT/CB = \frac{T}{B}$$

By combining these two relationships it follows that

$$P = -P^o + C_B \frac{T}{B}$$

If Q is the total concentration of antibody binding sites and Q_B is the concentration of bound or occupied binding sites, which antigen is in excess, $Q = Q_B = C_B$, since the reaction is assumed to have so to completion consequently.

$$P = -P^o + Q \frac{T}{B}$$

By plotting the concentration (P) of dose antigen (non radioactive or non labelled) as a function of the ratio of $\frac{T}{B}$ total to bound radioactivity, a linear relationship is obtained, the (Y) intercept is $-P^o$ and gives an apparent concentration of radioactive antigens. The slope gives the concentration of antibody sites. In the assay, $\frac{T}{B}$ is quantity measured and P is the quantity sought, for the example cited above.

$$P = -6 + 3 \frac{T}{B}$$

A plot of linear data is shown in the Fig. 24.1.

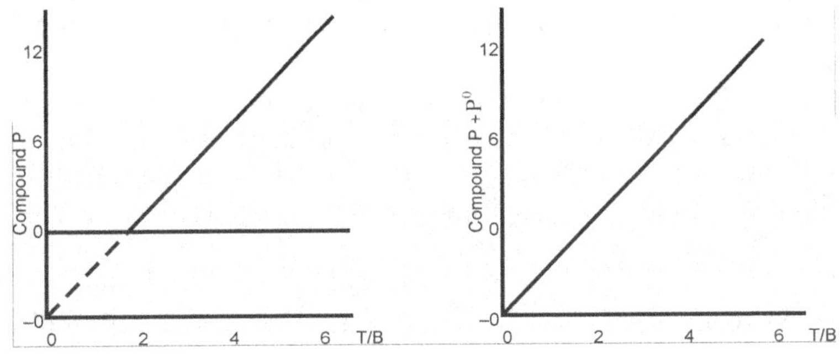

Fig. 24.1

Techniques used are :

1. Double antibody technique
2. Solid phase RIA.

3. Resin technique

4. Salting out or solvent precipitate.

Advantages

1. Immuneassays are sensitive, precise, rapid and convenient because they require sample sizes as small as 5-50 PM/ml (PM = Picomoles).

2. They possess good adaptability for the analysis of large number of sample and can be easily automated.

3. Sample pre-treatment step such as solvent extraction and hydrolysis are usually unnecessary.

Disadvantage

Cost for analysis is high.

Radioisotopes used to labelled drugs are as follows :

1. AC^{14-} labelled drug is preferred in RIA procedures, because it usually binds to the antibody in exactly the same manner as unlabelled drug. However, the specific activity attainable with C^{14} is generally so low that sensitivity of the assay is sacrificed. Another problem concerning the C^{14} as a label on to a drug structure, is that such synthesis usually provides low yields of radio labelled product. In case of macro-molecule analysis, C^{14} labelling may be difficult to achieve owing to lack of suitable synthetic pathways and of some of the necessary starting materials.

2. Drugs labelled with tritium (H^3) are usually employed in RIA procedures. A limited drug is stable, has a long half life (12.3 years) and represents minimal radiation hazard, tritium is usually introduced into a drug molecule by such methods as catalytic titration of double bonds, the Willbach techniques or by an exchange reaction such as halogen for tritium. The resulting labelled compound is then purified by an appropriate chromatographic procedure before use in assay.

3. Drug labelled as I^{125} have some advantages over H^3 labelled drugs. The samples from the assay can be counted directly in a gamma counter, which is more convenient, less expensive, and requires less counting time than liquid scintillation counting.

Applications

1. RIA is used in the analysis of pentazocaine, Diazepam, Chlorodiazapoxide and donazepam.

2. In the estimation of hormones like ACTH, Gastrin, FSH, growth hormones, glucogan, insulin, Thyroxine.

3. In the estimation of steroids such as aldosterone, testosterone, estrone, C.T.C

4. In the estimation of drugs such as Digoxin, Digitoxin amphetamine, morphine, barbiturates, L.S.D. etc.

CHAPTER 25

POLARIMETRY

Introduction

Rotation of plane polarized light which is known as 'optical rotation' is an important optical property of pharmaceutical liquids and solutions of solids. This measurement provides valuable insight regarding the molecular structure, purity of pharmaceutical compounds and also the composition of binary mixtures in pharmaceutical liquid dosage forms.

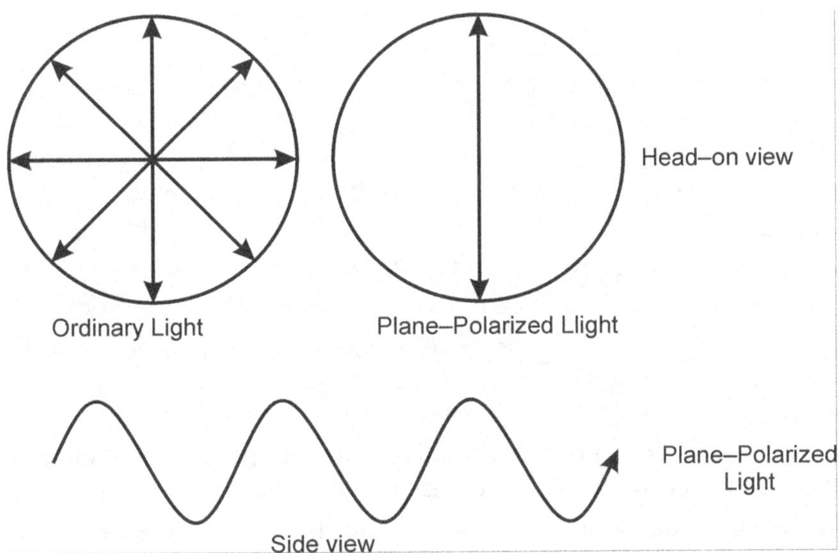

Fig. 25.1 Plane polarized light.

According to the wave theory of light, an ordinary ray of light is considered to be vibrating in all the planes at right angels to the direction of its propagation. If this ordinary ray of light is passed through a nicol prism, the emergent ray has its vibrations only in one plane. This light having wave motion in one plane is known as a 'Plane polarized light'. The plane along which vibrations are taking place is known as 'Plane of Polarization'.

Optical Activity

If the substances rotate the plane polarized light to the left (Anti Clock wise), they are known as 'Levo Rotatory' (–) and if they rotate light towards the right (Clock wise), they are known as 'Dextro Rotatory' (+). A mixture of these two varieties in equal proportions will be optically inactive and is called a 'Racemic form'.

When certain organic liquids and solutions like glucose are placed in the path of plane polarized light, the plane of polarization is rotated. This property is called 'Optical Activity' and the substance possessing this property is called 'Optically active'.

Optical Activity and Chemical Constitution

Optical activity is purely a constitutive property and it depends entirely on the arrangement of atoms in the molecule. In case of organic compounds, only those which contain an asymmetric carbon atom (a carbon atom whose four valencies are satisfied by four different atoms or radicals) have the power of rotating the plane of polarized light.

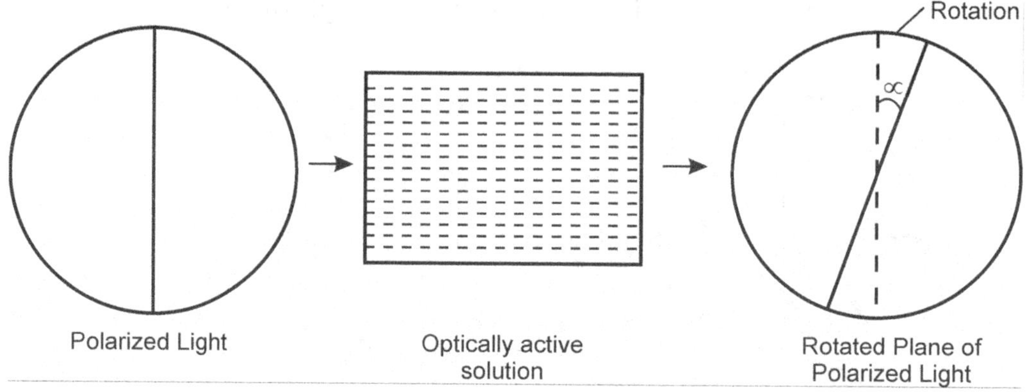

Fig. 25.2 Optical activity.

1. To be optically active, a compound must have a chiral center.
2. Depending on the orientation of these four different groups about the chiral carbon, the compound may rotate plane polarized light to the left or to the right.
3. If the compound does not have a chiral center, it will not rotate light at all.
4. No two groups attached to the central carbon atom are identical. Ex. Lactic Acid (Optically active compound).

According to Le Bel and Vant's Hoff theory, lactic acid molecule can be arranged in two different ways in space.

These two models are related to each other as an object to its mirror image and one cannot be superimposed over the other.

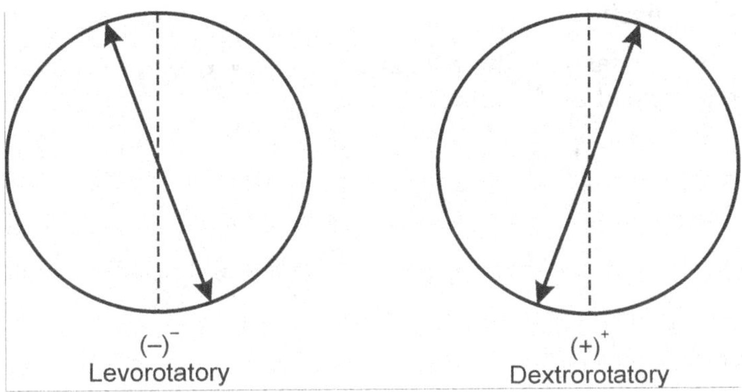

Fig. 25.3 Types of optical rotation.

- One of these models corresponds to l-acid other d-acid, but we cannot say exactly as to which model represents which form of the acid, because the internal mechanism by which a molecule rotates the plane of polarized light is not clearly understood.

- From the above model, it is evident that the groups in one case are arranged from left to right (clock wise) and in other case from right to left (anti clock wise).

- This probably explains that why one form rotates the plane of polarization to the left and the other to the right.

- Optical activity is seen not only in compounds which contain an asymmetric carbon atom but also in compounds which contain other asymmetric atoms like Silicon and Nitrogen etc.

There are two positions of maximum and minimum brightness in a complete rotation of analyzer, the setting of maximum and minimum brightness can be obtained by rotating the analyzer in either direction, left or right. According to universally accepted convention, the substance is said to be dextro rotatory if the analyzer has to be rotated through an angle less than $90°$ in order to get extinction.

Specific Rotation

The extent of optical rotation exhibited by a particular compound depends on several factors.

1. Nature of the substance.

2. Length of the column through which the light possess.

3. Wave length of the light used (the angle of rotation is inversely proportional to the square of wave length).

4. The temperature at which measurement is made.

5. The concentration of the solution if the substance is dissolved in a solvent.

6. Nature of the solvent.

For the purpose of comparison, the results are usually expressed in terms of 'specific rotation' and is represented by the relation.

$$[\alpha]_D^t = \alpha/ld$$

where,

$[\alpha]_D^t$ = The specific rotation at temperature 't' when D-line of sodium vapour lamp is used.

α = Observed angle of rotation

l = Length of liquid column (decimetre)

d = Density of liquid

The specific rotation of a substance in solution is represented by

$$[\alpha]_D^t = \frac{100 \times \text{observed angle of rotation}}{\text{Length in decimeters} \times \text{grams of substance in } 100\,\text{ml of solution}}$$

$$[\alpha]_D^t = \frac{100 \times \alpha}{l \times c}$$

Thus specific rotation of a substance may be defined as an angle of optical rotation when the length of the column through which the light possess is 1 decimeter and filled with a solution having 1 gram of the substance per ml.

In order to compare rotatory power of different substances, it is more convenient to consider the molar rotation, which is defined as

$$[M]_D^t = \frac{100 \times \alpha}{l \times c}$$

$$= \frac{100 \times \alpha}{l\rho p}$$

where,

c = Concentration of the substance in g per 100 ml of the solution

P = Concentration of the substance in g per 100 g of the solution

ρ = Density of the solution

In dilute solutions α is proportional to C, i.e., α/C is a constant. So specific rotation of a substance in solution is a constant value, independent of concentration (this is strictly true for dilute solutions only) however in concentrated solutions, specific rotation in found to be dependent on the concentration.

The limiting value of specific rotation, when 'C' approaches zero, is known as 'intrinsic rotation'. This can be determined by extrapolating [a] vs C graph to C = 0.

$$[\alpha] = (a) + kC$$

where,

(α) = Intrinsic Rotation

Instrumentation

Measurement of Angle of Rotation

The magnitude and direction of the rotation of polarization through an optically active substance or its solution is measured with a polarimeter. The instruments which are used now-a-days involve the half-shadow device, i.e., the field of view is divided into two halves of equal brightness. The important versions are:

1. Lippich Polarimeter
2. Biquartz Polarimeter

1. Lippich Polarimeter

It consists of two polarizing elements, one of which is fixed and the other is an analyzer. It can be rotated and mounted within a graduated circular scale in order to measure its orientation with respect to the polarizer.

- When the planes of polarization of two elements (prisms) are mutually perpendicular, no light is transmitted.
- Liquid can be directly filled in the sample tube.
- If the substance is a solid, accurately weighed portion is transferred into a volumetric flask and dissolved in water or other solvent, as specified.
- A portion of solvent is used for blank determination
- The sample solution is filled in the sample tube.
- Care should be taken so that end-windows will not be strained while screwing the caps.
- Any air bubble that may appear in the sample tube should be accommodated in the bubble trap at the centre of the tube.

- Complete filling of the sample tube is essential.

- It is better to use long sample tube to get maximum difference in the optical rotations between two samples.

- The light source is usually a sodium vapour lamp.

- On introducing an optically active sample between the polarizing elements, the balance is disturbed.

- It is necessary to rebalance by turning the analyzer.

- When the two halves are of equal intensity, it is in the balanced position. Then scale reading indicates the angle of rotation.

- The extent to which the scale is rotated is a direct measure of the sample's optical activity.

- This is normally obtained by the difference between the readings obtained with and without the sample.

- The direction of rotation and specific rotation is reported together for a given substance in a given solvent.

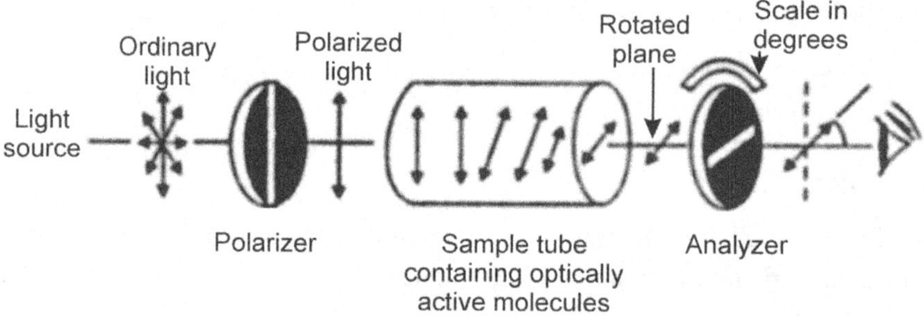

Fig. 25.4 Schematic diagram of Lippich polarimeter.

Smaller is the angle through which the analyzer has to be rotated to pass the shadow from one half to the other of the field of view, greater is the accuracy of the instrument. Thus, the sensitivity can be improved by decreasing the half shadow angle 2q. There is, however, a lower limit of the value of half shadow angle, for by diminishing the angle the illumination of the field of view becomes faint, and a difficulty arises in deciding the uniform brightness of the two halves. Thus there is an optimum value of the half shadow angle usually 4-5° which depends on the brightness of the source, the wavelength and the transparency of the solution. An arrangement is provided in the instrument by which this angle can be varied according to the conditions of the experiment.

Most modern polarimeters are fitted with two small prisms (Lippich prisms) each of which occupies one third apperature of the polariser and is placed immediately after it. This arrangement splits up the field of view into three parts and facilitates the matching, since if the eye is off the axis of the instrument involving half shadow device, the matching of the two portions is difficult.

Polarimeter Tube

The polarimeter tube or observation tube consists of a thick glass tube with accurately ground ends, covered with optical (plane parallel) glass disc. By means of screw caps and rubber washers these discs are pressed against the ends. These discs held in position must be perpendicular to the incident light. Otherwise the intensity of light emerging from it will be decreased. Caps must not be screwed too tightly, otherwise any strain in the glass plate will cause the light to be no more perfectly polarized.

In order to avoid the difficulty of removing any air bubble from getting in, a bulb is provided in the middle of the tube. The air will be trapped in the bulb and the path of light in the tube is completely occupied by the liquid or the solution. Since the length of the liquid or solution column in polarimetric measurements is measured in decimetres, the observation tubes are generally, 1 dm long or some multiple or some fraction of it. For controlling the temperature of the liquid under test, the observation tube is surrounded by a metal jacket, through which water from a thermostat can be circultated.

Applications

The important applications of the polarimetry are as follows :

- It is useful for the qualitative analysis of various drugs and Pharmaceuticals.
- Optical activity is used to identify chirality (asymmetry).
- Specific rotation is used whether a substance is optically active or not.
- The purity of the substance can be measured. It is an important pharmacopoeial test.
- The concentration of a substance dissolved in a solvent can be determined. This test is used as quality control test.
- Specific rotation is useful for the determination of purity of various drugs and Pharmaceuticals.
  - The sugar (+) glucose plays important role in the animal metabolism; where as (–) glucose is neither metabolized nor fermented by yeasts.
  - The hormonal activity of adrenaline (–) is many times that of its enantiomer.

- (+) Ephedrine not only has no activity, but also interferes with the action of its enantiomer.
- Only one stereoisomer of chloramphenicol is an antibiotic.
- Among amino acids, only one leucine and asparagines are sweet and only one glutamic acid increase the flavour of food.

- Polarimetry is widely used in quantitative analysis of sugars.
- It is also useful to distinguish dextro and levo isomeric forms.
- It is useful in analyzing molecular structure by plotting optical rotary dispersion curves over a wide range of wavelengths and helps in identifying and characterizing biopolymers of natural and synthetic origin.
- Polarimetry is used for inspecting the incoming raw materials, inspection of camphors, citric acid, lemon oil, gums, etc.
- It determines product purity by measuring specific rotation and optical rotation of amino acids, Antibiotics, Amino sugars, Diuretics, Dextrose, Vitamins, Steroids, Analgesics, etc.
- It ensures produce quality by measuring the concentration and purity of the following compounds in sugar based foods, cereals and syrups – Carbohydrates, Fructose, Glucose, Maltose, Lactose, Sucrose, Xylose and various starches.

CHAPTER 26

REFRACTOMETRY

Introduction

The measurement of Refractive Index is an important optical property and provides valuable information regarding the molecular structure and purity of Pharmaceutical compounds.

Refractometry is a technique that measures how light is refracted when it passes through a given substance (unknown compound). The amount by which the light is refracted determines the refractive index.

Definition of Refractive Index

When a ray of monochromatic light passes from one isotropic medium to another, it changes its path at the interface of the two media, except when it enters perpendicularly to the interface. If the ray enters from a rarer and less denser medium (air) to a more

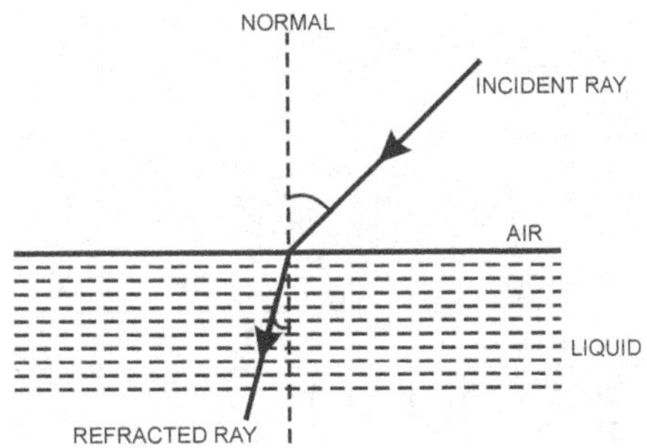

Fig. 26.1 Refraction of light through a denser liquid medium.

denser medium (liquid), it deviates towards the normal at the interface where as converse takes place if the light enters into the rarer medium. This phenomenon is known as "Refraction".

Snell's Law

It states that the ratio of the sine of the angle of incidence to and that of refraction is a constant and characteristic of that liquid which is equal to the ratio of velocity of light in the two media.

$$\frac{Sin\ i}{Sin\ r} = n = \frac{\text{Velocity of light in I medium}}{\text{Velocity of light in II medium}}$$

where,

i = Angle of incidence

r = Angle of refraction.

If medium I (rarer) is vacuum or air, the above ratio is known as the refractive index of the medium II, which is always greater then unity.

If the angle of incidence is increased, the angle of refraction also increases and attains the maximum value r' corresponding to the angle of incidence equal to $90°$.

$$n = 1/\sin r'$$

The angle r' is known as the critical angle.

At this angle r', the ray passing from the denser medium to rarer one would emerge along the boundary of separation. On increasing the angle greater than r', the ray will not emerge in the rarer medium but will be totally reflected in the same medium (denser I).

The refractometry refers to the measurement of refractive index. The refractive index of most of the liquids lies in between the range 1.3 to 2.5 or slightly more.

Refractive index is a ratio and hence it has no units of expression.

Refractive Index of some chemicals at 20 °C.

Liquid	Refractive Index/Range
Methyl Acetate	1.3615 – 1.3625
Nitrobenzene	About 1.380 (22°C)
Tetradecane	1.4280 – 1.4300
Trimethylene glycol	1.4550 – 1.4570
Ethyl Benzoate	1.5048 – 1.5058

Mechanism

When incident light strikes a liquid, the light photons interact with the molecules causing imbalance of electron cloud. Thus induced dipoles are generated. Since a part of the supplied energy is spent, the velocity of light in that liquid decreases. The greater the refractive index of a liquid, the greater is the dipolar induction.

Factors Influencing Refractive Index

The factors which usually affect the value of refractive index are temperature, wave length of light and pressure.

1. **Temperature**

   The refractive index of all the liquids varies with temperature. This is because of corresponding change in the density of liquid. (For every 1 °C increase in temperature, the refractive index decreases by $0.0004 - 0.0005$)

2. **Wavelength of Light Employed**

   For transparent substances, the refractive index usually decreases with a increase in the wavelength of light.

3. **Pressure**

   The refractive index of the substance is proportional to the pressure. This is because of the corresponding increase in the density of a substance.

Molar Refraction

It is also known as Molar Refractivity. Molar refraction is related to both the refractive index and molecular properties of substance being tested. It was expressed as per Lorentz and Lorentz in 1880 as

$$R_m = \frac{n^2 - 1}{n^2 + 2} \times \frac{M}{d}$$

where,

R_m = Molecular refraction or molecular refractivity

M = Molecular weight.

n = Refractive index

d = Density

R_m has the units of molar volume, $cm^3\ mol^{-1}$

Molar refractivity of a compound is the product of specific refractivity and the molecular weight of the compound.

- It is influenced by the arrangement of atoms in the molecule or by such factors as unsaturation and ring closure etc.
- The molar refractivity is a characteristic of liquid and independent of temperature.
- The atomic refractivity of O_2 has different values in alcohols, ethers and ketones.
- Most of the atomic and structural molar contributions were determined by Eisenolhr and later revised by Vogel in 1948.

Molar refractive contributions for D-line (Vogel)

Fragment	Vlaue
Hydrogen	1.028
Carbon	2.591
Chlorine	5.844
Bromine	8.741
Iodine	13.954
Oxygen	1.764
$-C = O$	4.601
$-OH$	2.546
Double bond	1.575
Triple bond	1.977

For   6-membered 'C'- ring   −0.15

5-membered 'C'-ring   −0.10

4-membered 'C' ring   0.317

Molar refraction of a compound which depends only on the wavelength is additive and constitutive property. It is thus possible to work out the refraction equivalents of atoms, groups, radicals and bonds by determining the molar refraction of a large number of compounds. The experimental determination of molar refraction is of utmost importance in elucidating the molecular structures.

The above constants can be employed to confirm the structure of a compound.

Ex. Benzene, C_6H_6

Calculate the molar refraction of Benzene

Solution

6- Carbons $6 \times 2.591 = 15.546$

6- Hydrogens $6 \times 1.028 = 6.168$

3- Double bonds $3 \times 1.575 = 4.725$

1-6 membered ring $= (-\,0.150)$

$$\therefore R_m = 25.289$$

The experimentally determined value 25.93 is in good agreement with the calculated value. From this example, it can be concluded that the determination of molecular refractivity of liquids affords an easy means of a ascertaining their chemical constitution.

- When a compound contains more than one double bond, the molecular refraction depends not only on the number of double bonds but also their relative positions in the molecule.

- Two double bonds when separated from each other by one single bond (conjugated double bonds) shows a marked increase in the observed molecular refraction.

- Two isomeric hydrocarbons of the formula C_6H_{10} with the following structures have different molecular refractions.

	R_m observed	R_m calculated
1. $CH_2 = CH - CH_2 - CH_2 - CH = CH_2$	28.77	28.99
2. $CH_3\_ CH = CH - CH = CH - CH_3$	29.87	28.99

The increase in the molecular refraction due to the presence of conjugated double bonds in the molecule is termed as 'Optical exaltation'. The conjugated double bonds when present in a ring compound (like Benzene) don't give rise to optical exaltation.

Measurement of Refractive Index

For the rapid and convenient measurement of the refractive index of liquids a number of instruments have been developed. They are called refractometers. Most of the refractometers make use of the principle of critical angle. The commonly employed instruments based upon the principle of critical angle are :

1. Abbe's Refractometer
2. Pulfrich Refractometer and
3. Immersion Refractometer

The choice of a particular refractometer depends upon the precision required, the amount of the sample available and the economy of time.

Abbe's Refractometer - Construction and Working

This is the most commonly used instrument for measuring the refractive indices of organic liquids which have widely different refractive indices. The main advantages of this instrument are:

1. Only a few drops of liquid is sufficient for measurements.

2. It is very convenient as the operation of the instrument is simple.

3. It covers a wide range of refractive indices ranging from 1.300 to 1.850 with an accuracy of 2 parts in 10,000.

4. Source of monochromatic light is not required.

5. The measurements can be made quickly.

Construction

- It consists of two Abbe prisms (A and B) of flint glass of high refractive index 1.75, cemented into a mounting hollow cases.

- The hypotenuse surface of B is polished and A is finely ground.

- The two prisms are housed in a metallic casing hinged at H.

- The two prism faces can be held in contact with clamp.

- A and B can be rotated about a horizontal axis immediately below a telescope T.

- An arm R is attached to metal case carrying the prisms, which moves along a graduated scale, the reading on which gives directly the refractive index value.

- Commercial refractometers are normally constructed for use with white light but are calibrated to give refractive index in terms of the D-line of sodium.

- The apparatus is provided with a water jacket to control the temperature of measurement.

Working

- A drop of liquid is placed upon the surface of prism A.

- On clamping the two prisms A and B, a thin film of the liquid spreads between them.

- The light reflected by a mirror M is then directed towards the prism.

- On reaching the ground surface of A, it is scattered into the liquid film.

- No ray can enter B with a greater angle of refraction than that of ray corresponding to 'grazing incidence'. (i.e. at an angle slightly less than 90°)

- When observed through a telescope, the field of view is divided into bright and dark portion.

- The edge of the bright portion which coincides with the cross wire of the telescope gives the refractive index on the scale.

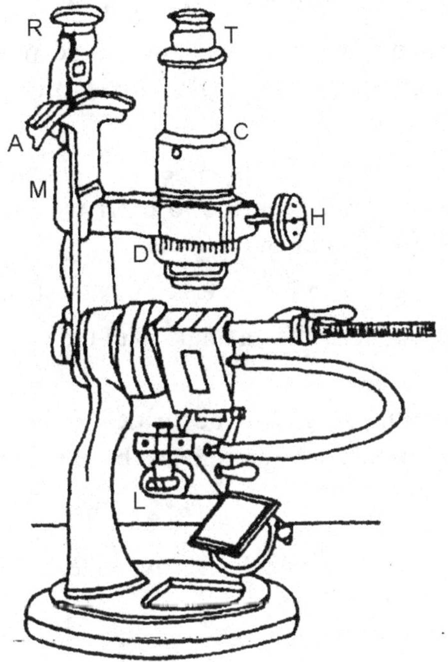

Fig. 26.2 Abbe's refractometer.

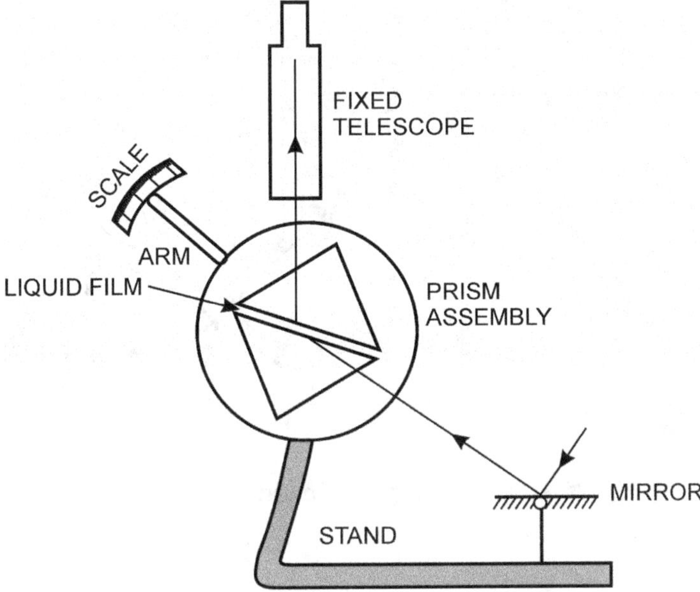

Fig. 26.3 Optical path of light in abbe's refracto meter.

Pulfrich Refractometer Construction and Working

- This instrument is highly accurate and gives good results. The essential part of pulfrich Refractometer is a right angled glass prism with a small glass cell cemented to its top.

- The liquid, whose refractive index is to be determined, is placed in the cell and a beam of monochromatic light is made to enter the liquid at 'grazing incidence' along the surface between liquid and the prism.

- It follows the path of ABCD and is observed in a telescope at D.

- If the telescope is moved to make an angle with the horizontal which is less than i, no light can reach it.

- A very accurate determination can be made of the angle i at which a sharp boundary between a dark and a light field can be seen through a telescope.

Refractive index of the liquid $(n_1) = n1 \sqrt{n^2 2 - \sin^2 i}$

$$n_2 = \text{Refractive index of glass}$$

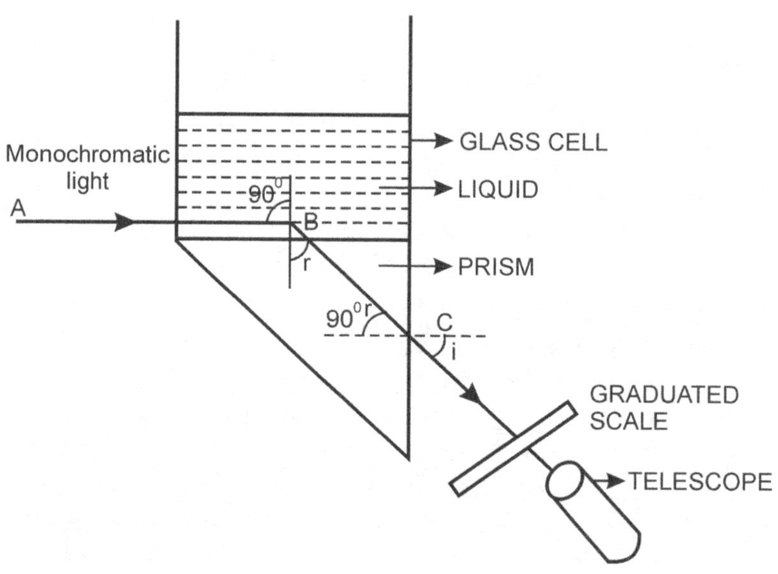

Fig. 26.4 Optical diagram of pulfrich refractometer.

Applications

Refractometer can be used for qualitative and quantitative analysis of various pharmaceutical dosage forms.

- It is useful for the determination of refractivity or molecular refractivity, thereby the chemical constitution can be easily ascertained.
- The technique is useful for the identification of conjugated double bonds in pharmaceutical compounds.
- It can also be used for the study of purity of various drugs and pharmaceuticals.
- It is used for the determination of alcohol content in fermentation broth.
- Similarly, it can be used for the determination of the concentration of sugar solutions.

APPENDIX - I

REAGENTS AND SOLUTIONS

Acetic acid: Contains approximately 33 percent w/w of CH_3COOH.

Dilute 315 ml of glacial acetic acid to 1,000 ml with water.

Acetic acid, dilute: Contains approximately 6 percent w/w of CH_3COOH. Dilute 57ml of glacial acetic acid to 1,000 ml with water.

Acetic acid, glacial: Contains not less than 99.0 percent w/w of CH_3COOH. About 17.5N in strength.

Acetic anhydride, $(CH_3CO)_2O$: Contains not less than 95.0 percent of $C_4H_6O_3$.

Alcohol: Contains not less than 94.7 percent v/v and not more than 95.2 percent v/v of C_2H_5OH.

Alcohol (90 percent): Dilute 947 ml of alcohol to 1,000 ml with water.

Alcohol (80 percent): Dilute 842 ml of alcohol to 1,000 ml with water.

Alcohol (50 percent): Dilute 526 ml of alcohol to 1,000 ml with water.

Alcohol (20 percent): Dilute 210 ml of alcohol to 1,000 ml with water.

Ammonium acetate solution: Dissolve 150g of ammonium acetate in 200 ml of water. Add 3 ml of glacial acetic acid and dilute to 100 ml with water.

Ammonium chloride solution: A 10.0 percent w/v solution of ammonium chloride in water.

Ammonia-cyanide solution Sp.: Dissolve 2g of potassium cyanide in 15 ml of strong ammonia solution and dilute with water to 100 ml.

Ammonium citrate solution Sp:. Dissolve 40 g of citric acid in 90 ml of water. Add two drops of phenol red solution then add slowly strong ammonia solution until the solution acquires a reddish colour. Remove any lead present by extracting the solution with 20 ml quantities of dithizone extraction solution until the dithizone solution retains its orange green colour.

Ammonia solution, dilute: Contains approximately 10 percent w/w of NH_3.

Ammonia solution, strong: Contains 25.0 percent w/w of NH_3 (limits 24.5 to 25.5). About 13.5 N in strength.

Ammonium carbonate solution: Dissolve 5 g of ammonium carbonate in a mixture of 7.5 ml of dilute ammonia solution and 50 ml of water; add sufficient quantity of water to produce 100 ml and filter, if necessary.

Ammonium Mercuric thiocyanate solution:(Mercuric ammonium thiocyanate solution) dissolve 30 g of ammonium thiocyanate and 27 g of mercuric chloride in water to produce 1,000 ml.

Ammonium molybdate solution: A 10.0 percent solution of ammonium molybdate, $(NH_4)_6 Mo_7O_{24}$ in water.

Ammonium Oxalate solution: A 2.5 percent w/v solution of ammonium oxalate, $(COONH_4)_2$, H_2O in water.

Ammonium Thiocyanate, 0.1N: Contains 7.612 g of NH_4SCN in 1,000 ml solution in water.

Arsenic solution AsT, dilute: Add sufficient water to 1 ml of strong arsenic solution to produce 100 ml. It must be freshly prepared, 1 ml contains 0.01 mg of arsenic, As.

Barfoed's reagent Dissolve: 13.3 g of crystallized neutral copper acetate in 200 ml of 1 percent acetic acid solution. The reagent does not keep well; it should be freshly prepared.

Barium chloride, 0.5M: Barium chloride dissolved in water to contain in 1,000 ml 122.1 g of $BaCl_2$, $2H_2O$.

Barium chloride solution: A 10.0 percent w/v solution of barium chloride, $BaCl_2$, $2H_2O$ in water.

Barium hydroxide, 0.1N solution: Barium hydroxide dissolved in water to contain in 1,000 ml 15.77 g of Ba $(OH)_2$ $8H_2O$.

Barium sulphate of the Indian pharmacopoeia.

Barium sulphate reagent: Mix 15 ml of 0.5M barium chloride, 55 ml of water, and 20 ml of sulphate-free alcohol, add 5 ml of a 0.0181 percent w/v solution of potassium sulphate, dilute to 100 ml with water, and mix. Barium sulphate reagent must be freshly prepared.

Bentonite of the Indian pharmacopoeia. Benzyl chloride $C_6H_5CH_2Cl$.

Borax: Contains not less than 99.0 percent and not more than the equivalent of 103.0 percent of $Na_2B_4O_7$, $10H_2O$.

Boric acid of the Indian pharmacopoeia.

Bromine solution AsT: Bromine 30 g; potassium bromide 30 g; water sufficient to produce 100 ml. It complies with the following test. Evaporate 10 ml on a water-bath nearly to dryness, add 50 ml of water, 10 ml hydrochloric acid AsT and sufficient stannous chloride solution AsT to reduce the remaining bromine and apply the general test; the strain produced is not deeper than a 1 ml standard stain, showing that the proportion of arsenic does not exceed 1 part per million.

Bromine solution: Dissolve 9.6 ml of bromine and 30 g of potassium bromide in sufficient water to produce 100 ml.

Bromine water: A freshly prepared saturated solution obtained by shaking occasionally during twenty-four hours 3 ml of bromine with 100ml of water, and allowing to separate. Store the solution over an excess of bromine.

Bromophenol blue solution: Warm 0.1g of bromophenol blue with 3 ml of 0.05N sodium hydroxide and 5 ml of alcohol (90 percent); after solution is effected add sufficient alcohol (20 percent) to produce 250 ml.

Bromothymol blue solution: Warm 0.1 g of bromothymol blue with 3.2 ml 0.05N sodium hydroxide and 5 ml of alcohol (90 percent); after solution is effected, add sufficient alcohol (20 percent) to produce 250 ml.

Calcium chloride solution A 10.0 percent w/v solution of calcium chloride in water.

Calcium gluconate of the Indian pharmacopoeia.

Ceric ammonium sulphate, 0.1 N: Contains 63.26 g of Ce $(SO_4)_2$, $2(NH_4)_2$ SO_4, $2H_2O$ in 1,000 ml solution in water.

Chlorine solution: A saturated solution of chlorine, Cl_2 in water. The chlorine may be generated by dropping concentrated hydrochloric acid upon potassium permanganate.

Chromotropic acid, sodium salt Disodium (4,5-dihydroxynaphthalene-2,7-disulphonate).

Chromotropic acid solution: Dissolve 50 mg of chromotropic acid (4,5-dihydroxynaphthalene-2,7-disulphonic acid), $C_{10}H_8O_8S_2$, $2H_2O$, or its sodium salt, $C_{10}H_6Na_2O_8,S_2$, in 100 ml of 75 percent v/v of N sulphuric acid.

Chloroform of the Indian Pharmacopoeia.

Citric acid, Iron-free: Citric acid which complies with the following additional test. Dissolve 0.5 g in 40 ml of water, and 2 drops of thcoglycolic acid, mix, make alkaline with iron-free ammonia solution, and dilute to 50 ml with water; no pink colour is produced.

Cobalt acetate $(CH_3CO_2)_2$ Co, $4H_2O$.

Cobalt chloride $CoCl_2$, $6H_2O$.

Copper: The pure copper, Cu, metal known commercially under the term 'electrolytic'. It is usually in the form of turnings or borings.

Copper sulphate solution: A 10.0 percent w/v solution of copper sulphate, $CuSO_4$, $5H_2O$ in water.

2,4-Dinitrophenylhydrazine Reagent: A dissolve 0.5 of the powdered 2,4-dinitrophenylhydrazine in a mixture of 80 ml of concentrated hydrochloric acid and 100 ml of distilled water by gently heating the mixture on a water-bath. Cool the solution and add 120 ml of water. If necessary, filter the pale yellow solution. The reagent should be stored in a cool place and preferably in the dark. It is stable for several weeks, but ultimately gives a brown deposit.

2,4-Dinitrophenylhydrazine reagent B: Suspend 1 g of the powdered 2,4-dintrophenylhydrazine in 30 ml of stirred methanol and cautiously add 2 ml of concentrated sulphuric acid. If necessary, filter the solution while it is still warm and cool the nitrate. The reagent should be stored in a cool in a cool place and preferably in the dark. It is stable for several weeks, but ultimately gives a brown deposit.

Diphenylcarbazide, 1, 5-Diphenylcarbazide, $(C_6H_5NHNH)_2\,CO$.

Diphenylcarbazide solution: A 2.0 percent w/v solution of diphenylcarbazide in a mixture of 10 ml of glacial acetic acid and 90 ml of alcohol (90 percent).

Disodium hydrogen phosphate solution: A 10.0 percent w/v solution of disodium hydrogen phosphate in water.

Disodium ethylenediaminetetraacctate edetate disodium of the Indian pharmacopoeia.

Dithizone extraction solution: Dissolve 30 mg of diphenylthiocarbazone in 1,000 ml of chloroform, and add 5 ml of alcohol. Store the solution in a refrigerator. Before use, shake a suitable volume of the solution with about half its volume of 1 percent v/v solution of nitric acid and discard the acid.

Dithizone solution, standard: Dissolve 10 mg of diphenylthiocarbazone in 1,000 ml of chloroform. Store the solution in a glass-stoppered, lead-free bottle, protected from light and store in a refrigerator.

Eriochrome black T (Mordant Black 11): Sodium 1-(hydroxyl-2-naphthylazo)-5-nitro-2-naphthol-4-sulphonate.

Ether, solvent: ether is diethyl ether, $(C_2H_5)_2O$. It contains a suitable stabilizer in a proportion not greater than 0.002 percent w/v.

Fehling's solution: See potassium cupri-tartrate solution.

Ferric ammonium sulphate solution: An 8.0 percent w/v solution of ferric ammonium sulphate in water.

Ferric chloride solution: Dissolve 135 g of ferric chloride, $FeCl_3$, $6H_2O$, in 1,000 ml of water containing 20 ml of concentrated hydrochloric acid. The I.P. reagent contains not less than 14.25 percent and not more than 15.75 percent w/v of $FeCl_3$.

Ferric chloride solution, neutral: Add drop by drop dilute ammonia solution to the ferric chloride solution until a slight permanent precipitate forms. Filter this off through a small fluted filter paper and used the filtrate.

Ferric chloride test solution: A 5.0 percent w/v solution of ferric chloride in water.

Ferrous fumarate of the Indian Pharmacopoeia.

Ferrous sulphate of the Indian Pharmacopoeia

Ferrous sulphate solution: A 2.0 percent w/v solution of ferrous sulphate, $FeSO_4$, $7H_2O$, in freshly boiled and cooled water. The solution must be freshly prepared.

Formaldehyde solution (Formalin): Formaldehyde solution is a solution of formaldehyde in water with methyl alcohol added to prevent polymerization. It contains not less than 34.0 percent w/w and not more than 38.0 percent w/w of HCHO.

Hydrochloric Acid: Contains not less than 35.0 percent w/w and not more than 38.0 percent w/w HCl. About 11.5 N in strength.

Hydrochloric acid, 0.01N: Contains 0.3646 g of HCl in 1,000 ml solution in water.

Hydrochloric acid, 0.1N: Contains 0.646 g of HCl in 1,000 ml solution in water

Hydrochloric aicd, 0.5N: Contains 18.23 g of HCl in 1,000 ml solution in water.

Hydrochloric acid, XN: Solutions of any normality xN may be prepared by diluting 85x ml of hydrochloric acid to 1,000 ml with water.

Hydrochloric acid, dilute: Contains approximately 10 percent w/w of HCl.

Hydrogen peroxide solution of the Indian Pharmacopoeia.

Hydrogen sulphide, H_2S: Prepared by action of hydrochloric acid, diluted with an equal volume of water; on iron sulphide; the resulting gas is washed by passing it through water.

Hydrogen sulphide solution: A recently prepared saturated solution of hydrogen sulphide in water.

Hydroxylamine hydrochloride solution: Sp.: Dissolve 20 g of hydroxylamine hydrochloride in sufficient water to produce about 65 ml. Transfer to a separator, add five drops of thymol blue solution until the solution becomes yellow. Add 10 ml of a 4 percent w/v solution of sodium diethyldithiocarbamate and allow it to stand for five minutes. Extract with successive quantities, each of 10 ml of chloroform until a 5 ml portion of the extract does not assume a yellow colour when shaken with dilute copper sulphate solution. Add dilute hydrochloric acid until the solution is pink and then dilute with sufficient water to produce 100 ml.

8-hydroxy-7-iodoquinoline-5-sulphonic acid: A yellow powder. Slightly soluble in cold water, more soluble in hot water.

Iodine of the Indian Pharmacopoeia.

Iodine: 0.1 N Contains 12.69 g I and 18.00 g Kl in, 1,000 ml solution in water.

Iodine: 0.01N Contains 1.27 g I and 1.80 g Kl in 1,000 ml solution in water.

Iodine solution: Dissolve 2.6 g of iodine, I and 3 g of potassium iodie, KI, in water to produce 100 ml.

Iron solution, standard: Weigh accurately 0.1726 g of ferric ammonium sulphate and dissolve in 10 ml of 0.1 N sulphuric acid and add sufficient water to produce 1,000 ml 1 ml contains 0.02 mg of Fe.

Lead acetate $(CH_3CO_2)_2$ pb, $3H_2O$.

Lead acetate paper: Pieces of thin filter-paper about 100 mm × 50 mm, soaked in solution of lead acetate and dried at 100°, avoiding dioxide contact with metal.

Lead acetate solution: A 10.0 percent w/v solution of lead acetate in carbon dioxide-free water.

Lead nitrate stock solution: Dissolve 0.1598 g of lead nitrate, $pb(NO_3)_2$, in 100 ml of water to which has been added 1 ml of nitric acid, then dilute to 1,000 ml with water. This solution must be prepared and stored in polyethylene or glass containers free from soluble lead salts.

Lime water: Shake 10 g of calcium hydroxide with 1,000 ml of water and allow to stand. Siphon out the upper solution for use.

Lithium carbonate of the Indian Pharmacopoeia

Litmus: Fragments of blue pigment, prepared from various species of Rocella, Lacanora or other lichens. It has a characteristic odour.

Litmus paper, blue: Made by impregnating unglazed with paper with a solution of litmus.

Litmus paper, red: Made by impregnating unglazed white paper with a solution of litmus, reddened by the previous addition of a very small quantity of sulphuric acid.

Litmus solution: Boil 25 g of coarsely powdered litmus with 100 ml of alcohol (90 pecent) under a reflux condenser for one hour, and pour away the clear liquid; repeat this operation using two successive quantities, each of 75 ml, of alcohol (90 percent). Digest the extracted litmus with 250 ml of water.

Magnesium sulphate of the Indian Pharmacopoeia.

Magnesium sulphate solution: A 10.0 percent w/v solution of magnesium sulphate, $MgSO_4$, $7H_2O$, in water.

Magnesium sulphate solution, ammoniacal: Dissolve 10 g of magnesium sulphate and 20 g of ammonium chloride in 80 ml of water and add 42 ml of 5N ammonia. Allow to stand for a few days in a well-closed container, decant and filter.

Magnesium trisilicate of the Indian Pharmacopoeia.

Methyl alcohol methanol, CH_3OH.

Methyl orange sodium 4'-dimethylminoazobenzene-4-sulphonate.

Methyl orange solution: A 0.1 percent w/v solution of methyl orange in alcohol (20 percent).

Methyl red solution: Warm 0.1 g of methyl red with 1.85 ml of 0.2 N sodium hydroxide and 5 ml of alcohol (90 percent); after solution if effected add sufficient quantity of alcohol (50 percent) to produce 250 ml.

Mercuric chloride, 0.2 M: Dissolve 54.30 g of mercuric chloride in sufficient water to produce 1,000 ml.

Mercuric chloride paper: Smooth white filter paper, not less than 25 mm in width, soaked in a saturated solution of mercuric chloride, pressed to remove superfluous solution, and dried at about 60° in the dark. The grade of the filter paper shall be such that the weight in g per sq. m shall be between 65 and 120 g, the thickness in mm of 400 papers shall be approximately equal, numerically, to the weight in g per sq. m.

Note: Mercuric chloride paper should be stored in a stoppered bottle in dark. Paper which has been exposed to sunlight or to the vapour of ammonia affords a lighter stain or no stain at all when employed in the limit test for arsenic.

Mercuric chloride solution: A 5.0 percent solution of mercuric chloride, $HgCl_2$ in water.

Mordant Black 11: See Eriochrome Back T.

β-naphthol solution: Dissolve 5 g of β-naphthol, (freshly recrystallized), in 8 ml of sodium hydroxide solution and 20 ml of water, and add sufficient water to produce 100 ml. β-naphthol solution must be freshly prepared.

Nitric acid: Contains 70.0 percent w/w of HNO3 (limits 69.0 to 71.0). About 16 N strength.

Nitric acid, dilute: Contains approximately 10 percent w/w of HNO_3. Dilute 106 ml of nitric acid to 1,000 ml with water.

Nitrobenzene $C_6H_5NO_2$.

4 Nitrobenzyl chloride p-nitrobenzyl chloride; $NO_2C_6H_4CH_2Cl$

1, 10-Phenanthroline o-phenanthroline; $C_{12}H_8N_2$, H_2O. White to cream-coloured crystals, or a crystalline powder.

Phenol carbolic acid of the Indian Pharmacopoeia.

Phenol red solution: Warm 0.1 g of phenol red (phenol sulphonphthalein) with 1.42 ml of 0.2 N sodium hydroxide and 5 ml of alcohol (90 percent); after solution is effected, add sufficient quantity of alcohol (50 percent) to produce 250 ml.

Phenolphthalein solution: A 1.0 percent w/v solution of phenolphthalein in alcohol (50 percent).

Phenolphthalein solution Dilute: A 0.1 percent w/v solution of phenolphthalein in alcohol (80 per cent).

Phenylhydrazine Hydrochloride $C_6H_5NHNH_2,HCl$.

Phosphoric acid of the Indian Pharmacopoeia.

Picric acid solution: A 0.1 percent w/v solution of picric acid in hot water.

Potassium Antimonate Solution: Boil 2 g of potassium antimonate, $KSbO_3$, $3H_2O$ with 95 ml of water, until dissolved. Cool rapidly and add 50 ml of potassium hydroxide solution and 5 ml of N sodium hydroxide. Allow to stand for twenty four hours, filter and add sufficient water to produce 150 ml. Potassium antimonite solution should be freshly prepared.

Potassium chromate solution: A 5.0 percent w/v solution of potassium chromate, K_2CrO_4, in water.

Potassium citrate of the Indian Pharmacopoeia.

Potassium dichromate $K_2Cr_2O_7$.

Potassium dichromate 0.1N: Contains 4.903 g of $K_2Cr_2O_7$ in 1,000 ml solution in water.

Potassium dichromate solution: A 7.0 percent w/v solution of potassium dichromate, $K_2Cr_2O_7$, in water.

Potassium Ferrocyanide solution: A 5.0 percent w/v solution of potassium ferrocyanide, $K_4Fe(CN)_6$, $3H_2O$, in water.

Potassium Iodide and Starch Solution Dissolve 10 g of potassium iodide in sufficient water to produce 95 ml and add 5 ml of starch solution. Potassium iodide and starch solution must be recently prepared.

Potassium Mercuri-iodide solution, Alkaline (Nessler's Reagent) To 3.5 g of potassium iodide add 1.25 g of mercuric chloride dissolved in 80 ml of water, add a old saturated solution of mercuric chloride in water, with constant stirring until a slight red precipitate remains. Dissolve 12 g of sodium hydroxide in the solution, add a little more of the cold saturated solution of mercuric chloride and sufficient water to produce 100 ml, Allow to stand and decant the clear liquid.

Potassium Iodide of the Indian Pharmacopoeia.

Potassium permanganate solution A 1.0 percent w/v solution of potassium permanganate, $KMnO_4$, in water.

Potassium Permanganate, 0.1N Cotains 3.161 g of $KMnO4$ in 1,000 ml solution in water.

Quinalizarin Cl 58500; 1, 2, 5, 8-Tetrahydroxyanthraquinone; $C_{14}H_8O_6$. A reddish brown powder.

Resorcinol Resorcin, Benzene-1, 3-diol; 1,3-Dihydroxybenzene; $C_6H_4(OH)_2$.

Schiffs Reagent Dissolve 1 g of rosaniline in 50 ml of water with gentle warming. Cool, Saturate with sulphur dioxide, add about 1 g of animal charcoal, shake and filter; make up to 1,000 ml with water. If the pink colour reappears on standing, add a few drops of sulphur dioxide-water carefully with stirring until the colour just disappears.

Silver Nitrate, 0.1N Contains 16.99 G of $AgNO_3$ in 1,000 ml solution in water.

Silver Nitrate solution A 5.0 percent w/v solution of silver nitrate, $AgNo_3$, in water.

Sodium Acetate CH_3COONa, $3H_2O$.

Sodium antimony gluconate of the Indian Pharmacopoeia.

Sodium Benzoate of the Indian Pharmacopoeia.

Sodium Bicarbonate of the Indian Pharmacopoeia.

Sodium Bicarbonate solution A 5 per cent w/v solution of sodium bicarbonate in water.

Sodium Carbonate contains not less than 99.0 per cent and not more than the equivalent of 105.0 percent of Na_2Co_3, $1OH_2O$.

Sodium Carbonate, Anhydrous Na_2CO3. Contains not less than 98.0 percent of Na_2CO_3.

Sodium Carbonate solution A 10.0 percent w/v solution of sodium carbonate in water.

Sodium Chloride of the Indian Pharmacopoeia. Sodium Cobaltinitrite $Na_3Co(NO^o_2)_6$.

Sodium Cobaltinitrile Solution A 30 percent w/v solution of sodium cobaltinitrite, $Na_3Co(NO_2)_6$ g in water.

Sodium Hydroxide of the Indian Pharmacopoeia.

Sodium Nitrite solution A 10 percent w/v solution of sodium nitrite, $NaNO_2$, in water.

Sodium Nitroprusside $Na_2[Fe(CN)_5 (NO)]$, $2H_2O$.

Sodium Nitroprusside solution A 1.0 percent w/v solution of sodium nitroprusside, $Na_2[Fe(CN)_5 (NO)]$, $2H_2O$, in water. Sodium Nitroprusside solution should be recently prepared.

Sodium Nitroprusside Solution, Alkaline Dissolve 1g of sodium nitroprusside, $Na_2[Fe(CN)_5 (NO)]$, $2H_2O$, and 1 g of sodium carbonate in sufficient water to produce 100 ml.

Sodium Potassium Tartrate Rochelle Salt; NaOOC, CH(OH) CH(OH) COOK, $4H_2O$.

Sodium Sulphide Na_2, $9H_2O$. Contains not less than 95.0 percent of Na_2S, $9H_2O$.

Sodium sulphide solution A 10.0 percent w/v solution of sodium sulphide in water.

Sodium Sulphite Na_2SO_3.

Sodium Thiosulphate, 0.1N Contains 24.82 g of $Na_2S_2O_3$, $5H_2O$ in 1,000 ml solution in water.

Starch Iodide Paper Made by impregnating unglazed paper with starch solution diluted with an equal volume of 5.0 percent w/v solution of potassium iodide in water.

Starch Paper Made by impregnating unglazed white paper with Starch solution.

Starch, soluble Starch which has been treated with hydrochloric acid until, after being washed it forms an almost clear limpid solution in hot water.

Starch solution Triturate 0.5 g of starch of soluble starch with 5 ml of water and add this, with constant stirring, to sufficient water to produce about 100 ml; boil for a few minutes, cool and filter. Starch solution must be recently prepared.

Sulphamic Acid NH_2SO_3H.

Sulphuric Acid Contains not less than 97.0 percent w/w of H_2SO_4. About 36 N in strength.

Sulphuric Acid, N Contains 49.04 g of H_2SO_4 in 1,000 ml solution in water.

Sulphuric Acid, 2N Contains 98.08 g of H_2SO_4 in 1,000 ml solution in water

Shulphuric Acid, 5N Contains 245.2 g of H_2SO_4 in 1,000 ml solution in water.

Sulphuric Acid, Dilute Contains approximately 10 percent w/w of H_2SO_4.

Tannic Acid solution A 10.0 percent w/v solution of tannic acid in water.

Tartaric Acid of the Indian Pharmacopoeia.

Thioacetamide CH_3CSNH_2.

Thioacetamide Reagent Add 1 ml of a mixture of 15 ml of N sodium hydroxide, 5 ml of water, and 20 ml of glycerine to 0.2 ml of a 4 percent w/v solution of thioacetamide in water. Heat on a water bath for twenty seconds and cool. Thioacetamide reagent should be prepared immediately before use.

Thiogloycollic Acid Contains not less than 89.0 percent w/v of $HSCH_2COOH$.

Thymol Blue Solution Warm 0.1 g of thymol blue with 4.3 ml of 0.05N sodium hydroxide and 5 ml of alcohol. (90 percent); after solution is effected, add sufficient alcohol (20 percent) to produce 250 ml.

Trinitrophenol solution See Picric Acid Solution.

Turmeric Paper Made by impregnating unglazed white paper with Turmeric Tincture.

Water, Carbon Dioxide-free water Which has been boiled vigorously for a few minutes and protected from the atmosphere during cooling and storage.

Zinc oxide of the Indian Pharmacopoeia.

Zinc powder Zn. Dense bluish-grey powder.

Zinc sulphate of the Indian Pharmacopoeia.

APPENDIX - II

pH Ranges and Colour changes of Indicators

Indicator	pH Range	Colour Change
Cresol Red	0.2 to 1.8 and 7.2 to 8.8	Red and Yellow Yellow to Red
Metacresol Purple	0.5 to 2.5 and 7.5 to 9.2	Red to yellow Yellow to Violet
Thymol Blue	1.2 to 2.8 and 8.0 to 9.6	Red to Yellow Yellow to Violet-blue
Metanil Yellow	1.2 to 3.2	Red to Yellow
Quinaldine Red	1.4 to 3.2	Colourless to Red
Naphthol Yellow	2.0 to 3.2	Colourless to Yellow
Dimethyl Yellow	2.8 to 4.6	Red to Yellow
Bromophenol Blue	2.8 to 4.6	Red to Yellow
Methyl Orange	2.9 to 4.0	Red to Yellow
Methyl Orange-xylene cyanol FF	2.9 to 4.6	Violet to Green
Congo Red	3.0 to 5.0	Blue to Red
Bromocresol Green	3.6 to 5.2	Yellow to Blue
Methyl red	4.2 to 6.3	Red to Yellow
Litmus	5.0 to 8.0	Red to Blue
Bromocresol Purple	5.2 to 6.8	Yellow to Blue-violet
Bromothymol Blue	6.0 to 7.6	Yellow to Blue
Neutral Red	6.8 to 8.0	Red to Orange
Phenol Red	6.8 to 8.4	Yellow to Red
1-Naphtholphthalein	7.3 to 8.7	Pale Red to Blue
Phenolphthalein	8.3 to 10.0	Colourless to Red
Thymolphthalein	9.3 to 10.5	Colourless to Blue
Alizarin Yellow GG	10.0 to 12.0	Colourless to Yellow
Titan Yellow	12.0 to 13.0	Yellow to Red

APPENDIX - III

Ethyl Alcohol Table

Specific Gravity at 25°	Ethyl Alcohol content (per cent v/v of the preparation at 15.56°)	Specific Gravity At 25°	Ethyl Alcohol content (per cent v/v of the preparation at 15.56°)
0.9695	96.88	0.9810	57.20
0.9700	95.20	0.9815	55.52
0.9705	93.52	0.9820	53.84
0.9710	91.84	0.9825	52.16
0.9715	90.12	0.9830	50.52
0.9720	88.44	0.9835	48.88
0.9725	86.72	0.9840	47.24
0.9730	85.00	0.9845	45.64
0.9735	83.28	0.9850	44.00
0.9740	79.80	0.9855	42.40
0.9745	78.00	0.9860	40.84
0.9750	76.24	0.9865	39.24
0.9760	74.48	0.9870	37.64
0.9765	72.72	0.9875	36.04
0.9770	70.96	0.9880	34.44
0.9775	69.20	0.9885	32.88
0.9780	67.48	0.9890	31.32
0.9785	65.76	0.9900	28.20
0.9790	64.00	0.9905	26.68
0.9800	60.60	0.9910	25.16
0.9920	22.16	0.9965	9.40
0.9925	20.68	0.9970	8.04
0.9930	19.24	0.9975	6.68
0.9935	17.80	0.9980	5.36

Specific Gravity at 25°	Ethyl Alcohol content (per cent v/v of the preparation at 15.56°)	Specific Gravity At 25°	Ethyl Alcohol content (per cent v/v of the preparation at 15.56°)
0.9940	16.36	0.9985	4.00
0.9945	14.96	0.9990	2.64
0.9950	13.56	0.9995	1.32
0.9955	12.16	1.0000	0.00
0.9960	10.80		

APPENDIX - IV

Dissociation Constants of Some Acids in Water at 25°C

Dissolution Constants are expressed as pK_a (= - log k_a)

Acid	pK_a	Acid		pK_a
Benzoic	4.21	Mandelic		3.41
Phenylacetic	4.31	1-Naphthoic		3.70
Sulphanilic	3.23	1-Naphthylacetic		4.24
Phenoxyacetic	3.17	2-Naphthylacetic		4.26
Formic	3.75	Succinic	K_1	4.21
Acetic	4.76		K_2	5.64
Propanoic	4.87	Glutaric	K_1	4.34
Butanoic	4.82		K_2	5.28
Fluoracetic	2.58	Methylmalonic	K_1	3.07
Chloroacetic	2.90	Ethylmalonic	K_1	2.96
Iodoacetic	3.17		K_2	5.90
Cyanoacetic	2.47	Dimethylmalonic	K_1	3.15
Diethylacetic	4.73		K_2	6.20
Lactic	3.86	Diethylmalonic	K_1	2.15
Pyruvic	2.49		K_2	7.47
Acrylic	4.26	Fumaric	K_1	3.02
Vinylacetic	4.34		K_2	4.38
Tetrolic	2.65	Maleic	K_1	1.92
Tans-Crotonic	4.69		K_2	6.23
Furoic	3.17	Tartaric	K_1	3.03
Oxalic K_1	1.27		K_2	4.37
K_2	4.27	Citric	K_1	3.13
Malonic K_1	2.85		K_2	4.76
K_2	5.70		K_3	6.40
2-Benzoylbenzoic	3.54	Trans-Cinnamic	4.44	
Phthalic K_1	2.95	Phenol		10.00
K_2	5.41	1-Nitroso-2-naphthol		7.77
Cis-cinnamic	3.88	2-Nitroso-1- naphthol		7.38
Trans-Cinnamic	4.44			

Acid	Ortho (2-)	Meta (3-)	Para (4-)
Aromatic acids			
Fluorobenzoic	3.27	3.86	4.14
Chlorobenzoic	2.94	3.83	3.98
Bromobenzene	2.85	3.81	3.97
Iodobenzoic	2.86	3.85	3.93
Hydroxybenzoic	3.00	4.08	4.53
Methoxybenzoic	4.09	4.09	4.47
Nitrobenzoic	2.17	3.49	3.42
Aminobenzoic	4.98	4.79	4.92
Toluic	3.91	4.24	4.34
Chlorophenol	8.48	9.02	9.38
Nitrophenol	7.23	8.40	7.15
Methylphenol (cresol)	10.29	10.09	10.26
Methoxyphenol	9.98	9.65	10.21

Acid		pK_a	Acid		pK_a
Inorganic acids					
Arsenious		9.22	Nitrous		3.35
Arsenic	K_1	2.30	Phosphoric	K_1	2.12
	K_2	7.08		K_2	7.21
	K_3	9.22		K_3	12.30
Boric		9.24	Phosphorous	K_1	1.8
Carbonic	K_1	6.37		K_2	6.15
	K_2	10.33	Sulphuric	K_2	1.92
Hydrocyanic		9.14	Sulphurous	K_1	1.92
Hydrofluoric		4.77		K_2	7.20
Hydrogen sulphide	K_1	7.00	Thiosulphuric	K_1	1.7
Hypochlorous	K_2	2.5		K_2	14.00
		7.25			

APPENDIX – V

Specific Gravities of Acids at 20°C

Percent by weight	Specific gravity H_2SO_4	HNO_3	CH_3COOH	H_3PO_4	HCl
1	1.0051	1.0036	0.9996	1.0038	1.0032
2	1.0118	1.0091w	1.0012	1.0092	1.0082
3	1.0184	1.0146	1.0025	-	-
4	1.0250	1.0201	1.0040	1.0200	1.0181
5	1.0317	1.0256	1.0055	-	-
10	1.0661	1.0543	1.0125	1.0532	1.0474
15	1.1020	1.0842	1.0195	-	-
16	1.1094	1.0903	1.0209	1.0884	1.0776
20	1.1394	1.1150	1.0263	1.1134	1.0980
24	1.1704	1.1404	1.0313	1.1395	1.1187
25	1.1783	1.1469	1.0326	-	-
30	1.2185	1.1800	1.0384	1.1805	1.1493
34	1.2515	1.2071	1.0428	-	1.1691
35	1.2599	1.2140	1.0438	1.216	-
36	1.2684	1.2205	1.0449	-	1.1789
40	1.3028	1.2463	1.0488	1.254	1.1980
45	1.3476	1.2783	1.0534	1.293	-
50	1.3951	1.3100	1.0575	1.335	-
55	1.4453	1.3393	1.0644	1.379	-
60	1.4983	1.3667	1.0642	1.426	-
65	1.5533	1.3913	1.0666	1.475	-
70	1.6105	1.4134	1.0685	1.526	-
75	1.6692	1.4337	1.0696	1.579	-
80	1.7272	1.4521	1.0700	1.633	-
85	1.7786	1.4686	1.0689	1.689	-
90	1.8144	1.4826	1.0661	1.746	-

Percent by weight	Specific gravity H_2So_4	HNO_3	CH_3COOH	H_3PO_4	HCl
92	1.8240	1.4873	1.0643	1.770	-
93	1.8279	1.4892	1.0632	-	-
94	1.8312	1.4912	1.0619	1.794	-
95	1.8337	1.4932	1.0605	-	-
96	1.8355	1.4952	1.0588	1.819	-
97	1.8364	1.4974	1.0570	-	-
98	1.8361	1.5008	1.0549	1.844	-
99	1.8342	1.5056	1.0524	-	-
100	1.8305	1.5129	1.0498	1.870	-

APPENDIX – VI

Specific Gravities of Alkaline Solutions at 20°C

Percent By weight	Specific gravity			Percent By weight	Specific gravity		
	KOH	NaOH	NH_3		KOH	NaOH	NH_3
1	1.0083	1.0095	0.9939	26	1.2489	1.2848	0.9040
2	1.0175	1.0207	0.9895	27	1.2592	-	-
3	1.0267	1.0318	-	28	1.2695	1.3064	0.8980
4	1.0359	1.0428	0.9811	29	1.2800	-	-
5	1.0452	1.0538	-	30	1.2905	1.3279	0.8920
6	1.0544	1.0648	0.9730	31	1.3010	-	-
7	1.0637	1.0758	-	32	1.3117	1.3490	-
8	1.0730	1.0869	0.9651	33	1.3224	-	-
9	1.0824	1.0979	-	34	1.331	1.3696	-
10	1.0918	1.1089	0.9575	35	1.3440	-	-
11	1.1013	-	-	36	1.3549	1.3900	-
12	1.1108	1.1309	0.9575	37	1.3440	-	-
13	1.1203	-	-	38	1.3769	1.4101	-
14	1.1299	1.1530	0.9430	39	1.3879	-	-
15	1.1396	-	-	40	1.3991	1.4300	-
16	1.1493	1.1751	0.9362	41	1.4103	-	-
17	1.1590	-	-	42	1.4215	1.4494	-
18	1.1688	1.1972	0.9295	43	1.4329	-	-
19	1.1786	-	-	44	1.4443	1.4685	-
20	1.1884	1.2191	0.9229	45	1.4558	-	-
21	1.1984	-	-	46	1.4673	1.4873	-
22	1.2083	1.2411	0.9164	47	1.4790	-	-
23	1.2184	-	-	48	1.4907	1.5065	-
24	1.2285	1.2629	0.1901	49	1.5025	-	-
25	1.2387	-	-	50	1.5143	1.5253	-

APPENDIX – VII

Data on the Strength of Aqueous Solutions of the Common Acids

Reagent	Approximate			Vol. required to make 1 dm^{-3} of approx. N solution (cm^3)
	Percent by weight	Specific gravity	Normality	
Hydrochloric acid	35	1.18	11.3	89
Nitric acid	70	1.42	16.0	63
Sulphuric acid	96	1.84	36.0	28
Perchloric acid	70	1.66	11.6	86
Hydrofluoric acid	46	1.15	26.5	38
Phosphoric acid	85	1.69	41.1	23
Acetic acid	99.5	1.05	17.4	58

MODEL QUESTION PAPERS

II/IV B.Pharma Examination

Pharmaceutical Analysis – I & II

Time : Three Hours   **Maximum Marks : 80**

Note : - (i) Answer any **FIVE** questions.

        (ii) All questions carry equal marks.

1. (a) Classifty the different types of solvents used in the non-aqueous titration with suitable examples.

   (b) How will you prepare and standardise N/10 sodium methoxide solution for non-aqueous titrations ?

   (c) Explain the principle involved in the assay of compounds using standard solution of sodium methoxide.

2. Write detailed notes on any *two* of the following :-
   (a) Complexometric titrations ;
   (b) GLC;
   (c) Gasometry.

3. (a) With the help of a schematic diagram, explain the working of a high performance liquid chromatography.

   (b) Outline the technique of oxygen flask combustion and its importance in pharmaceutical analysis.

4. Write the principle of polarographic methods of analysis. Describe the advantages of polarographic methods over the other methods of analysis. What type of products are analysed by polarography?

5. Write notes on any *three* of the following :
   (a) Kjeldahl's method of nitrogen estimation;
   (b) Two dimensional chromatography ;
   (c) Colourometric titrations ;
   (d) Dead stop end-point technique.

6. (a) Discuss the construction and working of a standard hydrogen electrode and calomel electrode.

   (b) Describe the analytical methods of evaluation in potentiometric titration.

7. (a) What are the different methods of solvent extraction? Explain their importance in pharm-analysis.

   (b) Explain the principles underlying the separation of components by paper chromatography and TLC. Discuss the advantages and disadvantages of the methods.

8. Describe the principles and procedures involved in the assay of the following :

   (a) Elphedrine HCl;

   (b) Calcium gluconate;

   (c) Folic acid.

II/IV B.Pharmacy (I Semester) Examination
Pharmaceutical Analysis – I & II

Time : Three Hours   **Maximum Marks :** 80

Note : - (i) Answer any **FIVE** questions.

(ii) All questions carry equal marks.

1. (a) Explain the theory of conductometric titrations with the help of different conductometric titration curves.

   (b) Enumerate the applications of conductometry in analysis.

2. Write detailed notes on any *TWO* of the following :
   (a) Complexometric titrations;
   (b) Different methods of solvent extraction;
   (c) HPTLC.

3. (a) Explain the principle and methodology of non-aqueous titrations. What are the various types of solvents used and their merits and demerits?

   (b) Describe the estimation of a weak basic pharmaceutical compound by this method.

4. (a) Explain the basic principle and instrumentation of gas chromatography using a diagrammatic sketch of the instrument.

   (b) Name the carrier gases and detectors used in gas chromatography

   (c) Give the applications of this technique in pharmaceutical analysis.

5. Write short notes on any *THREE* of the following :
   (a) Amperometric titrations;
   (b) Column Chromatography;
   (c) Calomel and glass electrodes;
   (d) Nernst equation and its significance in pharmaceutical analysis.

6. (a) What are the principles and techniques involved in paper chromatography?

   (b) What are the applications of paper chromatography in analysis?

7. Write the principle of polarographic method of analysis. Give the advantages of this method over other electro analytical methods. Add a note on applications of this technique in quantitative analysis.

8. Describe the principles and procedures involved in the assay of the following :
   (a) Acetazolamide;
   (b) Magnesium sulphate;
   (c) Sulphamethoxazole.

Pharmacy (I Semester) Examination
Pharmaceutical Analysis – I & II

Time : Three Hours   **Maximum Marks :** 80

Note : - (i) Answer any **FIVE** questions.

(ii) All questions carry equal marks.

1. (a) Explain the principle and methodology of complexometric titration using a suitable example of pharmaceutical product.

   (b) How will you standardise EDTA solution?

   (c) What are the common complexometric indicators?

2. Write detailed notes on any *two* of the following :

   (a) Diazotisation titrations;

   (b) GLC;

   (c) Gasometry.

3. (a) With the help of a schematic diagram explain the working of a high performance liquid chromatograph.

   (b) Write a note on applications of HPLC in quantitative analysis.

4. Explain the principle of polarography. Give the construction and working of a polarographic cell. Enumerate the applications of polarographic analysis.

5. Write short notes on any *three* of the following :

   (a) Two dimentional paper chromatography;

   (b) Kjeldahl's method of nitrogen determination;

   (c) Karl Fischer titration;

   (d) Colourometric titrations.

6. With a suitable diagrammatic sketch, describe a potentiometric titration unit. Explain the principle and different methods used to detect the end-point in such titrations. Add a note on applications of this technique in pharmaceutical analysis.

7. (a) Explain the principle and methodology of TLC.

   (b) What are the common absorbents used in TLC and the method of preparing chromatoplates.

   (c) Explain the different spraying reagents for different classes of natural products.

8. Describe the principles and procedures involved in the assay of the following :

   (a) Metronidazole ;

   (b) Calcium gluconate;

   (c) Folic Acid.

II/IV B.Pharmacy (I Semester) Examination
Pharmaceutical Analysis – I & II

Time : Three Hours   **Maximum Marks :** 80

Note : - (i) Answer any **FIVE** questions.

(ii) All questions carry equal marks.

1. (a) Write a detailed account of the principles involved in complexometric titrations.

   (b) Describe how magnesium is determined by EDTA solution.

   (c) Write a note on the indicators used in complexometric titrations.

2. (a) Explain the principles involved in the non-aqueous titrations. Discuss about the common titrants, indicators and various vehicles used in non-aqueous titrations.

   (b) Write about the analysis with oxygen flask combustion method.

3. Describe the principles and procedures involved in the assay of :

   (a) Ephedrine HCL;

   (b) Folic acid;

   (c) Ascorbic acid.

4. Write notes on any *THREE* of the following :

   (a) Different methods of photo-coating in T.L.C;

   (b) Kjeldahl method of Nitrogen estimation

   (c) Determination of water;

   (d) Columns used in H.P.L.C.

5. (a) Describe in brief about the principle and techniques involved in T.L.C. What are its advantages over other types of chromatography ?

   (b) Write notes on the following :

   (i)   Two dimensional and circular chromatography;

   (ii) Flame ionisation detector.

6. (a) Describe the construction, use, advantages and disadvantages of dropping mercury electrode.

   (b) What is half-wave potential ? Explain its significance in polarographic analysis.

7. Write a detailed account of any *TWO* of the following :
   (a) Potentiometry;
   (b) Solvent Extraction methods;
   (c) Conductometric titrations.

8. (a) Give an account of stationary and mobile phases used in gas chromatography.
   (b) Explain the importance of Reverse Phase Chromatography.
   (c) Explain various techniques used in Paper Chromatography.

II/TV B.Pharmacy (I Semester) Examination
Pharmaceutical Analysis

Time : Three Hours   **Maximum Marks :** 80

Note : – (i) Answer any **FIVE** questions.

      (ii) All questions carry equal marks.

1. With the help of a schematic diagram, explain the working of High performance liquid chromatography. What are its applications in pharmaceutical analysis?

2. (a) What are the different types of indicator electrodes used in neutralisation reactions by potentiometric titration method? Explain the working of any one of them.

   (b) Write briefly about the various methods used in the determination of end point in potentiometric titrations.

3. Describe the principles and procedures involved in the assay of the following :

   (a) Isoniazid;

   (b) Riboflavin;

   (c) Magnesium sulphate.

4. (a) Write the principles involved in the conductometric titrations.

   (b) Explain with the help of graphs how conductometric methods can be applied to the following :

      (i) Determination of mineral acids;

      (ii) Displacement titrations;

      (iii) Solubility of sparingly soluble compounds.

5. Write a detailed account of any *three* of the following :

   (a) Karl-Fischer titrations;

   (b) Retention time and Retention volume;

   (c) Various adsorbents used in chromatography;

   (d) Preparation and stadardisation of M/20 EDTA solution.

6. Write notes on any *TWO* of the following :

   (a) Polarography;

   (b) Amperometric titrations;

   (c) Paper Chromatography.

7. (a) Describe the working of a gas-liquid chromatogram and explain the functions of each part.

   (b) Explain different methods adopted for quantitative analysis by TLC.

8. (a) Classify the different types of solvents used in non-aqueous titrations with examples.

   (b) How will you prepare and standardise a solution of N/10 sodium methoxide for non-aqueous titrations?

   (c) Explain the principle involved in the assay of any compound using the above solution of N/10 Sodium Methoxide.

II/IV B.Pharmacy (I Semester) Examination

Pharmaceutical Analysis – I & II

Time : Three Hours   **Maximum Marks :** 80

Note : - (i) Answer any **FIVE** questions.

(ii) All questions carry equal marks.

1. (a) Describe the construction and working of a saturated calomel electrode.

    (b) How 0.1N Perchloric acid is prepared for use in non-aqueous titrations? How is it standardised?

    (c) What are the various methods of preparation of T.L.C. plates?

2. (a) Explain the principle of conductometric titrations.

    (b) What is conductivity cell ? How is it used?

    (c) Explain how solubility of sparingly soluble salt can be determined conductometrically.

3. Write notes on any *THREE* of the following :

    (a) Diazotisation titrations and their applications.

    (b) Gasometry and its importance in pharmaceutical analysis.

    (c) Various adsorbents used in chromatography.

    (d) Dead-stop method.

4. (a) Describe the principles of adsorption and partition chromatography. Write in brief the separation of mixtures by the above techniques giving suitable examples.

    (b) Briefly explain the important parts of an instrument used for isocratic operation in H.P.L.C.

5. Describe the principles and procedures involved in the assay of the following:

    (a) Phenobarbitone;

    (b) Sulphathiazole;

    (c) Calcium Gluconate.

6. Write a detailed note of any *TWO* of the following :

    (a) Polarography;

    (b) Non-aqueous titrations;

    (c) G.L.C.

7. (a) Explain the following terms used in complexometric titrations :
   (1) Ligand;
   (2) Sequestering agent;
   (3) Coordinate number;
   (4) Solubility constant.
   (b) Classify the different types of complexometric titrations with suitable examples and explain.
   (c) What are masking agents ? Explain their use in complexometric titrations.

8. (a) Explain the principle and importance of amperometric tritrations.
   (b) Discuss in brief about colorometric titrations and its applications in Pharmaceutical analysis.

II/IV B.Pharmacy (I Semester) Examination
Pharmaceutical Analysis – I & II

Time : Three Hours   **Maximum Marks :** 80

Note : - (i) Answer any **FIVE** questions.

      (ii) All questions carry equal marks.

1. (a) Explain the terms 'Reverse Phase Chromatography', 'Two dimensional Chromatography and "R_f Values'. What are their applications in chromatography?

   (b) Describe the process of thin layer chromatography.

   (c) Write a note on Kjeldahl method of nitrogen estimation.

2. Write the principles involved in the assay of the following :

   (a) Ephedrine hydrochloride;

   (b) Calcium Gluconate;

   (c) Sulphanilamide.

3. (a) With the help of a schematic diagram explain the working of Gas Chromatography.

   (b) Write a detailed account of different columns used in HPLC.

4. (a) Discuss the principle of polarography and mention its applications. Explain about DME.

   (b) Explain the principles of non-aqueous titrations. What do you mean by levelling and delevelling effect in Non-aqueous titrations?

5. (a) What is Nernst Equation ? How can we use it for quantitative estimations?

   (b) Explain the terms :

       (i) Reference electrode;

       (i) Half cell;

       (i) Standard electrode.

6. Write notes on any *FOUR* of the following :

   (a) Flame ionisation detector;

   (b) Standardisation of perchloric acid (N/10).

   (c) Separation of amino acids by paper chromatography;

   (d) Plate theory in chromatography;

   (e) Separation of drugs from excipients.

7. Write a detailed account of :

   (a) Absorbents used in gasometry;

   (b) Colourimetric titrations;

   (c) Diazotisation titrations.

8. (a) What do you mean by masking agents in complexometric titrations? Write a note on indicators used in complexometry.

   (b) Write a detailed account of the principles involved in Amperometric and conductometric titrations.

II/IV B.Pharmacy (I Semester) Examination

Pharmaceutical Analysis – I & II

Time : Three Hours   **Maximum Marks :** 80

Note : - (i) Answer any **FIVE** questions.

      (ii) All questions carry equal marks.

1. (a) Explain the theory of conductometric titrations.
   (b) Enumerate the applications of conductometry in analysis.

2. (a) Explain the principle and instrumentation of spectrophotometer using a diagrammatic sketch of the instrument.
   (b) Briefly explain about the applications of spectrophotometer in pharmaceutical analysis.

3. (a) Write about various types of solvents used in non-aqueous titrations and their merits and demerits.
   (b) Explain about the titrations involving perchloric acid.

4. (a) What are the principles and techniques involved in paper chromatography?
   (b) Explain about the method of separation of amino acids by paper chromatographic technique

5. Write short notes on :
   (a) Nernst equation and its significance in Pharmaceutical analysis;
   (b) HPTLC;
   (c) Oxygen flask combustion.

6. Describe the principles and procedures involved in the assay of the following :
   (a) Dapsone;
   (b) Aluminium hydroxide gel;
   (c) Actazolamide.

7. (a) Explain the basic principle and instrumentation of gas chromatography using a diagrammatic sketch of the instrument.
   (b) Write a brief note on the carrier gases used in gas chromatography.
   (c) Give the applications of this technique in pharmaceutical analysis.

8. Write notes on :
   (a) Column chromatography;
   (b) Applications of polarography in pharmaceutical analysis;
   (c) Karl Fischer titration.

II/IV B.Pharmacy (I Semester) Examination
Pharmaceutical Analysis – I & II

Time : Three Hours   **Maximum Marks :** 80

Note : - (i) Answer any **FIVE** questions.

(ii) All questions carry equal marks.

1. (a) Write a note on amperometric titrations.

   (b) Discuss oxidation-reduction electrodes and the method of determining redox potentials.

2. (a) Write a note on role of hydrogen ion concentration in Chelate formation and that of masking agents in complexometric analysis.

   (b) Give the principle and the procedure for analysis of a sulfa drug by sodium nitrite titration.

3. (a) Discuss the principles involved in non-aqueous titrimetry.

   (b) Discuss the general principles involved in solvent extractions and describe any one method.

4. (a) Write a note on TLC and describe the analysis of triple sulfa using TLC.

   (b) Describe the working of a Gas chromatograph fitted with an electron capture detector.

5. (a) Describe the construction of a polarographic cell and discuss the methods used in quantitative polarography.

   (b) Discuss the applications of conductometry in analysis.

6. Write a note on any *three* of the following :-

   (a) Column Chromatography;

   (b) Coulometric analysis;

   (c) Karl-Fisher titrations.

   (d) Reverse phase Chromatography.

7. Write informative note on :

   (a) HPLC and

   (b) Paper Chromatography.

8. Discuss the principles and describe the method involved in the assay of the following :

   (a) Pyridoxine hydrochloride ;

   (b) Magnesium sulphate ;

   (c) Chloral hydrate.